DRUGS, SYSTEMIC DISEASES, AND THE KIDNEY

ADVANCES IN EXPERIMENTAL MEDICINE AND BIOLOGY

Recent Volumes in this Series

Volume 247A
KININS V, Part A
Edited by Keishi Abe, Hiroshi Moriya, and Setsuro Fujii

Volume 247B
KININS V, Part B
Edited by Keishi Abe, Hiroshi Moriya, and Setsuro Fujii

Volume 248
OXYGEN TRANSPORT TO TISSUE XI
Edited by Karel Rakusan, George P. Biro, Thomas K. Goldstick, and Zdenek Turek

Volume 249
MINERAL ABSORPTION IN THE MONOGASTRIC GI TRACT:
Chemical, Nutritional, and Physiological Aspects
Edited by Frederick R. Dintzis and Joseph A. Laszlo

Volume 250
PROGRESS IN POLYAMINE RESEARCH:
Novel Biochemical, Pharmacological, and Clinical Aspects
Edited by Vincenzo Zappia and Anthony E. Pegg

Volume 251
IMMUNOBIOLOGY OF PROTEINS AND PEPTIDES V: VACCINES
Edited by M. Zouhair Atassi

Volume 252
DRUGS, SYSTEMIC DISEASES, AND THE KIDNEY
Edited by Alberto Amerio, Pasquale Coratelli,
Vito M. Campese, and Shaul G. Massry

Volume 253A
PURINE AND PYRIMIDINE METABOLISM IN MAN VI, Part A:
Clinical and Molecular Biology
Edited by Kiyonobu Mikanagi, Kusuki Nishioka, and William N. Kelley

Volume 253B
PURINE AND PYRIMIDINE METABOLISM IN MAN VI, Part B:
Basic Research and Experimental Biology
Edited by Kiyonobu Mikanagi, Kusuki Nishioka, and William N. Kelley

---

DRUGS, SYSTEMIC DISEASES, AND THE KIDNEY

Edited by

Alberto Amerio and
Pasquale Coratelli
University of Bari
Bari, Italy

Vito M. Campese and
Shaul G. Massry
University of Southern California
Los Angeles, California

PLENUM PRESS • NEW YORK AND LONDON

Library of Congress Cataloging in Publication Data

Bari Seminar in Nephrology (3rd: 1988)
Drugs, systemic diseases, and the kidney / edited by Alberto Amerio . . . [et al.].
p. cm. – (Advances in experimental medicine and biology; v. 252)
"Proceedings of the Third Bari Seminar in Nephrology, held April 20-23, 1988, in Bari, Italy" – T.p. verso.
Bibliography: p.
Includes index.

DOI 10.1007/978-1-4684-8953-8

1. Renal manifestations of general diseases – Congresses. 2. Kidneys – Effect of drugs on – Congresses. 3. Drugs – Side effects – Congresses. I. Amerio, A. II. Title. III. Series.
RC903.B36 1988 89-8494
616.6′1 – dc20 CIP

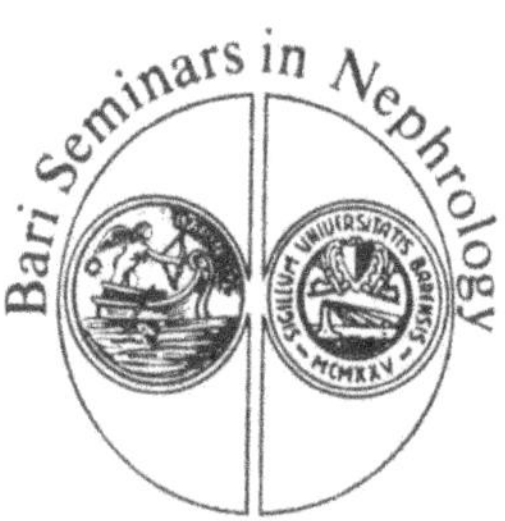

Proceedings of the Third Bari Seminar in Nephrology,
held April 20-23, 1988, in Bari, Italy

MyCopy version of the original edition 1989
A Division of Plenum Publishing Corporation
233 Spring Street, New York, N.Y. 10013

TO OUR WIVES

Pia Amerio
Liliana Coratelli
Stefania Campese
Meira Massry

AND OUR CHILDREN

PREFACE

We are pleased to present to our readers the proceedings of the Third Bari Seminars in Nephrology. The topic of these proceedings deals with effects of drugs and systemic diseases on the kidney.

The Bari Seminars in Nephrology are bi-annual meetings attended by a large international audience comprised of clinicians-scientists in the various displines of nephrology and related fields.

The next Bari Seminars of Nephrology will take place in April 1990 and the theme of the gathering will be **Interstitial Nephritidies and Obstructive Uropathy.** We are indebted for the generous financial support of the Centro Nazionale delle Richerche, Italy.

Alberto Amerio
Pasquale Coratelli
Vito M. Campese
Shaul G. Massry

CONTENTS

KIDNEY IN SYSTEMIC ABNORMALITIES AND DISEASES

LUPUS NEPHRITIS: PATHOGENESIS, COURSE AND MANAGEMENT

James E. Balow

Kidney Disease Section
National Institutes of Health
Bethesda, Maryland 20892

INTRODUCTION

Lupus nephritis contributes notably to the morbidity and mortality of systemic lupus erythematosus. Improved medical therapies have increased the median survival of patients with lupus to more than 15 years over the past several decades. Uremia was a rare cause of death in the era before steroids, anti-hypertensives and antibiotics. As longevity of patients with lupus improved in the second half of the twentieth century, renal disease became a key factor in the clinical expression and management of this disease. Today, renal involvement is expected in the majority of patients with systemic lupus erythematosus.

PATHOGENESIS

Lupus nephritis represents a complex illness with a broad spectrum of immunopathology. The deposition of immune complexes appears to be the inciting step in the pathogenesis of this disease. DNA and anti-DNA antibodies are among the most nephritogenic of circulating immune complexes and they are amassed in glomerular deposits (Koffler et al, 1969).

The factors which promote the deposition of immune reactants in different sites along the nephron are incompletely understood (Couser, 1985). Immune complexes appear earliest in the mesangium (Michael et al, 1980). Localization in the mesangium may not be governed by specific immunologic factors (such as complement or immunoglobulin receptors); experimental studies show that the mesangium is a clearing site for a host of macromolecules many of which have limited nephritogenicity. On the other hand, certain attributes of immune complexes appear to enhance their accumulation in the subendothelial region of glomerular capillaries. DNA antigen has been shown to have an affinity for the glomerular basement membrane (Izui et al, 1977). This characteristic of DNA could account for the deposition of preformed DNA/anti-DNA circulating immune complexes or cause in situ formation of complexes following the "planting" of DNA in the glomerulus.

The glomerular capillary is comprised of proteoglycans which confer an distinctively high density of anion charges (Stow et al, 1985). Nephritogenicity of immune complexes appears to be substantially augmented if there is a dominance of cationic charge groups on either the antigen (Border et al, 1982) or antibody (Gauthier et al, 1982). Immune complexes with a high isoelectric point have been reported to be concentrated in glomerular deposits in murine lupus nephritis (Ebling and Hahn, 1980).

The composition of subepithelial immune deposits in membranous lupus nephropathy is unknown; it is doubtful that DNA is a relevant antigen in these lesions. The prospect that the subepithelial deposits are formed in situ by reaction of an autoantibody with constituents of the basement membrane or of the epithelial cell podocytes has not been determined (Madaio et al, 1983).

COURSE AND PROGNOSIS

In a multicenter study of over 1000 patients, the mortality rate was 10% at one year and 29% at 10 years after diagnosis of lupus (Ginzler et al, 1982). Patients with evidence of lupus nephritis had a nominally worse death rate. In a study of over 600 patients at a single center (Wallace et al, 1981), 10 year patient mortality was 21% (11% without and 35% with nephritis). In a group of over 100 patients with lupus nephritis followed at the National Institutes of Health, the risk within 10 years of dying was 25%, of end stage renal failure 28%, and of doubling serum creatinine 38%.

Lupus nephritis is the cause of approximately 3% of cases of end stage renal failure requiring maintenance dialysis or transplantation. These patients experience a higher mortality rate than properly matched dialysis patients (Kramer et al, 1982; Jarratt et al, 1983); the subset of patients with rapid escalation of their renal disease and persistently active extra-renal lupus are at particular risk (Cheigh et al, 1983; Correia et al, 1985).

The course of lupus nephritis is intricate and cannot be easily defined for several reasons. Among others, the clinical characteristics of the patients are extremely heterogeneous, the onset of the disease (systemic lupus erythematosus, lupus nephritis, or the specific class of glomerulonephritis) is often difficult to pinpoint, transitions among several types of renal pathology are common, and several different outcomes of the renal disease must be considered. Thus, determination of the probable clinical course of the individual patient with lupus nephritis is usually based on crude estimations at best.

Prognosis undoubtedly depends on a large number of factors specific to each patient with lupus nephritis. It is difficult to define the single most important variable in estimating the prognosis of lupus nephritis. It is judicious to develop a composite of demographic, clinical, laboratory and pathologic parameters in estimating prognosis and in planning management.

Demographic features

Young age at onset of lupus and male gender are associated with an increased risk of renal failure (Austin et al, 1983; Cameron et al, 1979). Race has been thought to have an influence on the severity of lupus; but recent analyses suggest that when race is adjusted for socioeconomic factors, it does not appear to have a major influence on the clinical course of systemic lupus or lupus nephritis (Ginzler et al, 1982).

Clinical features

Numerous clinical and laboratory measurements have been assessed for their prognostic value in lupus nephritis. The presence of nephrotic syndrome at onset of proliferative lupus nephritis (especially refractory nephrotic syndrome) seems to signal an adverse prognosis (Baldwin et al, 1977; Wallace et al, 1982; Ginzler et al, 1982).

There is no doubt that renal function tests are useful in the overall assessment of the patient with lupus nephritis. It is also important to recognize their limitations. Renal function is affected by reversible perfusional and structural lesions, as well as by fixed scarring and atrophic processes. Furthermore, hemodynamic and hypertrophic compensatory mechanisms can result in an underestimation of the degree of permanent renal damage based on standard renal function tests (Shemesh et al, 1985). Analyzing renal function tests over time yields a better correlation of structure and function as well as a more reliable estimate of renal prognosis. Insidious progression of azotemia heralds the development of chronic irreversible disease, while rapid swings in renal function often indicate the presence of active, treatable and potentially reversible lupus nephritis.

Pathology

The prognostic usefulness of the World Health Organization classification of lupus nephritis is controversial (Churg et al, 1982; Appel et al, 1978). It is apparent that there are smaller differences in renal outcomes among these classes of lupus nephritis in recent times (Appel et al, 1987; Austin et al, 1986; Cameron et al, 1979; Platt et al, 1982; Wallace et al, 1982) than there were a few decades ago (Baldwin et al, 1970; Pollak et al, 1964).

Assessment of lupus nephritis has been facilitated by defining the types and degrees of reversible and permanent renal lesions (Austin et al, 1984; Balow and Austin, 1988). The activity index encompasses the following: glomerular cellularity, leucocyte exudation, fibrinoid necrosis, hyaline thrombi, cellular crescents, and interstitial inflammation. The chronicity index encompasses the following: glomerular sclerosis, fibrous crescents, tubular atrophy, and interstitial fibrosis. The chronicity index has been found to have a graded relationship to the risk of end-stage renal failure (Austin et al, 1984; Morel-Maroger et al, 1976). Glomerular sclerosis, fibrous crescents, interstitial fibrosis and/or tubular atrophy are attended by reduction of renal reserve capacity or ineffective compensatory mechanisms; the presence of these lesions appears to increase the risk of renal functional deterioration as a consequence of superimposed active glomerular disease. The risk of renal failure is highest in patients with nephritic and/or nephrotic syndrome associated with extreme histologic activity (i.e., crescents, necrosis) or with less severe glomerular lesions superimposed on a background of chronic irreversible disease (i.e., tubular atrophy, interstitial fibrosis). Although suggested from observations in certain experimental models, there is little evidence that sclerosing or atrophic lesions themselves perpetuate renal failure in the absence of concomitant immunological disease.

The activity index was found to be a relatively weak predictor of renal failure outcome (Austin et al, 1984). Mild to moderate elevations of this index usually represent reversible disease (under the influence of effective treatment). Marked elevations of the activity index usually reflect structural disruption of the glomerular capillaries which heal by scarring rather than by regression. Thus, extreme elevations of the activity index predict an increased risk of renal failure. Subendothelial electron dense deposits are considered to be evidence of active lupus nephritis. However, their occurrence in a renal biopsy need not portend an unfavorable outcome since they can be mobilized and reduced in patients who are receiving effective immunosuppressive therapy (Austin et al, 1984).

Serologic Parameters

The obvious limitations on repeated sampling of renal histology have prompted studies of the utility of serologic tests to predict the activity of the lupus nephritis, to guide therapy and to judge prognosis. The level of serum complement (CH50,as well as C3 and C4 components) have been found to correlate with the degree of activity of glomerular disease on renal biopsy (Feldman et al, 1982). Falling levels of complement components are felt to be rather strong predictors of a flare of lupus nephritis. Some have advocated that therapy should be adjusted according to the level of C3 complement (Garin et al, 1979). Our group has found a relatively weak correlation between the duration of abnormal C3 levels and the acquisition of chronic sclerosing lesions on serial renal biopsies (Pillemer et al, 1988). Immunosuppressive drugs often produce an improvement in levels of C3 components which seems to be associated with reduction of disease activity. In particular, cytotoxic drugs are effective in this process. However, it should be underscored that one risks serious overtreatment of some patients by attempting to increase persistently abnormal levels of complement components. Supporting evidence of disease activity should be present if one utilizes these serologic tests as therapeutic guidelines.

Other tests have been advocated by some for monitoring lupus nephritis, including anti-DNA antibodies, circulating immune complexes, immunoglobulin levels, cryoglobulins, C-reactive protein, and erythrocyte sedimentation rate. However, none of these tests alone have sufficient power in terms of specificity or sensitivity to support their use as strict guides to therapy, disease activity or prognosis.

MANAGEMENT

The diversity of renal involvement and the paucity of therapeutic trials have impeded the establishment of standard treatments for lupus nephritis. However, there is general acknowledgement that immunosuppressive drug therapies have contributed to the steady improvement in the prognosis of lupus nephritis over the past three decades.

Indications for therapy

Progressive azotemia in the face of worsening, nephritic urinary sediment is clearly an indication for therapy. Increasing or nephrotic range proteinuria, falling serum complement and increasing anti-DNA antibody levels lend weight to the decision to initiate or to intensify therapy. Search for poor indications for therapeutic intervention is also important if one is to minimize the risk-benefit ratio. Fixed azotemia, fixed proteinuria, as well as abnormal but fixed levels of anti-DNA antibodies or serum complement are weak criteria for treatment.

The World Health Organization classes of lupus nephritis are widely used as indications for treatment. Diffuse proliferative lupus nephritis is considered to be the strongest indication for therapy. The intensity of treatment is usually escalated if there are extensive fibrinoid necrosis, cellular crescents and heavy subendothelial immune complex deposits in the renal biopsy. Focal proliferative lupus nephritis is managed similarly to diffuse disease, although with somewhat less urgency and intensity. Mesangial nephropathy bears a low risk of renal failure, but patients must be diligently monitored for evidence of progression to other classes of lupus nephritis. Management of membranous nephropathy is controversial. Therapy is usually directed toward control of the morbidity of nephrotic syndrome. However, prevention of renal failure is a research issue which is only recently beginning to be addressed in patients with membranous nephropathy.

Specific treatment options

Therapeutic decisions should be based on estimates of the natural history of the specific form of lupus nephritis, the likelihood of progression or conversion, and whether or not the renal manifestations reflect reversible pathology. These considerations must be cautiously balanced against the risk of iatrogenic complications of treatment.

Corticosteroids and cytotoxic drugs. The introduction to clinical medicine of antibiotics and cortisone derivatives in the 1940's produced a dramatic change in the natural history of lupus. High morbidity and mortality from lupus crises of extrarenal disease and from uncontrolled infections were replaced by those from the complications of chronic glomerulonephritis (Muehrcke et al, 1957; Pollak et al, 1961;

Baldwin et al, 1970; Dubois et al, 1974). High doses of corticosteroids and nitrogen mustard provided modest improvement in risks of mortality and uremic complications (Pollak et al, 1964). The prospect of greater efficacy with cytotoxic drug treatment was ardently pursued in the 1960's. Anecdotal reports supported the use of azathioprine and cyclophosphamide (Cameron et al, 1970; Drinkard et al, 1970; Hayslett et al, 1972; Fries et al, 1973; Cade et al, 1973).

Controlled trials of the use of these agents in lupus nephritis were undertaken at the National Institutes of Health and at the Mayo Clinic in the 1970's. Donadio et al (1972) found no short-term benefit of azathioprine for treatment of lupus nephritis. The short-term results reported by Steinberg and Decker (1974) indicated that standard doses of daily oral cyclophosphamide afforded greater control of proteinuria and of nephritic urine sediment than either azathioprine or prednisone. Follow-up observations at approximately two years (Decker et al, 1975) and longer (Decker et al, 1979; Carette et al, 1983) indicated marginal advantage of either cytotoxic drug over prednisone and no significant difference in the risk of developing end stage renal failure during the limited follow-up period. Comparable results with azathioprine treatment were noted by Hahn et al (1975).

Donadio and colleagues (1978) reported a study of the efficacy of cyclophosphamide versus prednisone in patients with severe proliferative lupus nephritis. Most patients responded to either treatment within the first six months. Subsequently, the patients who received cyclophosphamide and prednisone maintained a stable renal course more frequently than did patients treated with prednisone alone. After a mean period of nearly four years, there were few renal failure outcomes in either group and the differences were not statistically significant.

Patients in the studies at the National Institutes of Health were re-evaluated by two different criteria for evidence of superiority of any of the treatment regimens. Repeat renal biopsies were obtained from patient volunteers after participation in the therapeutic trial for a median of four years (Balow et al, 1984). The biopsies were analyzed semi-quantitatively for the evolution of chronic, irreversible renal lesions. Patients receiving prednisone treatment alone tended to develop increasing numbers of sclerotic and atrophic lesions over time. On the other hand, patients receiving any of the cytotoxic drugs (daily azathioprine, daily cyclophosphamide, combined low-dose daily azathioprine and cyclophosphamide, or intermittent pulse cyclophosphamide) showed less tendency to develop sclerotic, atrophic and fibrotic lesions. These observations formed the basis for the speculation that the patients treated with cytotoxic drugs were likely to experience a lower frequency of progressive renal failure.

With continued follow-up (median 7 years), the probability of developing end stage renal failure was significantly higher in patients treated with prednisone alone than in patients treated with intermittent pulse cyclophosphamide (Austin et al, 1986; Klippel et al, 1987). There were trends toward more favorable outcomes in patients treated with the other regimens of cytotoxic drugs and it is possible that additional observation would reveal a significant difference between the oral cytotoxic drugs and prednisone; but consideration of the high rates of side-effects of daily oral cytotoxic drugs has prompted us to discontinue these therapeutic approaches regardless of their potential efficacy.

The risk of major infections did not differ among the treatment groups except for an increase in herpes zoster in patients receiving any form of cyclophosphamide (Klippel, 1987). No episodes of hemorrhagic cystitis occurred in patients receiving intravenous cyclophosphamide. Premature ovarian failure developed in 18 of 33 patients receiving cyclophosphamide. The lowest rate occurred with intermittent pulse cyclophosphamide. Overall, the risk was low within the first decade from menarche and highest in patients initiated on therapy after the third decade of life. Six malignancies have developed in the cohort of 111 patients: three received daily azathioprine, three received daily cyclophosphamide. Pulse cyclophosphamide appeared to have fewer major side effects than conventional cyclophosphamide therapy.

Other therapies. Pulse methylprednisolone therapy is currently widely used in treatment of severe lupus nephritis (Cathcart et al, 1976; Ponticelli et al, 1982; Yeung et al, 1985). However, to date there has been no formal comparison of the efficacy of pulse methylprednisolone with that of high-dose oral prednisone. As with cyclophosphamide, there is a perception that pulse steroids are equally or more effective, but less toxic than daily prednisone. There is concern that single courses of pulse methylprednisolone add marginally to therapy with standard prednisone. Repeated courses of pulse therapy may be more efficacious and are under study (Balow et al, 1987).

Cyclosporin A has been shown to be effective in preventing and in controlling progressive renal failure in murine lupus nephritis. Limited trials have been undertaken in human lupus; none has been controlled. Anecdotal reports have claimed both unfavorable (Isenberg et al, 1981) and favorable (Feutren et al, 1986) results. Insidious nephrotoxicity is of great concern in the use of cyclosporine in autoimmune diseases (Palestine et al, 1986).

Total lymphoid irradiation has been used successfully for prevention and for reversal of murine lupus nephritis; this novel therapeutic approach has been applied successfully to a limited number of patients with drug resistant lupus nephritis (Strober et al, 1987). Long-term toxicity appears to be less than originally feared, but there have been no prospective comparisons of this therapy with other immunosuppressive drugs.

Plasma exchange therapy has been utilized for treatment of several components of lupus. In a double-blind study of real or sham plasma exchange in patients with mild systemic lupus, little objective advantage of plasma exchange was found (Wei et al, 1983). In a multicenter study of patients with severe diffuse proliferative lupus nephritis, there was no difference between immunosuppressive therapy alone and immunosuppressive therapy combined with plasma exchange (Lewis et al, 1987).

New therapeutic approaches are desireable for optimal management of lupus nephritis, both from the perspective of increased efficacy and of reduced toxicity. Increasingly selective approaches to immunosuppressive therapy have been historical goals. However, one should be mindful that the polyclonal nature of the autoreactive processes in lupus may require broadly immunosuppressive therapies for effective management. Murine lupus nephritis has been shown to respond favorably to monoclonal antibodies to T cell activation antigens, such as Ia (Adelman et al, 1983), and to T helper phenotype (Wofsy and Seamon, 1987). Recently it has been reported that one of the biologic response modifiers (eg. recombinant tumor necrosis factor) has a salutary effect on murine lupus nephritis (Jacob and McDevitt, 1988). The potential use of biologic agents as primary or adjunctive therapies for lupus, or as new approaches to reduction of toxicity of standard pharmacologic therapy (e.g., colony stimulating factors to accelerate recovery of leukopoiesis) is under study.

Practical approaches to treatment

Aggressive induction therapy for major indications usually includes high-dose prednisone at 1.0 mg/kg/day for 4 to 6 weeks. Continuation of daily prednisone for longer periods of time greatly increases the risk of iatrogenic complications, which can be minimized by tapering to a maintenance alternate day schedule of 0.2-0.5 mg/kg of prednisone. Alternative immunosuppressive drugs should be considered in the following situations: partial response of the objective signs of lupus nephritis or flare of the lupus nephritis while tapering to alternate day prednisone therapy. At the present time, therapy with prednisone alone is acceptable only if a dramatic and complete clinical remission is achieved within two months and sustained on low-dose alternate day therapy.

Pulse methylprednisolone in doses up to 1.0 gm/square meter of body surface area is a widely used option for intensive induction therapy. Intravenous methylprednisolone is typically given on three consecutive days; this is followed by moderate amounts of prednisone (0.5 mg/kg/day) for approximately four weeks with subsequent taper to an alternate day schedule. There have been no objective comparisons between oral high-dose prednisone and methylprednisolone pulse therapy, but it is thought that pulse therapy is at least as effective and has fewer short-term side effects than conventional oral prednisone.

Rigid guidelines for the optimal use of intravenous pulse cyclophosphamide have not been defined. The approach is mainly empiric as criteria by which to individualize therapy are lacking. Intravenous cyclophosphamide is usually initiated at a dose of 0.75 grams per square meter body surface area in patients whose estimated glomerular filtration rate is greater than one-third of normal. For patients with poorer renal function, the initial dose of cyclophosphamide is 0.5 grams per square meter. Cyclophosphamide is administered intravenously in 150 ml of 5% glucose solution over 30-60 minutes. Diuresis and frequent voiding are induced to minimize exposure of the urinary bladder to the toxic metabolites of cyclophosphamide. Approximately 2 liters per square meter of dilute intravenous solution (eg. 0.25 normal saline) are infused over the ensuing 24 hours. Occasionally, bladder irrigation via a three-way Foley catheter is instituted in patients with severe nephrotic syndrome who cannot achieve an copious urine output with volume and diuretic challenges.

White blood counts are measured on days 10 and 14 after cyclophosphamide infusion. These values are the major determinants of the subsequent dose modifications of cyclophosphamide. The nadir white blood count should fall below 4000/microliter but not less than 1500/microliter. The maximum dose of cyclophosphamide used in the National Institutes of Health studies is 1.0 gram/square meter. If the white blood count falls below 1500/microliter, the dose is reduced to 0.5 gram/square meter. Antiemetic therapy is individualized according to the desires and experience of each patient. Hair loss following cyclophosphamide is highly variable, but alopecia totalis is distinctly uncommon at these doses.

The optimal frequency and duration of cyclophosphamide pulse therapy have not been determined. At the present time, a regimen of monthly pulses for six months followed by quarterly pulses is preferred. Treatment is continued beyond evidence of remission for a period of one year. Earlier discontinuation of therapy appears to be associated with high risk of relapse of lupus nephritis.

REFERENCES

Adelman NE, Watling DL and McDevitt HO: Treatment of [NZB/NZW] F1 disease with anti-Ia monoclonal antibodies. J Exp Med 158:1350-1355, 1983

Appel GB, Cohen DJ, Pirani CL, Meltzer JI and Estes D: Long-term follow-up of patients with lupus nephritis. A study based on the classification of the World Health Organization. Am J Med 83:877-885, 1987

Appel GB, Silva FG, Pirani CL, Meltzer JI and Estes D: Renal involvement in systemic lupus erythematosus (SLE): a study of 56 patients emphasizing histologic classification. Medicine 57:371-410, 1978.

Austin HA III, Klippel JH, Balow JE, leRiche NGH, Steinberg AD, Plotz PH and Decker JL: Therapy of lupus nephritis: controlled trial of prednisone and cytotoxic drugs. N Engl J Med 314:614-619, 1986.

Austin HA III, Muenz LR, Joyce KM, Antonovych TT and Balow JE: Diffuse proliferative lupus nephritis: identification of specific pathologic features affecting renal outcome. Kidney Int 25:689-695, 1984.

Austin HA III, Muenz LR, Joyce KM, Antonovych TT, Kullick ME, Klippel JH, Decker JL and Balow JE: Prognostic factors in lupus nephritis. Contribution of renal histologic data. Am J Med 75:382-391, 1983.

Baldwin DS, Gluck MC, Lowenstein J and Gallo G: Lupus nephritis: clinical course as related to morphologic forms and their transitions. Am J Med 62:12-30, 1977.

Baldwin DS, Lowenstein J, Rothfield NF, Gallo G and McCluskey RT: The clinical course of the proliferative and membranous forms of lupus nephritis. Ann Intern Med 73:929-942, 1970

Balow JE and Austin HA III: Renal disease in systemic lupus erythematosus. Rheumatic Dis Clin North Am 14:117-133, 1988

Balow JE, Austin HA III, Muenz LR, Joyce KM, Antonovych TT, Klippel JH, Steinberg AD, Plotz PH and Decker JL: The effect of treatment on the evolution of renal abnormalities in lupus nephritis. N Engl J Med 311:491-495, 1984.

Balow JE, Austin HA III, Tsokos GC, Antonovych TT, Steinberg AD and Klippel JH: Lupus nephritis. Ann Intern Med 106:79-94, 1987

Border WA, Ward HJ, Kamil ES and Cohen AH: Induction of membranous nephropathy in rabbits by administration of an exogenous cationized antigen. Demonstration of a pathogenetic role for electrical charge. J Clin Invest 69:451-461, 1982.

Cade R, Spooner G, Schlein E, Pickering M, DeQuesada A, Holcomb A, Juncos L, Richard G, Shires D, Levin D, Hackett R, Free J, Hunt R and Fregly M: Comparison of azathioprine, prednisone, and heparin alone or combined in treating lupus nephritis. Nephron 10:37-56, 1973

Cameron JS, Boulton-Jones M, Robinson R and Ogg C: Treatment of lupus nephritis with cyclophosphamide. Lancet 2:846-849, 1970.

Cameron JS, Turner DR, Ogg CS, Williams DG, Lessof MH, Chantler C and Leibowitz S: Systemic lupus with nephritis: a long-term study. Q J Med 48:1-24, 1979

Carette S, Klippel JH, Decker JL, Austin HA III, Plotz PH, Steinberg AD and Balow JE: Controlled studies of oral immunosuppressive drugs in lupus nephritis: a long-term follow-up. Ann Intern Med 99:1-8, 1983

Cathcart ES, Idelson BA, Scheinberg MA and Couser WG: Beneficial effects of methylprednisolone pulse therapy in diffuse proliferative lupus nephritis. Lancet 1:163-166, 1976.

Cheigh JS, Stenzel KH, Rubin AL, Chami J and Sullivan JF: Systemic lupus erythematosus in patients with chronic renal failure. Am J Med 75:602-606, 1983

Churg J and Sobin LH: Lupus nephritis. In, Renal Disease. Tokyo, Igaku-Shoin. 1982, pp 127-149.

Correia P, Cameron JS, Lian JD, Hicks J, Ogg CS, Williams DG, Chantler C and Haycock DG: Why do patients with lupus nephritis die? Br Med J 290:126-131, 1985

Couser WG: Mechanisms of glomerular injury in immune-complex disease. Kidney Int 28:569-583, 1985.

Decker JL, Klippel JH, Plotz PH and Steinberg AD: Cyclophosphamide or azathioprine in lupus glomerulonephritis. A controlled trial: Results at 28 months. Ann Intern Med 83:606-615, 1975.

Decker JL, Steinberg AD, Reinertsen JL, Plotz PH, Balow JE and Klippel JH: Systemic lupus erythematosus: evolving concepts. Ann Intern Med 91:587-604, 1979

Donadio JV Jr, Holley KE, Ferguson RH and Ilstrup DM: Treatment of diffuse proliferative lupus nephritis with prednisone and combined prednisone and cyclophosphamide. N Engl J Med 299:1151-1155, 1978.

Donadio JV Jr, Holley KE, Wagoner RD, Ferguson RH and McDuffie

FC: Treatment of lupus nephritis with prednisone and combined prednisone and azathioprine. Ann Intern Med 77:829-835, 1972

Drinkard JP, Stanley TM, Dornfield L, Austin RC, Barnett EV, Pearson CM, Vernier RL, Adams DA, Latta H and Gonick HC: Azathioprine and prednisone in the treatment of adults with lupus nephritis. Medicine 49:411-432, 1970

Dubois EL, Wierzchowiecki M, Cox MB and Weiner JM: Duration and death in systemic lupus erythematosus. JAMA 227:1399-1402, 1974

Ebling J and Hahn BH: Restricted subpopulations of DNA antibodies in kidneys of mice with systemic lupus erythematosus: comparison of antibodies in serum and renal eluates. Arthritis Rheum 23: 392-403, 1980.

Feldman MD, Huston DP, Karsh J, Balow JE, Klima E and Steinberg AD: Correlation of serum IgG, IgM, and anti-native-DNA antibodies with renal and clinical indexes of activity in systemic lupus erythematosus. J Rheumatol 9:52-58, 1982

Feutren G, Querin S, Tron F, Noel LH, Chatenoud L, Lesavre P and Bach JF: The effects of cyclosporine in patients with systemic lupus. Transplant Proc 18:643-644, 1986.

Fries JF, Sharp GC, McDevitt HO and Holman HR: Cyclophosphamide therapy in systemic lupus erythematosus and polymyositis. Arthritis Rheum 16:154-162, 1973

Garin EH, Donnelly WH, Shulman ST, Fernandez R, Finton G, Williams RL and Richard GA: The significance of serial measurements of serum complement C3 and C4 components and DNA binding capacity in patients with lupus nephritis. Clin Nephrol 12:148-155, 1979

Gauthier VJ, Mannik M and Striker GE: Effect of cationized antibodies in preformed immune complexes on deposition and persistence in renal glomeruli. J Exp Med 156:766-777, 1982.

Ginzler EM, Diamond HS, Weiner M, Schlesinger M, Fries JF, Wasner C, Medsger TA, Ziegler G, Klippel JH, Hadler NM, Albert DA, Hess EV, Spencer-Green G, Grayzel A, Worth D, Hahn BH and Barnett EV: A multicenter study of outcome in systemic lupus erythematosus. I. Entry variables as predictors of prognosis. Arthritis Rheum 25:601-611, 1982

Hahn BH, Kantor OS and Osterland CK: Azathioprine plus prednisone compared to prednisone alone in the treatment of systemic lupus erythematosus: reports of a prospective controlled trial in 24 patients. Ann Intern Med 83:597-605, 1975

Hayslett JP, Kashgarian M, Cook CD and Spargo BH: The effect of azathioprine on lupus glomerulonephritis. Medicine 51:393-412, 1972.

Isenberg DA, Snaith ML, Morrow WJ, Al-Khader AA, Cohen SL, Fisher C and Mowbray J: Cyclosporin A for the treatment of systemic lupus erythematosus. Int J Immunopharmacol 3:163-169, 1981

Izui S, Lambert PH and Miescher PA: In vitro demonstration of a particular affinity of glomerular basement membrane and collagen for DNA: a possible basis for a local formation of DNA-anti-DNA complexes in systemic lupus erythematosus. J Exp Med 145:1115-1130, 1977.

Jacob CO and McDevitt HO: Tumour necrosis factor-alpha in murine autoimmune lupus nephritis. Nature 331:356-358, 1988

Jarrett MP, Santhanam S and Del Greco F: The clinical course of end-stage renal disease in systemic lupus erythematosus.

Arch Intern Med 143:1353-1356, 1983
Klippel JH: Morbidity and mortality, pp 89-92. In: Balow JE, moderator. Lupus nephritis. Ann Intern Med 106:79-94, 1987
Klippel JH, Austin HA III, Balow JE, leRiche NG, Steinberg AD, Plotz PH and Decker JL: Studies of immunosuppressive drugs in the treatment of lupus nephritis. Rheum Dis Clin North Am 13:47-56, 1987
Koffler D, Agnello V, Carr I and Kunkel HG: Variable patterns of immunoglobulin and complement deposition in the kidneys of patients with systemic lupus erythematosus. Am J Pathol 56:305-319, 1969.
Kramer P, Broyer M, Brunner FP, Brynger H, Donckerwolcke RA, Jacobs C, Selwood NH and Wing AJ: Combined report on regular dialysis and transplantation in Europe. XII. Proc Eur Dial Transplant Assoc 19:29-31, 1982
Lewis E and Lachin J: Primary outcomes in the controlled trial of plasmapheresis therapy (PPT) in severe lupus nephritis (Abstract). Kidney Int 31:208, 1987.
Madaio MP, Salant DJ, Cohen AJ, Adler S and Couser WG: Comparative study of in situ immune deposit formation in active and passive Heymann nephritis. Kidney Int 23:498-505, 1983.
Michael AF, Keane WF, Raij L, Vernier RL and Mauer SM: The glomerular mesangium. Kidney Int 17:141-154, 1980.
Morel-Maroger L, Mery JP, Droz D, Godin M, Verroust P, Kourilsky O and Richet G: The course of lupus nephritis: contribution of serial renal biopsies. Adv Nephrol 6:79-118, 1976
Muehrcke RC, Kark RM, Pirani CL and Pollak VE: Lupus nephritis: a clinical and pathologic study based on renal biopsies. Medicine 36:1-145, 1957
Palestine AG, Austin HA III, Balow JE, Antonovych TT, Sabnis SG, Preuss HG and Nussenblatt RB: Renal histopathologic alterations in patients treated with cyclosporine for uveitis. N Engl J Med 314:1293-1298, 1986
Pillemer S, Austin HA III, Tsokos GC and Balow JE: Lupus nephritis: association between serology and renal biopsy measures. J Rheumatol 15:284-288, 1988
Platt JL, Burke BA, Fish AJ, Kim Y and Michael AF: Systemic lupus erythematosus in the first two decades of life. Am J Kidney Dis 2:212-222, 1982
Pollak VE, Pirani CL and Kark RM: Effect of large doses of prednisone on the renal lesions and life span of patients with lupus glomerulonephritis. J Lab Clin Med 57:495-511, 1961.
Pollak VE, Pirani CL and Schwartz FD: The natural history of the renal manifestations of systemic lupus erythematosus. J Lab Clin Med 63:537-550, 1964
Ponticelli C, Zucchelli P, Moroni G, Cagnoli L, Banfi G and Pascuali S: Long-term prognosis of diffuse lupus nephritis. Clin Nephrol 28:263-271, 1987
Shemesh O, Golbetz H, Kriss JP and Myers BD: Limitations of creatinine as a filtration marker in glomerulopathic patients. Kidney Int 28:830-838, 1985
Steinberg AD and Decker JL: A double-blind controlled trial comparing cyclophosphamide, azathioprine and placebo in the treatment of lupus glomerulonephritis. Arthritis Rheum 17:923-937, 1974.
Stow JL, Sawada H and Farquhar MG: Basement membrane heparan sulfate proteoglycans are concentrated in the laminae rarae

and in podocytes of the rat renal glomerulus. Proc Natl Acad Sci (USA) 82:3296-3300, 1985.
Strober S, Farinas MC, Field EH, Solovera JJ, Kiberd BA, Myers BD and Hoppe RT: Lupus nephritis after total lymphoid irradiation: persistent improvement and reduction of steroid therapy. Ann Intern Med 107:689-690, 1987
Wallace DJ, Podell TE, Weiner JM, Cox MB, Klinenberg JR, Forouzesh S and Dubois EL: Lupus nephritis. Experience with 230 patients in a private practice from 1950 to 1980. Am J Med 72:209-220, 1982
Wallace DJ, Podell TE, Weiner JM, Klinenberg JR, Forouzesh S and Dubois EL: Systemic lupus erythematosus--survival patterns. JAMA 245:934-938, 1981
Wei N, Klippel JH, Huston DP, Hall RP, Lawley TJ, Balow JE, Steinberg AD and Decker JL: Randomized trial of plasma exchange in mild systemic lupus erythematosus. Lancet 1:17-22, 1983
Wofsy D and Seamon WE: Reversal of advanced murine lupus in NZB/NZW F1 mice by treatment with monoclonal antibody to L3T4. J Immunol 138:3247-3253, 1987
Yeung CK, Wong KL, Wong WS, Ng MT, Chan KW and Ng WL: Crescentic lupus glomerulonephritis. Clin Nephrol 21:251-258, 1984

PROGNOSTIC DETERMINANTS IN LUPUS NEPHRITIS

P.Coratelli, R.Rizzi, G. Pannarale, A.Ramunni
M. Giannattasio, and G. Passavanti

Institute of Medical Nephrology
University of Bari, Bari, Italy

The prognostic of SLE has progressively improved, especially during the past decade (1), and considerable advance has been made in the prognosis of lupus nephritis as well.

Recent series have reported overall survival rates greater than 70% at five years (2-6) and have failed to confirm the gloomy prognosis initially accorded to the diffuse proliferative class (3,7 - 10).

This remarkable improvement is due to general amelioration in medical care and particularly to increased sophistication in the application of corticosteroid and immunosuppressive therapy (11).

Because of the substantial toxicity of the immunosuppressive drugs, that can partially outweigh the beneficial effects of treatment, aggressive pharmacological immunosuppression is now reserved for patients considered at risk of developing end-stage renal failure.

Accordingly, in order to develop rational approaches to treatment in such a pleiomorphic disease, investigators in a number of centres have sought to improve the understanding of prognostic indicators, that would permit identification of those patients at high risk of poor outcome (12-16).

Although certain clinical and histological features have correlated with a higher likelihood of a poor response to treatment, the factor or factors which are of special importance as determinants of the long-term course of lupus nephritis have not been established.

In this paper the clinical course of 47 patients with lupus nephritis was reported and an attempt was made with different statistical methods to identify the clinical features, renal histological changes, and serological parameters which offered the best correlation with the long-term outcome and which could serve, therefore, as prognostic indices.

PATIENTS AND METHODS

Fourty seven patients with SLE and clinical evidence of renal involvement were followed at the Institute of Medical Nephrology, University of Bari, between 1974 and 1987.

All patients had sufficient clinical and laboratory findings to satisfy the criteria of the American Rheumatism Association for classification of SLE (17).

The following informations were analysed:

Clinical data

Age, sex, mode of presentation and outcome.

Laboratory tests

Serum creatinine levels, urinary protein excretion, urinary erythrocyte count, serum complement (C_3,C_4) and anti DNA titer by Farr assay or Crithidia luciliae method.

Histology

Renal biopsy specimens were obtained from 41 patients.

On 18 patients a second renal biopsy was done 6-12 months after treatment was begun, to assess results of therapy.

Histological findings were categorized according to World Health Organitation classification (18)

In addition biopsies were scored semiquantitatively using the method described by Morel-Maroger (2)

Composite scores derived from the sum of scores for individual active lesions (activity index), chronic lesions (chronicity index) and activity and chronicity indices (total pathologic score) were calculated. For total phatological score calculation, the chronicity index was arbitrarly weighted for a factor of 4, to balance the activity values.

Treatment

All patient had prednisone treatment:high dose (defined as 1 mg/Kg/day for a period of two months), or low dose (20 mg or less per day).

In 13 patients low doses of prednisone were associated with cyclophosphamide or azathioprine (50-100 mg/day). Recently metylprednisolone pulses were used for the treatment of renal flare-ups.

Follow-up

Patients were seen at regular intervals according to clinical indications and were followed until death or end stage renal failure, or for a minimun of one year.

Statistical analysis

For life-table analysis, "EPILOG" STATISTICAL SOFTWARE (Epicenter Software, Pasadena, California, USA) was employed. Survival curves were presented as actuarial life-table (Kaplan-Meier), to compare graphically the patient and the kidney survival. Patient survival included patient who where not undergoing dialysis or had not received a renal transplant and did not die. Except the latters, the same patients were included in the kidney survival.

The Kaplan-Maier survival curves for n groups were utilized using the log-rank Statistic, which is distributed as CHI-SQUARE with n-1 degree of freedom.

Disposing of observations, that is the measurements of the variables at the beginning of the follow-up period, and knowing the exit of the disease, we employed a stepwise discriminant analysis program (SPSS Inc., Chicago, IL, USA) to determine the best combination of variable for predicting survival.

As a check of the power of the found discriminant function we classified the original set of cases to see how many were correctly classified by the variables being used.

A probability of membership in the respective group was supplied.

RESULTS

Onset data

Of 47 patients with lupus nephritis 41 were female and 6 male, giving a female to male ratio of 6.8/1.

Table I. LUPUS NEPHRITIS: MODE OF PRESENTATION

	PATIENTS
NEPHROTIC SYNDROME	18 (38%)
NEPHRITIC SYNDROME	2 (4%)
ISOLATED URINARY ABNORMALITIES	22 (47%)
RAPIDLY PROGRESSIVE RENAL FAILURE	5* (11%)
	47 (100%)

* Three patients also had nephrotic syndrome, an other one had nephritic syndrome.

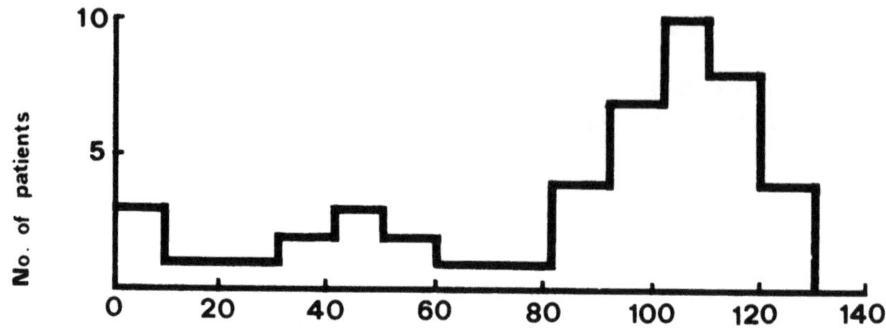

Fig. 1 Glomerular filtration rates of the 47 patients at clinical onset of nephritis

The mean age was 24 ± 11 years (ranging from 12 to 56) at onset of SLE, and 26 ± 11 years (ranging from 13 to 60) at onset of nephritis.

In 17 patients (36%) renal disease was detected as an initial manifestation of SLE.

The mode of presentation of renal disease itself is shown in table I and the glomerular filtration rates (GFR) at onset in Fig. 1.

Thirthy-two of 45 patients (71%) were hypocomplementemic at onset of nephritis; low C_3 levels were found in 19 of them (42%), low C_4 in 27 of 39 patients who were tested.

High titers of anti-ds-DNA antibodies were present in 14 of 39 patients (36 %) in whom were available.

The histological patterns on the initial renal biopsies are shown in Tab. II; diffuse proliferative glomerulonephritis was the most common finding.

Table II. LUPUS NEPHRITIS: HISTOLOGICAL PATTERNS

CLASS	DESCRIPTION	PATIENTS
I and II	Minimal change and mesangial proliferative	5 (12%)
III	Focal proliferative	6 (15%)
IV	Diffuse proliferative	25 (63%)
V	Membranous	4 (10%)
		41

Table III. LUPUS NEPHRITIS: MOST RECENT STATUS

	PATIENTS
DEATH	4 (8%)
END STAGE RENAL DISEASE	9 (19%)
CHRONIC RENAL FAILURE (GFR 80 ml/m')	5 (11%)
PERSISTENT PROTEINURIA (0.5 g/24h)	8 (17%)
COMPLETE REMISSION	21 (45%)
	47 (100%)

Follow-up data

At the end of follow-up period patients had SLE for 8.4 ± 5.7 years (range 1-31) and nephritis for 6.3 ±3.6 years (range 1-15).

During a cumulative follow-up of 295 years, 46 exacerbations occurred; so the risk of flare-up in this series was 1/6.2 years.

The most recent status of patients is summarized in Tab.III

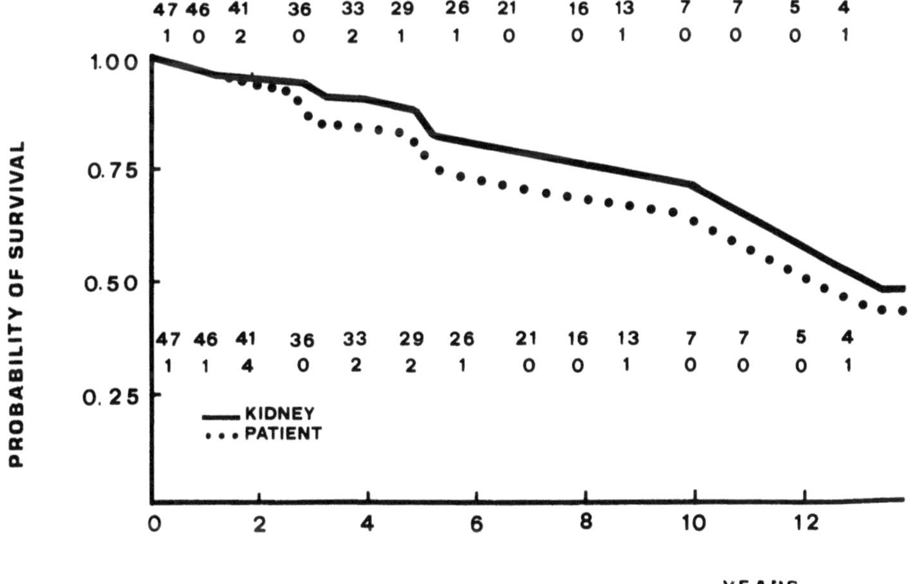

Fig. 2 Survival of the whole group of patients from the first clinical evidence of renal disease

The survival of the whole group of patients, from the first clinical evidence of renal disease, is shown in Fig. 2. Overall patient survival was calculated as 81% at five years and 66% at 10 years, kidney survival was respectively 87% and 73%.

Survival by clinical features

Figures 3,4,5 present analysis of survival from onset of lupus nephritis comparing patients with different sex (fig. 3), age at onset (fig. 4), and with and without nephrotic syndrome at onset (fig. 5)

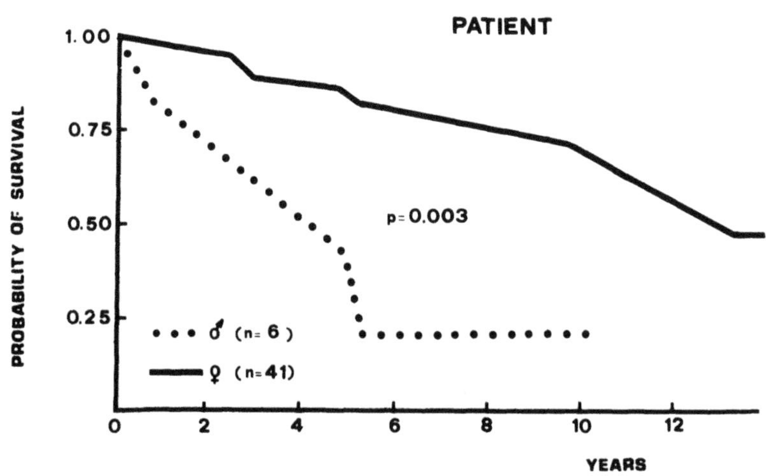

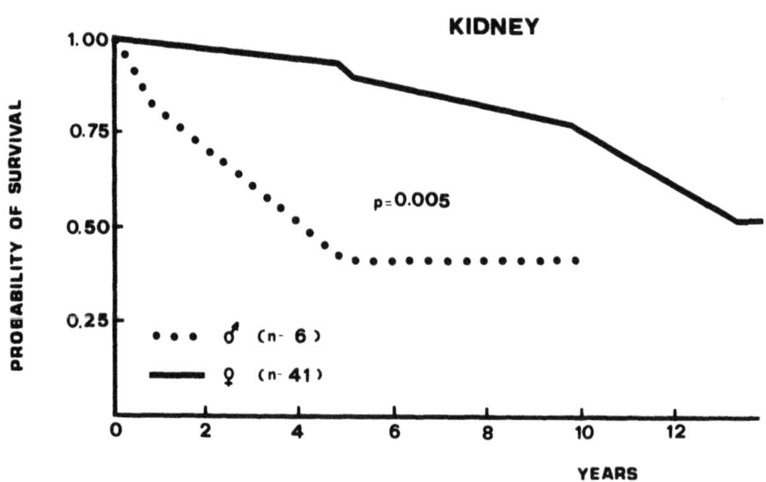

Fig. 3 Survival from clinical onset of lupus nephritis for female and male patients.

The overall male survival was significantly worse than the overall female survival (p = 0.003), furthermore male gender was associated with increased rate of renal failure (p = 0.005).

Patients younger than 16 years had a significantly worse outcome (p = 0.02),by contrast,kidney survival was unaffected by age.

As regard to nephrotic syndrome, althoug there was no significant difference in patient survival between patients with and without nephrotic syndrome, the presence was associated with an increased probability of renal failure developing (p = 0.0005).

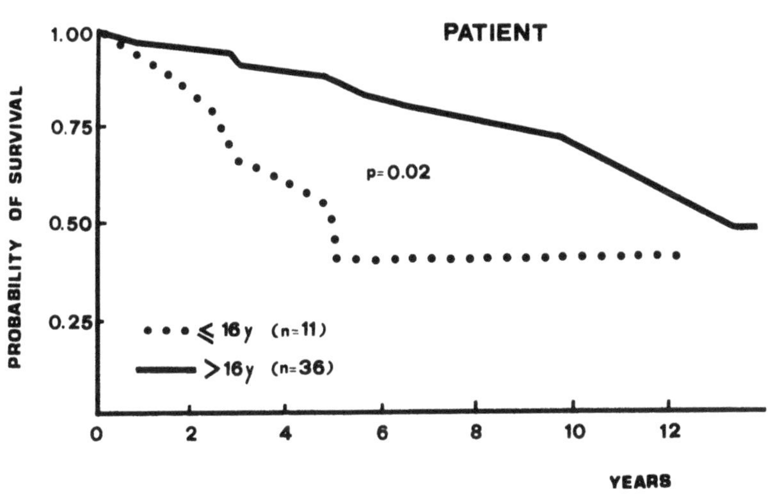

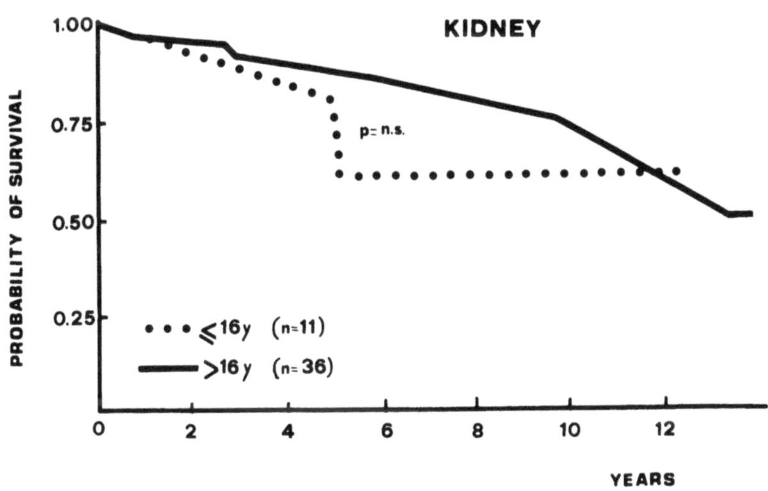

Fig. 4 Survival for patients with clinical onset of nephritis below and above 16 years of age

Renal disfunction did not appear to influence the long-term outcome for patient survival or the development of renal failure.

Immunological parameters (serum complement, anti-ds-DNA antibodies levels) were not predictive for different outcome, both for patients and kidney survival.

Survival by histological features

The survival for patients with mild (class II and V) or severe (class III and IV) histology on renal biopsy was not significantly different, although no deaths occurred in patients with mild nephritis.

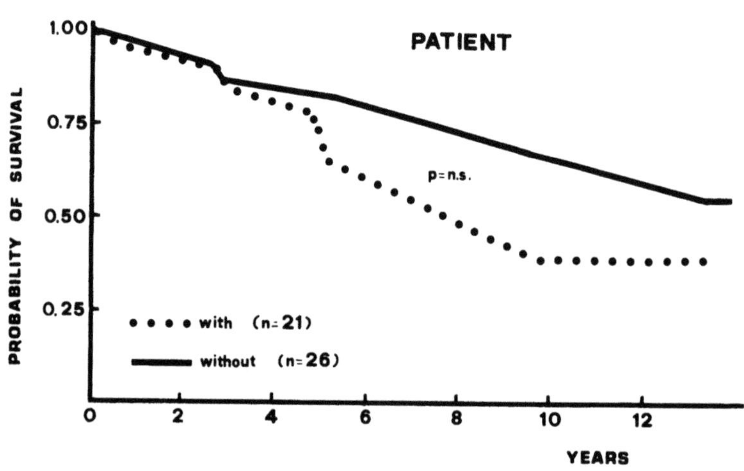

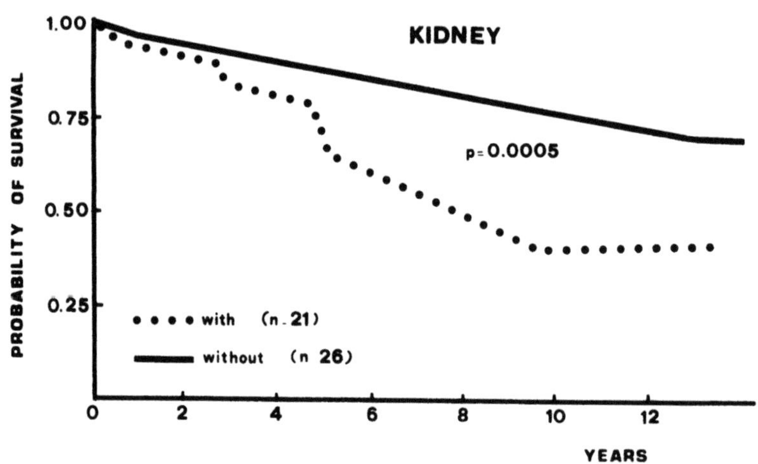

Fig. 5 Survival for patients with and without nephrotic syndrome at onset

Figures 6 and 7 present analysis of survival comparing patients with different degrees of chronicity index and total pathological score.

Patients and kidney survival was significantly worse both for patients with high ($\geqslant$2) chronicity index (patient survival p = 0.0004, kidney survival p = 0.01) and for patients with the highest ($\geqslant$19) total pathological score (patient survival p = 0.0003, kidney survival p $<$ 0.0001).

By contrast high ($>$10) activity index did not identify patients at high risk of poor outcome or end stage renal disease.

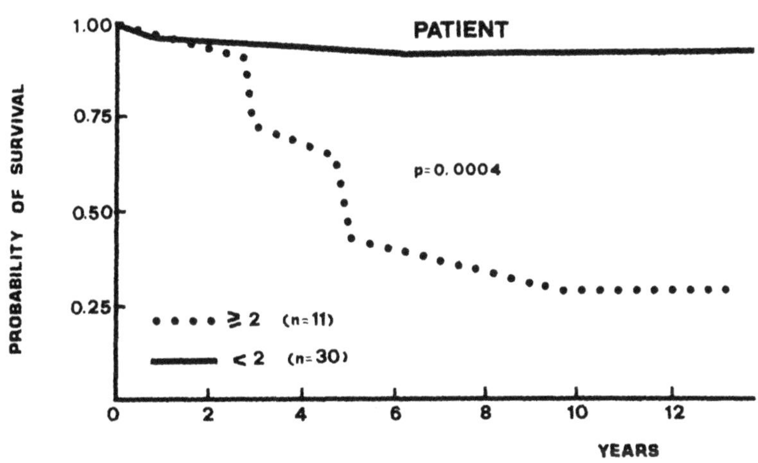

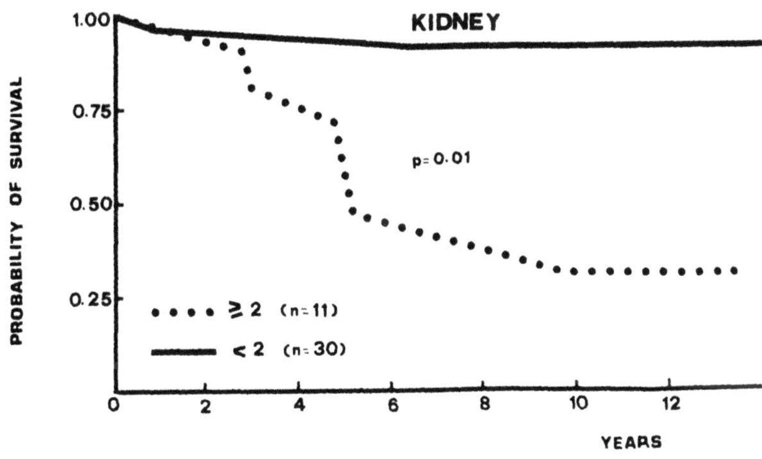

Fig. 6 Survival for patients with lupus nephritis comparing those with high chronicity index at renal biopsy versus rest.

Fig. 8 shows changes in chronicity score found at second renal biopsy of patients with low (⩽10) and high (>10) activity index at first biopsy. Chronicity score was no different between the two groups at first biopsy.

However, patients with high activity index at first biopsy had higher chronicity score at second biopsy (fig.8 botton). Furthermore, significant correlation was found in these patients between activity score at first biopsy and changes in chronicity score at second (fig.8 top)

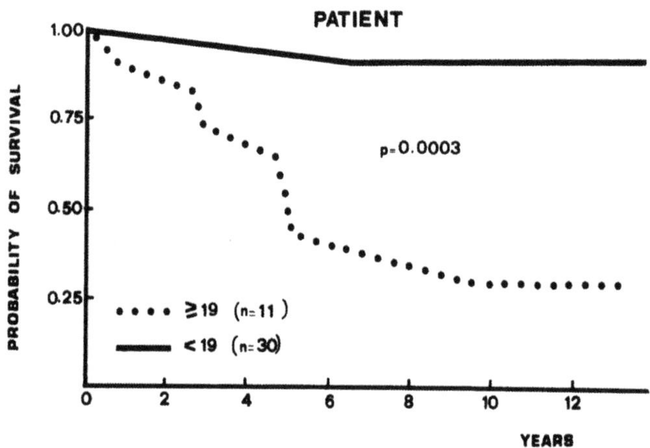

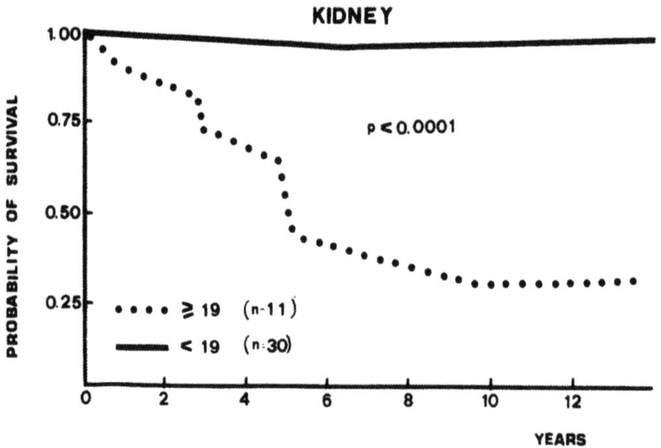

Fig. 7 Survival by total pathological score at renal biopsy

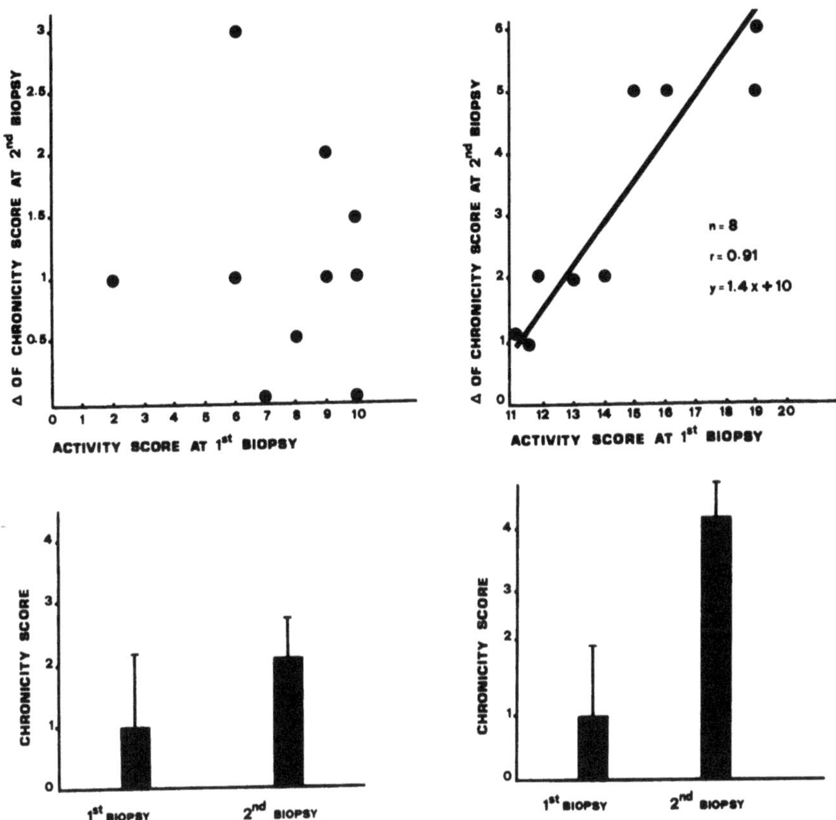

Fig. 8 Changes in chronicity score at second biopsy in patients with low (left side of figure) and high (right side) activity score at first biopsy.

Discriminant analysis

Using variables available at the onset of the lupus nephritis, the purpose of the discriminant analysis was to find the minimun subset of these variables which will best distinguish the patients divided into two classes (first: dead or hemodialyzed patients; second: alive patients). The descriptors introduced in the analysis were: sex, age, nephrotic syndrome, nephritic syndrome, isolated urinary abnormalities, rapidly progressive renal failure, serum creatinine, C3, C4, histological classes, activity score, chronicity score and total pathological score.

Table IV presents the results of stepwise discriminant analysis. As shown, sex, nephrotic syndrome and histological scores were selected. The standardized weights attached to each variable represent the relative contribution of their associated variable to the discriminant functions. The functions are formed in such a way to maximize the separation of the two classes: so their values are similar for individuals belonging to the same group, while present the highest differences among subjects belonging to different groups.

The high value attributed to histological scores enphasize their shrong weight in the separation of the two classes.

In order to validate the found discriminant functions we classified the original set of cases, according to the discriminant functions shown in table IV.

The estimated probability of correct classification was of 87%, because only two of 13 patients in the group 1 and 4 of 34 in the group 2 were misclassified (table V).

Table IV. DISCRIMINANT ANALYSIS

Standardized Canonical Discriminant Function Coefficients

X	W
SEX	.48102
NEPHROTIC SINDROME	.57150
ACTIVITY SCORE	5.25797
CHRONICITY SCORE	5.28239
TOTAL PATHOLOGICAL SCORE	8.01850

Table V. DISCRIMINANT ANALYSIS

Classification Results

Actual Group	No. of Cases	Predicted 1	Group Membership 2
Group 1	13	11 84.6%	2 15.4%
Group 2	34	4 11.8%	30 88.2%

Percent of "grouped" cases correctly classified: 87.23%

DISCUSSION

The purpose of this study was to identify a number of clinical, laboratory and pathologic variables which offered the best correlation with long-term outcome and which could serve, therefore, as prognostic indices, in a group of patients with lupus nephritis.

While similar to some previous studies in purpose, the present one differs from these in two important aspects. First, we report on a set of patients seen at a single center with relatively limited referral area and managed by the same medical staff for all the follow-up period, that allowed omogeneous evaluation of all clinical and histological findings

Second, two different statistical methods were employed: the first one to identify the clinical features, serological parameters and histological changes which could be of prognostic importance, the second one to weight and combine the different variables examined in order to individuate the smallest set of variables able to identify patients with poor outcome.

In the present study the overall survival rate of 81% at five years for patients and 87% for kidney is similar to other recent series (2-5). By contrast, Leaker and coll. (6) report analogous patient survival of 83% at five years with only 4% of renal deaths. Such a difference in renal failure rate may be partly explained by the varying severity of the disease seen in different parts of the world, but principally by different methods of patients management. Aggressive treatment may prevent the development of renal failure but lead to complications, particulary sepsis. In our series extrarenal deaths occurred predominantly within the first few years after diagnosis, as also reported by Balow (20), in that expression of more active lupus, whereas renal deaths occurred through the course of SLE.

Turning to prognostic determinants, with respect to clinical features our study suggests that sex, age and nephrotic syndrome are significant prognostic factors in lupus nephritis.

The overwhelming preponderance of female patients in nearly all the studies has made difficult to compare accurately survival of male patients with that of female patients, therefore results are often controversial. Our study, as Austin (15), shows that male gender is associated with increased rate of renal failure and furthermore that overall male survival is significantly worse than the overall female survival. By contrast, other investigators, as Cameron (3) and Leaker (6) have found that survival is unaffected by sex.

The prognostic value of age too remains controversial. Previous reports (4) showed that childhood nephritis tends to be severe and carry a worse prognosis than adult nephritis. Other investigators (3,6) were not able to find any difference. Other studies have shown that younger people have a better prognosis (21). These conflicting results preasumably come from differences either in geographic and racial composition of the groups or in age limits used for analysis. In our series, well-defined from the geographical viewpoint, patients younger than 16 years had a significantly worse outcome, by contrast kidney survival was unaffected by age.

With respect to mode of presentation, some studies (4,5,14) have found the presence of heavy proteinuria predictive of an unfavorable prognosis, others (3,6,22) have found no significant differences in long-term outcome. In our study the presence of nephrotic syndrome is associated with an increased probability of renal failure developing. These data are in agreement with Appel (5) who found furthemore that persistence of the nephrotic syndrome appears to be an unfavorable sign and defines a subset of patient who warrant consideration for vigorous treatment.

In contrast to many previous reports (4,6,14,15,22) in our series renal disfunction at onset doesn't appear to influence the long term outcome for patients or kidney survival. The reasons for this discrepancy are not apparent, but it is possible that differences in histological characteristics of our patients may account in part for them. Renal function may be altered by acute reversible disease as well as by various forms of irreversible pathologic changes. On the other hand renal functional compensatory mechanisms quickly reverse the effects of loss of renal mass. So glomerular filtration rate is not adequate measure of renal damage (23).
Therefore, although as many as 30% of our patients had renal disfunction at onset of nephritis, in the majority of these it was substained by active histological lesions, reversed by treatment with no or little residual damage. By contrast, other studies may have included patients with more advanced renal involvement and presumably less reversible forms of renal disfunction.

The value of renal biopsy in lupus nephritis is still matter of debate (24).
With respect to histologic classification most studies have found that renal biopsy in SLE provides useful information on the future clinical course (5,8,18,20). In the recent study of Appel (5) evaluation of renal biopsy using the WHO classification continued to provide valuable information concerning the risk of renal failure even 10 years after initial biopsy. However, many others studies have been unable to demonstrate a significant difference in outcome among different histological groups as defined by WHO classification (3,13,21,25,26). Some investigators (26,27) have examined critically the questions of whether the biopsy results provide information in addition to clinical and laboratory data obtained before biopsy.
They concluded that based on renal biopsy histologic classification

does not provide significant information for predicting renal death.

In the present study the survival for patients with mild (class II and V) or severe (class III and IV) histology on renal biopsy was not significantly different but it is possible that both the small number of patients with mild nephritis and the variable outcomes observed in patients with histologically severe nephritis may account for these results. In fact no deaths occurred in patients with mild nephritis. Therefore we exclude any comment based on our own experience.

For the conflicting and in some instances disappointing results obtained with the WHO classification various investigators have sought alternative measures to more accurately describe the histologic changes of lupus nephritis. In order to overcome the inflexibility of conventional classification, based entirely on certain glomerular abnormalities, namely proliferation and capillary loops tickening, they have proposed semiquantitative scoring systems, based on a broad range of tubular, interstitial and vascular changes. Their use as a source of prognostic information has been emphasized by many studies (2,15,20, 27, 28). Sclerosing lesions consistently emerged as ominous prognostic indicators that tend to progress regardless of therapeutic intervention.

In the present study the chronicity index appears to have a striking predictive value. By contrast, activity score alone does not necessarly identify patients with high risk of renal failure. However in our experience some patients with markedly elevated activity index showed increase of chronicity index at a second biopsy performed 6-12 months later. The changes of chronicity index showed significant correlation with the initial activity index, so indicating that severely active lesions are likely to heal by sclerosis. Consequently, total pathological score appears to enhance the prediction of an unfavorable outcome, in agreement with Balow (20).

The results of discriminat analysis support and extend those of survival analysis.

This multivariate statistical method, with a stepwise procedure, selected from a broad range of variables the smallest set that most contributes to differentiate among the dead and the living patients. Sex, nephrotic sindrome and histological scores were selected, that is the same, except the age, detected by analysis of survival curves.

The coefficients attributed to histological scores were higher than those of clinical parameters, emphasizing the strong predictive value of pathologic findings. Therefore, although clinical parameters may provide useful informations, prognosis of patients with lupus nephritis cannot adequately be addressed without pathological data, analyzed by scoring system.

It is apparent that a detailed description of renal histology can provide the most sensitive prognostic determinant and may contribute to develop a rationale approach to treatment in lupus nephritis.

ACKNOWLEDGMENT

We are grateful to Prof. Floriana Esposito for her invaluable statistical consulence and to miss Caterina Serafino for her excellent secretary assistance.

REFERENCES

1. Schwartz RS, Immunologic and genetic aspects of systemic lupus erythematosus, Kidney Int. 19: 474 (1981).
2. Morel Maroger L, Mery JPH, Droz D, Godin M, Verroust P, Kourilsky O, Richet G, The course of lupus nephritis: contribution of serial renal biopsies, Adv. Nephrol. 6: 79 (1976).
3. Cameron JS, Turner DR, Ogg CS, Williams DG, Lessof MH, Chantler C, Leibowitz S, Systemic lupus with nephritis: A long-term study, Quart.J.Med. 48: 1 (1979).
4. Wallace DJ, Podell T, Weiner J, Klinenberg JR, Forouzesh S, Dubois EL, Systemic lupus erythematosus-survival patterns JAMA 245: 934 (1981).
5. Appel GB, Cohen DJ, Pirani CL, Meltzer JI, Estes D, Long-term follow-up of patients with lupus nephritis. A study based on the classification of the World Health Organization, Am.J.Med. 83: 877 (1987).
6. Leaker B, Fairley KF, Dowling J, Kincaid-Smith P, Lupus nephritis: clinical and pathological correlation, Quart. J. Med. 62: 163 (1987).
7. Muehrcke RC, Kark RM, Pirani CL, Pollak VE, Lupus nephritis: a clinical and pathologic study based on renal biopsies, Medicine 36: 1 (1957).
8. Baldwin DS, Lowenstein J, Rothifield NF, Gallo G, McCluskey RT, The clinical course of the proliferative and membranous forms of lupus nephritis, Ann.Intern.Med. 73: 929 (1970).
9. Decker JL, Klippel JH, Plotz PK, Steinberg AD, Cyclophosphamide and azathioprine in lupus glomerulonephritis: A controlled trial: results at 28 months , Ann.Intern. Med. 83: 606 (1975).
10. Ponticelli C, Zucchelli P, Moroni G, Cagnoli L, Banfi G, Pasquali S, Long-term prognosis of diffuse lupus nephritis, Clin.Nephrol. 22: 263 (1987).
11. Steinberg AD, The treatment of lupus nephritis, Kidney Int. 30: 769 (1986).
12. Zweiman B, Kornblum J, Cornog J, Hildret EA, The prognosis of lupus nephritis. Role of clinical pathological correlations, Ann.Intern.Med. 69:441 (1968).

13. Hecht B, Siegel N, Adler M, Kashgarian M, Ayslett JF, Prognostic indices in lupus nephritis, Medicine 55: 163 (1976).
14. Ginzler EH, Diamond HS, Weiner M, Schlesinger M, Fries JF, Wasner C, Medsger TA, Ziegler G, Klippel JH, Hadler NM, Albert DA, Hess EV, Spencer-Green G, Grayzel A, Worth D, Hahn BH, Barnett EV, A multicenter study of outcome in systemic lupus erythematosus I. Entry Variables as predictors of prognosis, Arth.Rheum. 25: 601 (1982).
15. Austin HA, Muenz LR, Joyce KM, Antonovych TA, Kullick ME Klippel JN, Decker JL, Balow JE, Prognostic factors in lupus nephritis. Contribution of renal histologic data, Am.J.Med. 75: 382 (1983)
16. Banfi G, Mazzucco G, Barbiano di Belgiojoso G, Bestetti Bosisio M, Stratta P, Confalonieri R, Ferrario F, Imbasciati E, Monga G, Morphological parameters in lupus nephritis: their relevance for classification and relationship with clinical and histological findings and outcome, Quart.J.Med. 55: 153 (1985).
17. Tan EM, Cohen AS, Fries IF, Masi AJ, McShane DJ, Rothfield NF, Schaller JG, Talal N, Winchester JR: The 1982 revised criteria for the classification of systemic lupus erythematosus, Arthiritis Rheum. 25: 1271 (1982)
18. Appel GB, Silva FG, Pirani CL, Meltzer JI, Estes D: Renal involvement in systemic lupus erythematosus. A study of 56 patients emphasizing histologic classification, Medicine 57: 371 (1978).
19. Lachenbruch PA, Clarke WR: Discriminant analysis and its application in epidemiology. Meth.Inform.Med. 19: 220 (1980).
20. Decker JL, Steinberg AD, Reinertsen JL, Plotg PH, Balow JE, Klippel JH, Systemic lupus erythematosus: evolving concepts. Ann.Intern.Med. 91: 587 (1979).
21. Fish AJ, Blau EB, Westburg NG, Burke BA, Vernier RL, Michael AF, SLE within the first two decades of life, Am.J.Med. 62: 99 (1977).
22. Magil AB, Ballon HS, Chan V, Lirenman DS, Rac A., Sutton RAL, Diffuse prolipherative lupus glomerulonephritis. Determination of prognostic significance of clinical, laboratory and pathologic factors. Medicine 63: 210 (1984).
23. Balow JE, Therapeutic trials in lupus nephritis. Problems related to renal histology, monitoring of therapy and measures of outcome. Nephron 27 : 171 (1981)
24. McCluskey RT, The value of the renal biopsy in lupus nephritis. Arthr.Rheum. 25: 867 (1982).
25. Wallace DJ, Podell TE, Weiner JM, Cox MB, Klinenberg JR, Forouresh S, Dubois EL, Lupus nephritis. Experience with 230 patients in a private pratice from 1950 to 1980.Am.J.Med. 72:209 (1982)

26. Fries JF, Porta J, Liang MH, Marginal benefit of renal biopsy in systemic lupus erythematosus. Arch.Intern.Med. 138: 1386 (1978).
27. Whiting-O'Keafe Q, Heuke JE, Shearn MA, Hopper J, Biava CG, Epstein WV, The information cntent from renal biopsy in systemic lupus erythematosus, Ann.intern.Med. 96:718 (1982).
28. Austin HA, Muenz LR, Joyce KM, Antonovych TT, Balow, Diffuse proliperative lupus nephritis: identification of specific pathologic features affecting renal outcome. Kidney Int. 25: 689 (1984).

THROMBOTIC MICROANGIOPATHY IN LUPUS NEPHRITIS

M.T. Porri, **M.I. Quareghi, F. Ferrario, G. Colasanti,
**R. Rossi, *E. Schiaffio, *G. Toia, and G. D'Amico

Dept. of Nephrology and *pathology, S. Carlo Hosp, Milano-
**Dept. of Nephrology, S. Anna Hosp., Como, Italy
S. Carlo Hosp, Via Pio II, 3 - Milano - Italy

INTRODUCTION

Renal involvement in Systemic Lupus Erythematosus (SLE) mainly consists of inflammatory glomerular lesions, possibly due to immune-complex deposition. A considerable number of microscopic vascular changes related to an immune-complex pathogenesis have also been identified : necrotizing arteritis and arteriolitis, with or without fibrinoid necrosis, mucinous and/or onion-skin intimal thickening (1,2). More recently, several lines of evidence have indicated the importance of coagulation mechanisms and of platelets as mediators of glomerular injury in SLE (3,4,5). Nonetheless, the picture of "pure" thrombotic microangiopathy is very rare in SLE (6,7).

We report here two cases of SLE admitted to our Units for hemolytic-uremic syndrome with acute renal failure.

Table 1 - Laboratory data at onset and after treatment

	sCreat mg/dl	uProt g/24h	anti-DNA u/ml	ANF	LE	C I C ug/ml	C3/C4 %	LAC
L.A.	5.7	1.7	103	1/1280	++	174	32/ 5	neg
F,24y	2.4	2.3	51	1/ 160	+	157	46/25	neg
C.G.	10.6	3.0	90	1/ 80	++	130	44/ 6	neg
M,20y	12.2	-	64	1/ 40	+	90	42/ 8	neg

Table 2 - Hematological data at onset and after treatment

	Hb g/dl	PLT n/mm^3	HAPT mg/dl	SCHIST %	RETIC %	F mg/dl	FDP s/u ug/ml
L.A.	6.3	38,000	30	3	15	440	30/10
F,24y	8.5	151,000	150	0	6	200	8/ 2
C.G.	6.9	78,000	42	2	11	280	30/ 8
M,20y	7.0	90,000	140	0	5	300	25/ 7

CASE n° 1 = A 24-year-old woman, with SLE since 1982, was admitted to our Hospital because of abrupt onset of renal involvement, characterized by renal failure (sCr 5.7 mg/dl), proteinuria (2 g/24 hrs) and hypertension (200/100 mmHg).
The serum anti-double-stranded DNA level (Farr method) and the antinuclear factor titer were elevated (101 U/ml and 1/1280). LE cell preparation was positive. Serum levels of Complement fractions C3, C4 and C1q were extremely low while circulating immune complexes (C1q solid phase method) were 174 ugEq/AHG/ml (n.v. 3). At the time of admission, facial erythema and pleuropericarditis, systemic manifestations of the disease, were present.

Hematological investigation showed anemia (Hb 6.3 g/dl) and thrombocytopenia (38,000/mm^3). Serum haptoglobin was persistently low (35 mg/dl, n.v.70-380). Plasma Fibrinogen was high (440 mg/dl) as were serum and urinary Fibrin Degradation Products (30 and 10 ug/ml). The picture of hemolytic microangiopathic anemia was completed by the presence of 3% fragmented erythrocytes in the blood smear and by 15% reticulocytes. Prothrombin time was normal (11.3") and the search for "Lupus anticoagulant" activity and the Coombs' test were negative.

Renal biopsy showed massive arteriolar thrombosis with no evidence of fibrinoid necrosis or perivascular cell infiltration. The glomeruli showed widespread thickening of capillary walls, mainly caused by swelling between the endothelial cells and the overlying basement membrane. There were double contours, with light fibrillar material in the subendothelial space (8). Mild proliferation of mesangial cells and some inflammatory cells in the capillary lumina could also be observed (Fig.1). There were patchy areas of tubular atrophy and edema in the interstitium. By immunofluorescence microscopy, endoluminal deposits of Fibrin were seen in small and medium- sized arterioles while focal and segmental deposits of IgG, IgA, IgM and Complement were seen in the glomeruli, along the capillary walls.

A short course of i.v. pulse methylprednisolone and of i.v. Vincristine was prescribed, associated with administration of antiplatelet drugs, fresh frozen plasma and plasma exchanges.

Complete recovery of renal function was obtained in a few weeks and patient's serum creatinine is still 1.2 mg/dl after 18 months of follow-up.

CASE n° 2 = A 20-year-old man with SLE for 3 months, was admitted because of acute oliguric renal failure (serum creatinine 10.6 mg/dl) associated with anemia (Hb 6.9 g/dl)and thrombocytopenia (78,000 mm^3). Schistocytes were found in the blood smear.Haptoglobin was 42 mg/dl. Fibrinogen and Fibrin Degradation Products were elevated.

Antinuclear antibody level was 1/80 and anti-DNA antibodies 1/640 (Crythidia Luciliae, immunofluorescence method). Hypocomplementemia for C3 (44 mg/dl) and C4 (6 mg/dl) and elevated levels of circulating immunocomplexes (C1q solid phase test) were also present. Prothrombin and partial thromboplastin time were normal. There was no "Lupus anticoagulant" activity in his serum. Facial erythema and leg thrombophlebitis were the only extrarenal manifestations.

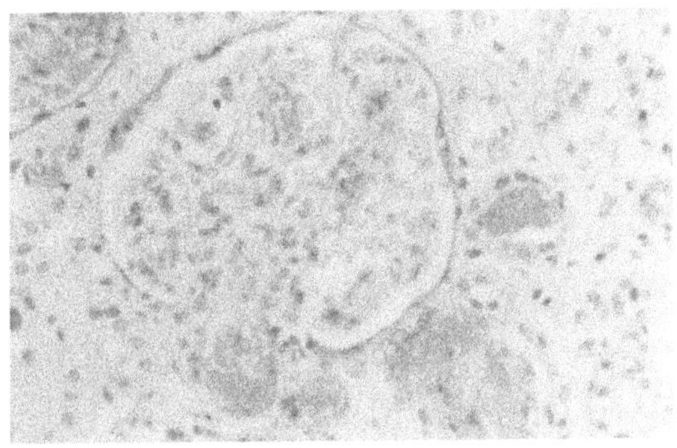

Fig. 1 - Massive arteriolar thrombosis. Thickening of capillary walls with double contours. Mild and segmental proliferation of mesangial cells.

At renal biopsy, massive thrombosis of all arterioles, especially the afferent ones, with complete lumina occlusion, was observed. Glomeruli contained typical ischemic lesions, with collapsed tufts and enlarged Bowman's spaces; the capillary walls were thickened and had double contours (Fig. 2). The interstitium was diffusely edematous. Immunofluorescence was positive for Fibrinogen in the arteriolar lumina but completely negative for Complement and Immunoglobulins in the glomeruli.

The patient was treated by i.v. pulses of methylprednisolone, anticoagulant drugs, fresh frozen plasma infusions, plasma exchanges and hemodialysis. Although the microangiopathic anemia disappeared, no improvement was observed in the renal failure and the patient is still on regular hemodialytic treatment 6 months after the onset of acute renal failure.

DISCUSSION

In Lupus nephritis many renal histological lesions might be due to intraglomerular coagulation (microaneurysms, focal areas of necrosis, intraluminal thrombi). On the contrary, ischemic glomerular changes secondary to massive arteriolar thrombosis are rarely seen.

We have observed "pure" thrombotic microangiopathy with the clinical features of hemolytic-uremic syndrome in only two of 92 patients with histological evidence of Lupus nephropathy.

Although a chance association cannot be entirely ruled out, two mechanisms might explain the occurrence of such microangiopathic lesions in Lupus nephropathy. "Lupus anticoagulant" activity (or related proteins) might directly trigger intravascular coagulation in

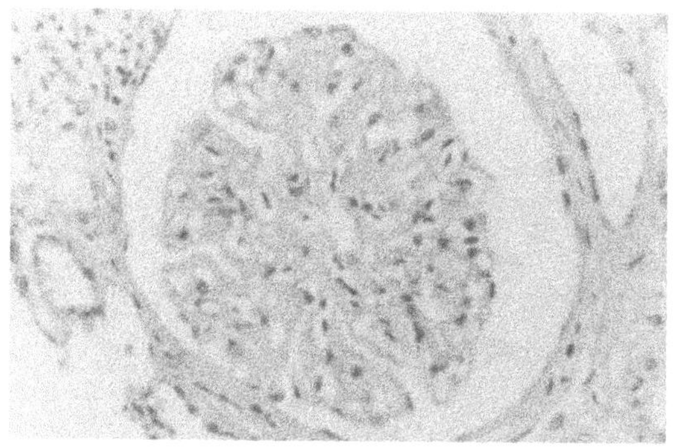

Fig. 2 - Ischemic glomerular lesions with collapsed tufts and enlarged Bowman's space; capillary walls are thickening with double contour appearance.

the kidney (2), as it frequently does in other vascular beds (cerebral, for instance) (9) or circulating immune complexes with particular physico-chemical properties might induce endothelial damage, inhibit prostacyclin synthesis and cause subsequent thrombotic microangiopathy (7,10,11), a mechanism which has been suggested for idiopathic cases of hemolytic uremic syndrome.

Our data indicate that acute renal failure in patients with SLE should be extensively studied before beginning treatment, since it is not invariably associated with crescentic glomerulonephritis.

ACKNOWLEDGEMENTS

The Authors wish to thank Mrs M.Marchesini and Miss V.Baretto for secretarial help.

REFERENCES

1. R.H. Heptinstall, Systemic Lupus Erythematosus, in: "Pathology of the kidney", R.H. Heptinstall ed., Little Brown and Company Boston (1983), p. 907.
2. T. Tsumagari and S. Fukumoto, Incidence and significance of intrarenal vasculopathies in patients with Systemic Lupus Erythematosus, Hum. Pathol. 16: 43 (1985).
3. K.S. Kant and U.E. Pollak, Glomerular thrombosis in Systemic Lupus Erythematosus: prevalence and significance. Medicine 60: 71 (1981).
4. W.F. Clark and M.L. Lewis, Intrarenal platelet consumption in the diffuse proliferative nephritis of systemic Lupus Erythematosus, Clin. Sci. (Mol. Med.) 49: 247 (1975).
5. C.L. Pirani, Coagulation and renal disease, in: "Glomerular injury 300 years after Morgagni", T. Bertani and G. Remuzzi eds., Wichtig, Milano (1983), p. 119.
6. A.B. Magil and D. Mc Tadden, Lupus glomerulonephritis with thrombotic microangiopathy, Hum. Pathol. 17: 192 (1986).
7. D.B. Bhathena and B.J. Sobel, Non inflammatory renal microangiopathy of Systemic Lupus Erytrhematosus, Am. J. Nephrol. 1: 114 (1981).
8. D.S. Baldwin and M.C. Gluck, Lupus nephritis, Am. J. Med. 62: 12 (1977).
9. M. Elias and A. Eldor, Thromboembolism in patients with the Lupus-Type Circulating Anticoagulant, Arch. Int. Med. 144: 510 (1984).
10. W.F. Clark and A.L. Liuton, Immunologic findings, thrombocytopenia and disease activity in Lupus nephritis. Can. Med. Assoc. J. 118: 1391 (1978).
11. U.N. Bhuyan and A.N. Malaviya, Prognostic significance of renal angiitis in Systemic Lupus Erythematosus, Clin. Nephrol. 20: 109 (1983).

VASCULITIS AND THE KIDNEY

Giovanni M. Frascà, Barbara Stagni, Concettina Raimondi, Alba Vangelista, and Vittorio Bonomini

Institute of Nephrology - St. Orsola Univ. Hospital
Bologna - Italy

The term "vasculitis" denotes a heterogeneous group of diseases characterized by inflammation and necrosis of blood vessels and a variable clinical picture, according to the organs or tissues mainly involved by the vasculitic lesions.

Renal involvement, often characterized by progressive impairment of renal function, frequently occurs in these patients where it represents one of the most pronounced clinical features, and a frequent cause of death [1].

The prevalence of renal vasculitis is difficult to assess since diagnosis may not be obvious owing to the variable clinical picture and possibly unspecific clinical features. Moreover, typical vasculitic lesions may be absent in renal biopsy material where more frequently a focal segmental necrotizing glomerulonephritis is observed [2]. This histological picture, particularly when scanty or no deposits are present at immunofluorescence, is considered strongly suggestive of vasculitis and deserves careful examination of the patients to identify signs confirming the diagnosis.

It has been suggested that most crescentic glomerulonephritis with negative immunofluorescence, which accounts for approximately 40% of extracapillary glomerulonephritis [3], may actually represent the renal consequences of systemic vasculitis. Among the renal biopsies carried out over 30 years in our Institute, vasculitis accounts for 7.4% of vascular nephropathies, but it is likely that the actual prevalence is higher, on account of the increased carefulness nowadays used in diagnosis.

CLASSIFICATION

No satisfactory classification exists of the various form of vasculitis because their etiology and pathogenesis are still largely unknown and there is a large overlap among the various diseases. It is clear that the ultimate classification will depend on identification of the various antigens responsible.

TABLE I. Classification of vasculitis

A) Systemic vasculitis

a) Non granulomatous vasculitis

1) Polyarteritis Nodosa
- Classic Polyarteritis Nodosa
- Microscopic Polyarteritis Nodosa
- Overlap syndrome

2) Hypersensitivity Vasculitis

3) Associated with other systemic diseases
- Schonlein-Henoch purpura
- Systemic lupus erythematosus
- Cryoglobulinemia
- Rheumatoid arthritis
- Relapsing polychondritis
- Malignancies

b) Granulomatous vasculitis

1) Wegener's granulomatosis
2) Allergic granulomatosis (Churg-Strauss syndrome)
3) Lymphomatoid granulomatosis

c) Giant cell arteritis

1) Temporal arteritis
2) Takayasu's disease

B) Renal vasculitis

- Associated with renal transplant rejection

The table I reports a possible classification which includes some well-defined clinical pictures that can be considered discrete nosographic entities (such as Wegener's granulomatosis) and other diseases whose separation in distinct categories could be questionable.

The distinction between hypersensitivity vasculitis and the microscopic form of polyarteritis nodosa, for example, is not always easy and the two forms are hardly distinguishable from each other on a pathological basis, the former being now generally applied to cutaneous vasculitis where an allergic reaction to an antigen (most commonly drugs) is evident.

Likewise, the separation between granulomatous and non granulomatous vasculitis, on the assumption that histological features may reflect different pathogenetic mechanisms, could be a matter of controversy.

The following discussion will focus on the main features of vasculitis of the Polyarteritis Nodosa group, Wegener's granulomatosis, and vasculitis associated with renal graft rejection since they are among the most frequent forms of renal vasculitis and their course is often characterized by irreversible renal damage leading to end stage renal failure.

A) SYSTEMIC VASCULITIS

Pathogenesis

The pathogenesis of vasculitis has not yet been clarified, but several data suggest that it is immunologic in nature.

One hypothesis is that they are mediated by the deposition of circulating immunecomplexes in the vessel wall with consequent activation of complement components and accumulation of polymorphonuclear leukocytes. The release of lysosomal enzymes eventually results in tissue damage [4] Some experimental evidence of this mechanism has been provided in animals by studies on acute serum sickness in rabbits, where vasculitic lesions resembling those of polyarteritis nodosa appear when circulating immunecomplexes in antigen excess are formed. Complement and neutrophils are required, since their depletion can prevent the lesion from occurring [5].

Some observations seem to suggest that in situ formation of immunecomplexes within vessels may be the primary mechanism in the vascular lesions of acute serum sickness [5], while the mere presence of large amounts of circulating immunecomplexes is not sufficient to produce vasculitis [6].

Data in human pathology are less convincing, resting mainly on the frequent observation of circulating immunecomplexes in the acute phase of the disease [7] with all the limitations that the assays for immunecomplex detection imply, while immunoglobulins and complement are rarely seen in the affected vessels [4,8]. The only convincing association with an antigen is that with the hepatitis B surface antigen which has been reported in 6 to 41% of cases [5,9,10] and demonstrated in vasculitic lesions.

Impairment of the reticulo-endothelial system has been observed in patients with vasculitis [11] but it is not clear whether it may contribute to the vascular damage or is merely the result of large amount of circulating immunecomplexes.

A pathogenetic role of cell-mediated immunity has been postulated, at least for granulomatous vasculitis. Sensitized lymphocytes may react with antigen and release lymphokines which cause monocyte-macrophage accumulation. The latter can directly induce vessel wall damage by releasing their lysosomal enzymes and transforming themselves into epithelioid and multinucleated giant cells leading to granuloma formation [1]. Recent immunohistochemical investigations of renal tissue from patients with Wegener's granulomatosis, have demonstrated that perivascular infiltrates are composed of T lymphocytes (mainly T helper/inducer) [12], consistent with a delayed type hypersensitivity reaction.

No experimental model of cell mediated vasculitis has been provided. However granulomatous vascular lesions can occasionally be observed in rabbits with serum sickness [4], and it is possible that cell mediated immunological mechanisms coexist with immunecomplexes.

Recently antibodies against cytoplasmic components of neutrophils have been identified both in patients suffering from Wegener's granulomatosis [13] and in patients with the microscopic form of Polyarteritis Nodosa [14]. These antibodies were found to correlate with the acute phase of the disease, thus confirming that immunological mechanisms play an important role in the pathogenesis of vasculitis. The possibility that the affected polymorphonuclear leukocytes can release their lysosomal enzymes within vessels could explain the polymorphism of the clinical picture of vasculitis and shed some light on their pathogenesis.

The glomerular damage can be a consequence of ischemia or cellular immune mechanisms. In fact, immunohistochemical evaluation of renal tissue has revealed a large number of monocyte/macrophages along with T cells in glomeruli from patients studied during the acute phase of the disease [15], while immunological deposits are rarely seen by immunofluorescence or electron microscopy.

Clinical and histological features

1) Polyarteritis Nodosa Group.. The Polyarteritis Nodosa group of vasculitis includes: the classic form; the microscopic form; and the overlap syndrome.

The differentiation is based on the size of the vessels involved, the classic form affecting the small and medium sized arteries, while in the microscopic form the smaller vessels and capillaries are involved. The overlap syndrome includes all cases where a clearcut difference in the level of vasculature involved does not exist.

The clinical picture of the classic form is characterized by a combination of general aspecific symptoms such as fever, weakness and weight loss, and variable organ involvement including polyneuropathy, central nervous system alterations, cardiac manifestations

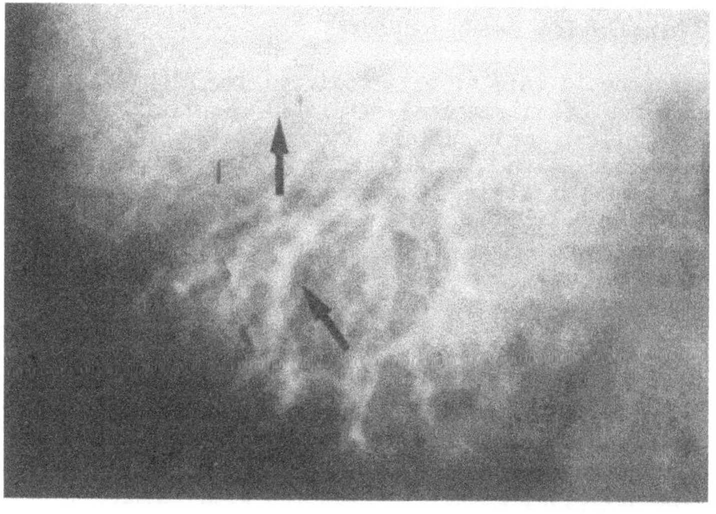

Fig.1. Renal arteriogram in a patient with the classic form of Polyarteritis Nodosa showing aneurysmal dilatations in medium sized arteries

TABLE II. Light microscopy findings in 43 renal biopsies from patients with systemic vasculitis studied at the Institute of Nephrology of the Bologna University.

	Classic Pan (3 pts)	Microscopic Pan (27 pts)	Overlap Syndrome (6 pts)	Wegener's Granulomatosis (7 pts)
Segmental Proliferative GN	1	3 (11%)	2 (33%)	2 (29%)
Diffuse Proliferative GN	/	5 (18%)	1 (17%)	1 (14%)
Necrotizing GN	2	19 (70%)	3 (50%)	5 (71%)
Crescents >60%	/	12 (44%)	2 (33%)	4 (57%)
Renal Angiitis	/	13 (48%)	2 (33%)	3 (43%)

varing from congestive heart failure to myocardial infarction, and infarction of viscera [1]. Typically, allergic histories and eosinophilia are uncommon and lung and spleen are not involved. Hypertension is frequently present and renal involvement is generally manifested by variable urinary findings, according to the site of vascular involvement. Renal failure frequently occurs in untreated patients [9].

A characteristic feature is the finding of aneurysmal dilatation in medium-sized arteries which may be seen by arteriogram in the renal, hepatic, and visceral vasculature (fig. 1) and may help the diagnosis in cases where a biopsy of the involved organs is not possible or negative.

Both vascular and glomerular changes characterize the renal involvement. The vascular alterations involve mainly segments of the arcuate and interlobular arteries, which typically show lesions of all ages: early lesions are characterized by neutrophilic infiltration of the vascular wall, fibrinoid necrosis, disruption of the elastic lamina and thrombosis. Ischemic lesions and infarction of varying severity may ensue. Late changes are characterized by fibrous thickening of the vascular wall with narrowing of the lumen without inflammatory infiltrates or scattered mononuclear cells which may resemble renal histological changes induced by chronic hypertension. The extensive disruption of the elastic lamina caused by the vasculitic process helps in the differential diagnosis. Since the vascular lesions are segmental and are generally limited to the larger arteries, they are frequently missed in renal biopsy. Immunofluorescence examination of renal tissue may show granular deposits of IgG and/or IgM and complement in the involved vessels.

The glomerular lesions of classic Polyarteritis Nodosa are characterized by segmental areas of fibrinoid necrosis and sclerosis and are a consequence of ischemia. Cell proliferation is normally minimal or absent and no deposits can be demonstrated either by immunofluorescence or electron microscopy.

In the <u>microscopic form</u> of Polyarteritis Nodosa the pathologic process is similar to the classic form, except that smaller vessels are affected and the glomerular damage is more prominent.

The systemic involvement resembles the classic form but is highly variable; cutaneous lesions and pulmonary haemorrhage may sometimes be present; by contrast with the classic form, hypertension is relatively rare.

In the kidney lesions involve the distal interlobular arteries and afferent glomerular arterioles which show inflammatory infiltrates of neutrophils and eosinophils along with fibrinoid necrosis (fig. 2a). A focal segmental necrotizing glomerulonephritis is typically seen in these patients, with areas of fibrinoid necrosis and crescents, associated with a variable degree of mesangial and endothelial cell proliferation. This histological picture was present in 19 out of 27 patients (70%) in our case material (tab. II). Only minimal abnormalities of glomerular basement membrane are seen, and in few cases does immunofluorescence demonstrate glomerular and vascular deposits, which are generally scanty or located on necrotic areas.

2) Wegener's granulomatosis Wegener's granulomatosis is characterized by a necrotizing granulomatous vasculitis of the upper and lower respiratory tract, associated with necrotizing glomerulonephritis. Systemic symptoms, whether unspecific (fever, weight loss, weakness) or related to eyes, ears, joints and skin, are frequently observed [1]

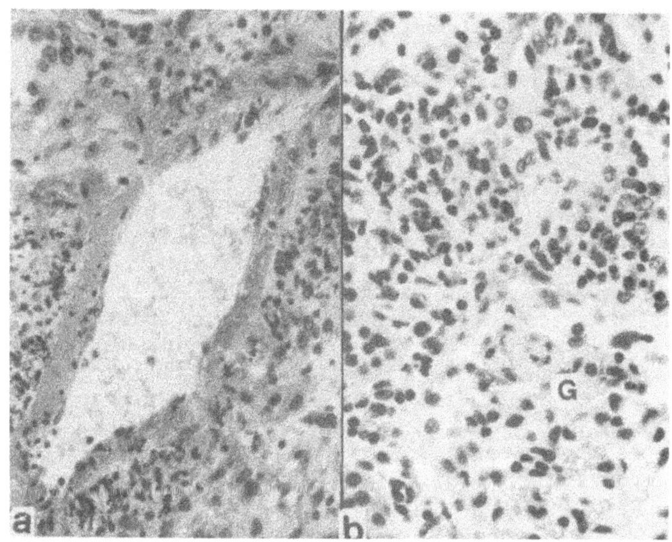

Fig.2.a) Renal biopsy from a patient with the microscopic form of Polyarteritis Nodosa: fibrinoid necrosis and inflammation of a distal interlobular artery (HE x330).
b) Renal biopsy from a patient with Wegener's granulomatosis showing a periglomerular granuloma (G = glomerulus) (HE x330).

and nearly always precede clinical renal involvement. Rhinorrhea, sinus pain, pulmonary haemorrhage and dyspnea are the most suggestive symptoms of Wegener's granulomatosis.

Renal involvement, manifested by proteinuria and hematuria in early stages, is associated with varying degrees of renal insufficiency as the disease progresses.

Frequently renal biopsy demonstrates focal segmental areas of fibrinoid necrosis and thrombosis of the glomerular tuft with crescent formation and varying degree of hypercellularity [16]. Sometimes a typical periglomerulitis can be appreciated in renal biopsy. It consists of a periglomerular granuloma mainly composed of polymorphonuclear leukocytes with a variable number of eosinophils and destruction of Bowman's capsule (fig. 2b). Occasionally renal angiitis can be observed in biopsies: it was present in 3 out of 7 patients we studied (43%; tab. II).

Course and Treatment

The course of patients with vasculitis of the Polyarteritis Nodosa group is extremely variable, according to the organ systems mainly involved, and is often very aggressive. The mortality rate reported varies from series to series, according to the features of the patients included, and it can be as high as 66% [2]. Extrarenal complications generally account for most deaths in patients suffering from the classic form of Polyarteritis Nodosa [9,17], while renal failure is the major cause in the microscopic form [18].

If untreated, vasculitis of the Polyarteritis Nodosa group are associated with poor prognosis, with a survival rate of 30-40% at 1 year and around 10% at 5 years [9,19]. Corticosteroids significantly improve the outcome of these patients, increasing the survival rate to 60-80% and around 50% respectively at 1 and 5 years [9,17,19]. Cytotoxic therapy seems somewhat to improve these figures [9,10,20,21], but there is still some controversy as to its role, considering its potential toxicity. Cyclophosphamide however should be considered for patients who run an aggressive course, particularly when major organs are involved by the vasculitic process, and when steroids do not induce a satisfactory improvement or are associated with unacceptable complications.

In patients with a clear association between vasculitis and HBsAg, encouraging results have been reported with the use of Vidarabin, an anti-viral agent, combined with plasmaexchange which seems to allow a good control of the disease without steroids or cytotoxic drugs [22].

Wegener's granulomatosis, when untreated, is associated with an extremely poor prognosis [23]. By contrast with the Polyarteritis Nodosa group, the use of corticosteroids has little benefit in these patients [24] inducing only occasional and temporary remission. On the other hand cyclophosphamide can induce a complete and long-lasting remission with a patient survival rate above 80% at 1 year in most series [25].

From the analysis of the literature and our experience, some features of the course of vasculitis are to be considered for appropriate treatment: 1) early deaths occur for inadequate control

TABLE III. Outcome of 21 patients with systemic vasculitis of the PAN group and GFR < 50 ml/min at biopsy, studied at the Institute of Nephrology of the Bologna University. The patients were divided into two groups according with their treatment (with or without plasmaexchange).
(* $p < 0.05$)

	Group A (PE)	Group B (non PE)
Patients (n.)	11	10
S. creat. at biopsy (mg/dl)	9.3±2.9*	6.2±3.5*
Follow-up (months)	29±14	26±12
Deaths (n.)	1	3
Regular dialysis (n.)	1	2
Chronic renal failure (n.)	6	6
S. creat. at follow-up (mg/dl)	2.6±1.3	2.4±1.5

of the disease or infections due to over-immunosuppression; 2) late deaths are due to relapses of the disease or residual morbidity owing to chronic vascular alterations which result from the pathologic process; 3) frequent relapses can occur; 4) the incidence of end stage renal failure in survivors is unacceptably high in some series.

Thus guidelines for treatment should consider: 1) The necessity of inducing complete remission early in the course of the disease which should reduce both early and late mortality as well as the incidence of end stage renal failure. 2) Optimization of immunosuppression to avoid life-threatening infections. 3) Prolonged treatment to reduce the risk of relapses (at least 1 year after remission has been achieved). 4) Careful follow-up of patients.

Whether plasmaexchange has a role in the treatment of vasculitis has not yet been clarified. On a theoretical basis, this technique, by enhancing the immunosuppressive therapy, should reduce both the mortality and the morbidity of vasculitis, by controlling the disease in a shorter time and reducing the need for steroids and cytotoxic agents. However it is not clear whether such treatment is of real benefit.

Although some patients with microscopic Polyarteritis Nodosa running an aggressive course have been reported to benefit from plasmaexchange [26], it does not seem that the treatment improves patient or kidney survival in larger series [21].

Similar results have been observed in Wegener's granulomatosis [27] although a quicker rise in GFR has been reported in patients treated with plasmaexchange, compared with those who received drug therapy alone [27].

To clarify this topic we analysed retrospectively the course and outcome of 21 patients with vasculitis of the PAN group and severe reduction in renal function at presentation, who were treated with steroid and cyclophosphamide combined or not with plasmaexchange. Although patients who underwent plasmaexchange therapy showed a more severe impairment of renal function before treatment, the renal outcome was not worse compared with the other group, and a lower number of deaths was observed among patients treated by plasmaexchange (tab. III). Moreover, a quicker improvement in renal function occurred in these patients (fig. 3).

Although some aspects, such as patient selection and length of treatment, need to be further clarified, it seems reasonable to reserve plasmaexchange treatment for those patients who run an aggressive course, particularly if oliguric acute renal failure is present.

B) VASCULITIS ASSOCIATED WITH RENAL GRAFT REJECTION

The occurrence of vasculitic lesions in renal graft rejection is well known, although their prevalence has not been precisely assessed. Our observations in over 300 patients in the last 10 years suggest that at least 25 to 30% of acute rejection episodes are associated with these lesions.

They involve vessels from medium size arteries to small capillaries and are characterized by inflammatory changes along with endothelial damage, necrosis and thrombosis. The endothelial changes are often very prominent and represent a distinguishing feature of this vasculitis: the endothelium is swollen and detached from the

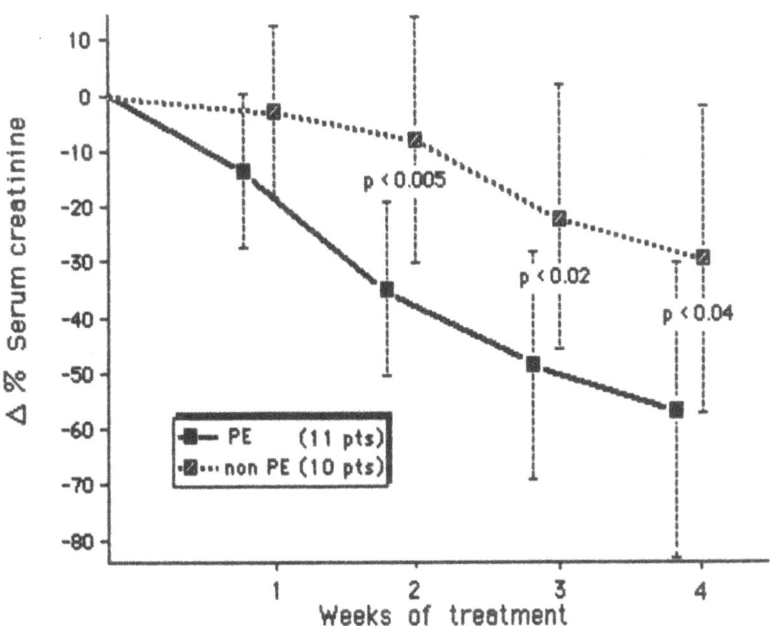

Fig.3. Per cent changes in serum creatinine during the first month of treatment in patients with vasculitis of the PAN group treated with drug therapy alone (non PE) or combined with plasmaexchange (PE)

basement membrane with mononuclear cells infiltrating the subendothelial space (fig. 4a). The media shows focal fibrinoid necrosis with fragmentation of the internal elastic lamina and polymorphonuclear leukocyte infiltrates sometimes associated with thrombosis. Interstitial changes, with extensive hemorrhage are always observed and later on glomerular lesions, characterized by necrosis and blood stasis, take place.

In contrast with systemic vasculitis, immunofluorescence examination of renal tissue reveals extensive deposits of immunoglobulins and/or complement which involve all the vessel wall in most cases (fig.4b).

These lesions are mainly mediated by humoral immunologic mechanisms [28], including specific anti-HLA antibodies against the donor's mismatched antigens [29], which, along with the typing of peripheral lymphocyte subpopulations, can be used to differentiate these cases from acute cellular rejection.

Vasculitis occurring during acute rejection episodes is associated with progressive impairment in renal function and poor prognosis, since it is usually unresponsive to conventional anti-rejection treatment [30].

These considerations prompted us some years ago to try plasmaexchange for treatment of these lesions. Our preliminary results in selected patients showed that plasmaexchange was effective in removing these antibodies from circulation and that the reduction in antibody titer was associated with an improvement in renal function in most

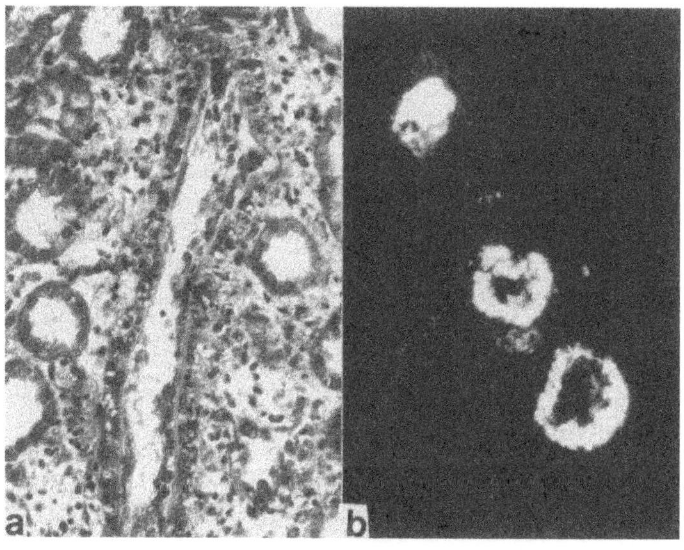

Fig.4. a) Graft biopsy during acute rejection episode showing vascular inflammatory changes along with swelling and detachment of endothelium (Masson's trichrome, x420). b) Graft biopsy during acute rejection: intense vascular deposits of IgM (I.F. x420).

patients [31]. A subsequent controlled study in 44 patients confirmed the efficacy of this approach, showing that the graft survival of these patients could be improved by more than 40%, provided that an early diagnosis and institution of therapy was made [32].

Our observations suggest the need for careful evaluation of the imunological status in transplanted patients undergoing acute rejection episodes, if necessary associated with graft biopsy, since appropriate treatment could significantly improve the results of renal transplantation.

REFERENCES

1. A.S. Fauci, B.F. Haynes, P. Katz, The spectrum of vasculitis. Clinical, pathologic, immunologic and therapeutic considerations, Ann. Intern. Med. 89:660 (1978).
2. J.E. Balow, Renal vasculitis, Kidney Intern. 27:954 (1985)
3. W.G. Couser , Idiopathic rapidly progressive glomerulonephritis, Am.J.Nephrol. 2:57 (1982).
4. R.T. McCluskey, R. Fienberg, Vasculitis in primary vasculitides, granulomatoses and connective tissue diseases, Hum. Pathol. 14:305 (1983).
5. C.L. Christian, J.S. Sergent, Vasculitis syndromes: clinical and experimental models, Am. J. Med. 61:385 (1976)
6. C.G. Cochrane, Mechanisms involved in the deposition of immune complexes in tissues, J. Exp. Med. 134:75s (1971).
7. G.M. Kamer, N.A. Soter, P.J. Schur, Circulating immunecomplexes in patients with necrotizing vasculitis, Clin. Immunol. Immunopathol. 15:658 (1980).
8. P. Ronco, P. Verroust, F. Mignon, O. Kourilsky, P. Vanhille, A. Meyrier, J-P Mery, L. Morel-Maroger, Immunopathologic studies of polyarteritis nodosa and Wegener's granulomatosis: A report of 43 patients with 51 renal biopsies, Q.J.Med. 52:212 (1983).
9. E.S. Leib, C. Restivo, H.E. Paulus, Immunosuppressive and corticosteroid therapy of polyarteritis nodosa, Am. J. Med. 67:941 (1979).
10. A.S. Fauci , P. Katz, B.F. Haynes, S.M. Wolff, Cyclophosphamide therapy of severe systemic necrotizing vasculitis, N. Engl. J. Med. 301:245 (1979).
11. C.M. Lockwood , S. Worlledge, A. Nicholas, C. Cotton, D.K. Peters, Reversal of impaired splenic function in patients with nephritis or vasculitis (or both) by plasma exchange, N. Engl. J. Med. 300:524 (1979).
12. I.J.M. Ten Berge, J.M. Wilmink, C.J.L.M. Meyer, J. Surachno, K.H. ten Veen, T.G. Balk, P.T.A. Schellekens, Clinical and immunological follow-up of patients with severe renal disease in Wegener's granulomatosis, Am. J. Nephrol. 5:21 (1985).
13. F.J. Van der Woude, N. Rasmussen, S. Lobatto, A. Wiik, H. Permin, L.A. van Es, M. van der Giessen, T.H. The, Autoantibodies against neutrophils and monocytes: tool for diagnosis and marker of disease activity in Wegener's granulomatosis, Lancet 1:425 (1985).
14. J. Freehally, D.C. Wheeler, J. Walls, S. Jones, C.M. Lockwood, C.O.S. Savage, A case of microscopic polyarterits associated with antineutrophil cytoplasmic antibodies (letter), Clin. Nephrol.27:214 (1987).

15. F. Nolasco, J.S. Cameron, B. Hartley, T lymphocyte and macrophage involvement in the glomerular lesions of microscopic polyarteritis, Proc. EDTA-ERA 22:752 (1985).
16. M.A. Weiss, J.D. Crissman, Renal biopsy findings in Wegener's granulomatosis: segmental necrotizing glomerulonephritis with glomerular thrombosis, Hum. Pathol. 15:943 (1984).
17. R.D. Cohen, D.L. Conn, D.M. Ilstrup: Clinical features, prognosis and response to treatment in polyarteritis, Mayo Clin. Proc. 55:136 (1980).
18. A. Serra, J.S. Cameron, D.R. Turner, B. Hartley, C.S. Ogg, G.H. Neild, D.G. Williams, D. Taube, C.B. Brown, J.A. Hicks, Vasculitis affecting the kidney: Presentation, histopathology and long-term outcome, Q.J. Med 53:181 (1984).
19. P.P. Frohnert, S.G. Sheps, Long-term follow-up study of periarteritis nodosa, Am. J. Med. 43:8 (1967)
20. R.A. Coward, N.A.T. Hamdy, J.S. Shortland, C.B. Brown, Renal micropolyarteritis: a treatable condition, Nephrol. Dial. Transplant 1:31 (1986).
21. C.O. Savage, C.G. Winearls, D.J. Evans, A.J. Rees, C.M. Loockwood, Immunosuppressive treatment of 34 patients with microscopic polyarteritis, Proc EDTA-ERA 22:720 (1985)
22. D. Ouzan, P.J. Tremisi, E. Strauss, P. Chossegros, J. Pasquier, P. Zech, P. Dujardin, J. Delmont, C. Trepo, Superiority of plasmaexchange combined with vidarabin over classic therapy in the management of polyarteritis nodosa associated with hepatitis B virus, Plasma Ther. Transfus Technol. 6:487 (1985).
23. E.W. Walton, Giant-cell granuloma of the respiratory tract (Wegener's granulomatosis). Br. Med. J. 2:265 (1958).
24. M.A. Aldo, M.D. Benson, F.R. Comerford, A.S. Cohen, Treatment of Wegener's granulomatosis with immunosuppressive agents. Arch. Intern. Med. 126:298 (1970).
25. A.S. Fauci, B.F. Haynes, P. Katz, S.M. Wolff, Wegener's granulomatosis: prospective clinical and therapeutic experience with 85 patients for 21 years, Ann. Intern. Med. 98:76 (1983).
26. F. Chenais, J.L. Debru, L. Baret, J. Faure, J.M. Chalopin, G. Rifle, Plasmaexchange in the treatment of Polyarteritis Nodosa, in: "Plasmaexchange", Sieberth HG, ed., F.K. Schattauer, Stuttgart (1980), pag.285.
27. A.J. Pinching, C.M. Lockwood, B.A. Pussell, A.J. Rees, P. Sweny, D.J. Evans, N. Bowley, D.K. Peters, Wegener's granulomatosis: Observations on 18 patients with severe renal disease, Q. J. Med. 208:435 (1983).
28. M.R. Garovoy, P. Gailiunas, C.B. Carpenter, G.J. Busch, Immunologic monitoring of transplant rejection: correlation of in vitro assays with morphologic changes on transplant biopsy, Nephron 22:208 (1978).
29. R. Roy, J.G. Lachance, Y. Fradet, J. Hebert, Characterization of lymphocytotoxic antibodies in renal transplantation. Transplantation 31:31 (1981).
30. A. Magil, J. Rubin, L. Ladewig, M. Johnson, M.B. Goldstein, R.A. Bear, Renal biopsy in acute allograft rejection. Nephron 26:180 (1980).
31. A. Vangelista, G.M. Frascà, A. Nanni Costa, S. Stefoni, V. Bonomini, Value of plasmaexchange in renal transplant rejection induced by specific anti-HLA antibodies, Trans. Am. Soc. Artif. Intern. Organs 28:599 (1982).
32. V. Bonomini, A. Vangelista, G.M. Frascà, A. Di Felice, G. Liviano D'Arcangelo, Effect of plasmapheresis in renal transplant rejection. A controlled study, Trans. Am. Soc. Artif. Intern. Organs 31:698 (1985).

MIXED CONNECTIVE TISSUE DISEASE AND RENAL DISEASE

Mohammad Akmal

University of Southern California School of Medicine

2025 Zonal Ave., Los Angeles, CA 90033

Mixed connective tissue disease (MCTD) was described in 1972 by Sharp et al (1) as a syndrome of overlapping features of systemic lupus erythematosus (SLE), progressive systemic sclerosis (PSS), and myositis. The serum of MCTD patients characteristically contained high titers of antibody to nuclear ribonucleoprotein (RNP) (2,3). While the initial report stressed the paucity of renal involvement in MCTD, subsequent studies of adults (4-13) and children (14-18) noted a higher prevalence of nephropathy (10-50%).

CLINICAL FEATURES (1,13,19,20)

The disease may appear at any age but the mean age at onset in our study of thirty patients was 32.0 ± 2.2 years with a range of 16-60 years (13). The mean disease duration was 13.2 ± 1.4 years (range 4-41 years). Twenty eight of our thirty patients were female. In general no racial or ethnic susceptibility is noted. The most common clinical manifestations in our study (Table 1) and previous studies include polyarthralgias, plyarthritis, Raynaud's phenomenon, sclerodactyly, myositis with myalgias, and esophageal hypomotility, scleroderma like features of the skin of face and hand may be prominant. Joint involvement may at times be severe, erosive and deforming but subcutaneous nodules are uncommon. Pulmonary dysfunction may be common and includes diminished diffusing capacity associated with diffuse interstitial infiltrates, and pleuritis. These pulmonary abnormalities may not be clinically apparent. Varying degrees of pulmonary hypertension in the absence of left ventricular failure have been reported with MCTD. Mediastinal lymphadenopathy may rarely be encountered. Pericarditis with or without pericardial effusion is the most common cardiac finding in MCTD and has been noted in about one third of the patients. Mitral valve prolapse is also a common cardiac finding in MCTD and was noted in 10 of 38 patients. Other cardiac manifestations include chest pain, systolic or diastolic murmurs, midsystolic and pulmonary ejection clicks, right ventricular enlargement and conduction disturbances such as premature atrial contractions and short P-R interval. Hematologic abnormalities found in half of the patients, manifested mainly by an anemia of chronic disease. However leukopenia and positive coomb's test are not infrequent but thrombocytopenia and autoimmune hemolytic anemia are less common. Splenomegaly may be detected in about 20% of the patients. Neuropsychiatric manifestations are not infrequent. The most common finding is an aseptic meningitis like syndrome which is very responsive to glucocorticoid therapy. Other features include psychosis, peripheral and/or trigeminal neuropathy, convulsions, and cerebral ataxia. The cerebrospinal fluid may show pleocytosis, and elevated protein content. Unlike patients with SLE, the neurological involvement in MCTD does not seem to be a cause of mortality. Organic obstruction of both small and medium size vessel detected by angiography is not infrequent. Patients with MCTD may present with manifestations of either one or multiple connective tissue diseases and evolve through a disease course which at times had indisputable features of three or four overlapping diseases or resembles more closely on distinct connective tissue disease entity. MCTD indeed seems to be the chameleon of connective tissue disease entity. The available data suggest that the majority of patients with MCTD may subsequently evolve into a scleroderma dominant pattern and lesser numbers may evolve into SLE or rheumatoid arthritis dominant patterns.

Table 1. Systemic Involvement in 30 Patients with MCTD

	No.	(%)
Arthritis	16	(97)
Raynaud	25	(83)
Cutaneous	25	(83)
Pulmonary	23	(77)
Swollen hands	18	(60)
Sclerodactyly ± proximal scleroderma	18	(60)
Esophageal hyomotility	18	(60)
Myositis	16	(53)
Serositis	16	(53)
Hematologic abnormalities	16	(53)
Nephropathy	12	(40)
Tendinitis	7	(23)
Sjorgren	7	(23)
Nerologic manifestations	6	(20)
Lymphadenopathy	5	(17)
Splenomegaly	2	(7)

LABORATORY FINDINGS (1,13,24-26)

The laboratory finding which sets MCTD apart from the other overlap syndromes is the presence of very high titer (Frequently greater than 1:1 million) of antibody to a ribonuclease sensitive, saline extractable nuclear antigen (RNase-sensitive anti-ENA) by hemagglutination and antibody to ribonucleoprotein. Some patients, during exacerbation of MCTD, become negative for RNP antibody, and with remission develop high titers. This may occur because of massive organ deposition of antigen antibody complexes leaving undetectable amount in the serum and/or massive proteinuria may lead to loss of the antibody in the urine. The fluorescent antinuclear antibody test very frequently reveals a high titer speckled fluorescent pattern. In addition, 20% of patients have LE cells tests, 40% free circulating DNA, 16% antibody to heat denatured DNA; and 16% have antibody to native DNA. The levels of C_3 and C_4 complements are usually normal or elevated, but depressed levels have been reported as well.

Circulating immune complexes and free RNP have been detected in MCTD and may have a role in it's pathogenesis. Rheumatoid factor occurs in 14-50% of patients and 75% have hypergammaglobulinemia. The erythrocyte sedimentation rate may be markedly elevated. The presence of antibodies against nuclear matrix antigen (M.W. 7000), detected by immunoblotting technique, is strongly suggestive of MCTD. Antilymphocytoxic antibodies are lower in patients with MCTD than those in SLE. Nailfold capillary microscopy could provide additional tool for the diagnosis of MCTD. Branched bushy capillary formation is the pattern seen in these patients. This pattern displays 72% sensitivity, 80% specificity and 87% negative predictive valve. Further longitudinal studies of both clinical and laboratory features of these patients hopefully will place MCTD in it's proper place in the spectrum of connective tissue diseases and shed lights in it's pathogenesis. Till then, the most appropriate way to diagnose MCTD seems to be finding the coexisting features of SLE, scleroderma, and polymyositis, with a high titer antibody to RNP preferably to the exclusion of other antinuclear antibodies.

RENAL DISEASE (13,14,25,29-31)

The renal involvement in patients with MCTD is less than in patients with SLE. A prevalence of renal manifestations of 10-50% has been reported in patients with MCTD. The renal involvement may be silent or clinically overt. There may be mild renal abnormalities consisting of asymptomatic proteinuria and/or hematuria, or the patient may manifest nephrotic syndrome or variable degrees of renal insufficiency or may even present with oliguric acute renal failure. We have studied 30 patietns with MCTD and seventeen were found to have various degrees of proteinuria. In 19 patients the proteinuria was transient and less than < 0.5 mg/ld. The remaining 11 patients folowed for a mean of 30 years presented with, or subsequently developed proteinuria of > 0.5 gm/d with nine of these with nephrotic syndrome, and an additional patient without clinical or biochemical evidence of renal disease at the time of death was found to have membranous nephropathy at autopsy. Renal tissue was available in 10 of 11 patients (five membranous, two mesangial, one membranoproliferative, and one focal sclerosing glomerulonephritis). Of 76 patients reported previously who had adequate description of renal pathology including ours (10 patients), 34% had membranous lesions, 30% mesangial, 17% focal or diffuse proliferative nephropathy, 5% had a mixed lesion with membranous change, and 7% were normal. Four of these 76 patients had vascular sclerosis (17%), and 3% had glomerular sclerosis. There were four transitions to a more severe histologic class (5%), including one of our patients (13) whose initial biopsy showed membranous nephropathy and subsequent autopsy histology revealed focal proliferative nephritis with crescents, necrotizing arteritis, and subintimal sclerosis of renal vessels. One of our patients with membranous nephropathy and nephrotic syndrome (31) presented initially with multisystem disease and oliguric acute renal failure requiring dialysis who had dramatic recovery with high dose steroids. However, the patient relapsed 2 months after discontinuation of steroid therapy and the patient was admitted with recurrence of oliguria, renal insufficiency and nephrotic syndrome. The renal biopsy showed membranous glomerulonephropathy and immunologically mediated tubulo-interstitial disease. She again responded to reinstitution of aforementioned therapy. She has remained in remission with prednisone 15 mg/d for about 9 years. Germain et al (25) also described a patient with long standing membranous nephropathy, who developed ARF, pulmonary hemorrhage, and cerebritis. The repeat renal biopsy in this case showed findings of MGN and tubulo-interstitial disease similar to what we found in our patient. This patient responded to dialysis and high dose steroid treatment and after 1 year of follow up remained stable with nephrotic syndrome and creatinine clearance of 41 ml/mm. The skin biopsy for immunofluorescent study was negative in these two patients. In some cases the review of the literature suggests that closer the serological profile resembles SLE, the more likely it is that the prevalence of histological renal involvement in MCTD is much higher than one would estimate from examination of clinical parameters alone, at least if the experience with SLE is applicable to MCTD.

THERAPY (13,22,32)

The treatment of MCTD is principally with glucucorticoids and nonsteroidal anti-inflammatory agents. The use of latter may be complicated with hyperkalemia with or without acute renal failure, and occasionally with aseptic meningitis (32). For severe extrarenal involvement and for diffuse, and progressive focal GN, high dose glucocorticoid therapy (1 mg/kg/day), followed by slow tapering to a maintenance level over several weeks to months is recommended. Maintenance glucocorticoid therapy is likely to be required for those with severe life threatening manifestations such as pericarditis, aortic valve involvement, serious central nervous system disease, nephrotic syndrome or renal failure. Severe exacerbations may appear following too rapid discontinuation of glucocoid therapy. In general, the response of the renal disease to glucocorticoid has been favorable, although occasionally steroid refractory progressive renal disease has been noted. The finding of widespread intimal and medial vascular lesions in renal biopsies may be poor prognostic feature even in the absence of hypertension. The role of adjunctive cytotoxic drug therapy is not established in MCTD, but anecdotal reports have suggested that in selected cases with severe renal or extrarenal involvement, the addition of cyclophosphamide or azathioprine to a program of oral glucocorticoids may permit a reduction in the dosage of glucorticoids at a safer and more tolerable level without risking a severe exacerbation.

OUTCOME OF OUR PATIENTS (13)

Renal function remained normal in seven of 12 (58%) of our patients. However, hypertension developed in 42%, trasient ARF in 8% and chronic renal failure in 17% of these 12 patients. The prevalence of latter was not significantly different from that observed in the 76 patients including our 10 patients with adequate biopsy (14%) (13). Three patients died, two of pulmonary hypertension with acute cor pulmonale and one of overwhelming sepsis.

REFERENCES

1. Sharp GC, Irvin WS, Tan EM, Gordon RG, Holman HR: Mixed connective tissue disease. An apparently distinct rheumatic disease syndrome associated with a specific antibody to an extractable nuclear antigen (ENA). Am J Med 52:158-159,1972.

2. Northway JD, Tan EM: Differentiation of antinuclear antibodies giving speckled staining patterns in immunofluorescence. Clin ImmunoImmunopathol 1:140-154, 1972.

3. Reichlin M, Mattiolo M: Correlation of prcipitin reaction to an RNA protein antigen and low prevalence of nephritis in patients with systemic lupus erythematosus. N Engl J Med 286:908-911, 1972.

4. Hence PK, Edgington TS, Tan EM: The evolving clinical spectrum of mixed connective tissue disease (MCTD). Arthritis Rheum 18:404, 1975 (abstr).

5. Sharp GC, Irvin WS, May CM, et al.: Association of antibodies to ribonucleoprotein and Sm antigens with mixed connective-tissue disease, systemic lupus erythematosus and other rheumatic disease. N Engl J Med 295:1149-1154, 1976.

6. Leibfarth JH, Persellin RH: Characteristics of patients with serum antibodies to extractable nuclear antigens. Arthritis Rheum 19:851-865, 1976.

7. Bennett RM, Spargo BH: Immune complex nephropathy in mixed connective tissue disease. Am J Med 63:534-541, 1977.

8. Hamburger M, Hodes S, Barland P: The incidence and clinical significance of antibodies to extractable nuclear antigens. Am J Med Sci 273:21-28, 1977.

9. Singsen BH, Landing B, Wolfe JF, et al: Histologic evaluation of mixed connective tissue disease in children and adults. Arthritis Rheum 21:593, 1978 (abstr).

10. Prystowsky SD: Mixed connective tissue disease. West J Med 132:288-293, 1980.

11. Silverstein R, Vergne-Marini P: The kidney in mixed connective tissue disease and Sjorgen's syndrome, in Suki WN, Eknoyan G (eds): The Kidney in Systemic Disease (ed 2). New York, Wiley & Sons, 1981, pp 77-97.

12. Grant KD, Adams LE, Hess EV: Mixed connective tissue disease - A subset with sequential clinical and loboratory features. J Rheumatol 8:587-598, 1981.

13. Kitridou RC, Akmal M, Turkel SB, Ehresman GR, Quismorio FP Jr, Massry SG: Renal involvement in mixed connective tissue disease: A longitudinal clinicopathologic study. Seminars in arthritis and Rheumatism. Vol 16:135-145, 1986.

14. Singsen BH, Bernstein BH, Kornreich HK, et al: Mixed connective tissue disease in childhood. A Clinical and serologic survey. J Pediatr 90:893-900, 1977.

15. Singsen BH, Swanson VL, Berstein BH, et al: A histologic evaluation of mixed connective tissue disease in childhood. Am J Med 68:710-717, 1980.

16. Mundy TM, Landing BH, Hanson V, et al: Renal involvement in mixed connective tissue disease in childhood. Arthritis Rheum 23:724, 1980 (abstr).

17. Baldassare A, Weiss T, Auclair R, et al: Mixed connective tissue disease (MCTD) in childhood. Arthritis Rheum 19:788, 1976 (abstr).

18. Eberhardt K, Svansesson H, Svensson B: Follow-up study of 6 children presenting with a MCTD-like syndrome. Scand J Rheumatol 10:62-64, 1981.

19. Guit GL, Shaw PC, Ehrlich J, Kroon HM, Oudkerk M: Mediastinal lymphadenopathy and pulmonary arterial hyperteinsion in pulmonary arterial hypertension in mixed connective tissue disease. Radiology 154:305-306, 1980.

20. Alpert MA, Goldberg SH, Singsen BH: Cardiovascular manifiestations of mixed connective tissue disease in adults. Circulation 68:482-1193, 1983.

21. Oetgen WJ, Mutter ML, Lawless OJ, Davia JE: Cardiac abnormalities mixed connective tissue disease. Chest 83:185-188, 1983.

22. Bennett RM, Bong DM, Spargo BH: Neuropsychiatric problems in mixed connective tissue disease. Am J Med 65:955-962, 1978.

23. Peller JS, Gabor GT, Porter JM, Bennett RM: Angiographitic findings in mixed connective tissue disease. Arth and Rheumatism 28:768-774, 1985.

24. Notman DD, Kurata N, Tan EM: Profiles of antinuclear antibodies in systemic rheumatic disease. Ann Int Med 83:464-469, 1975.

25. Germain MJ, Davidman M: Pulmonary hemorrhage and acute renal failure in a patient with mixed connective tissue disease. Am J Kidney Dis III:420-424, 1984.

26. Habets WJ, Derooij DJ, Salden MH, Verhagen AP, Van Eekelen CA, Vandeputte LB, Vanvanrooij WJ: Antibodies against distinct nuclear matrix proteins are characteristic for mixed connective tissue disease. Clin Exp. Immunol. 54:265-276, 1983.

27. Koike T, Suishi M, Tomioka H: Antlympocytotixic antibodies in mixed connective tissue disease and systemic lupus erythematosus. Arthritis and Rheumatism 26:570, 1983.

28. Granier F, Vayssairat M, Priollet P, Housset E: Nailfold capillary micorscopy in mixed connective tissue disease. Arthritis and Rheumatism 29:189-195, 1986.

29. Kobayashi S, Nagase M, Kimura M, Ohyama K, Ikeya M, Honda N: Renal involvement in mixed connective tissue disease. Am J Nephrol 5:282-289, 1985.

30. Bennett RM, Spargo BH: Immune complex nephropathy in mixed connective tissue disease. 63:534-541, 1977.

31. Glassock RJ, Goldstein DA, Akmal M, Kitridou R, Koss M: Recurrent acute renal failure in patients with mixed connective tissue disease. Am J Nephrol 2:282-290, 1982.

32. Gaeton D, Lorino MD, Hardin JG Jr: Sulindac-induced meningitis in mixed connective tissue disease. So Med J 76:1185-1187, 1983.

ATHEROEMBOLIC RENAL DISEASE: CLINICO-PATHOLOGIC CORRELATIONS

F.Antonucci*, S.Pizzolitto**, M.Travaglini***, G.F.Marrocco***, G.Boscutti*, M.Messa*, G.B.Fogazzi****, and E.Rivolta****

Servizio Nefrologia*, Istituto Anatomia Patologica**, III Divisione Chirurgica Ospedale Civile Udine***, Divisione Nefrologica Policlinico Milano****

INTRODUCTION

It has been known for long time that the course of atherosclerotic disease may be complicated by systemic manifestations of cholesterol embolism (1). The kidney is frequently involved in this phenomenon (2) which may give rise to diverse clinical pictures. The clinical diagnosis of atheroembolic renal disease may be easy in the presence of other embolic manifestations (livedo reticularis, digital ischemic necrosis, retinal emboli) and a clinical history of angiography, angioplasty and recent abdominal aortic surgery. In these cases, the cutaneous and muscular biopsies may provide valid and not invasive diagnostic support (3). When atheroembolism appears spontaneously, in the absence of causal events, and the clinical history is of acute or chronic renal failure of unknown origin, only renal biopsy with pathognomonic findings of needle-shaped cholesterol crystals within the vessel lumen permits diagnosis, distinguishing atheroembolic lesions from those of nephroangiosclerosis or other pathologies.

In our study we have attempted to assess the frequency of atheroembolism and possible clinico-pathologic correlations in a sample of patients with variable impairement of the renal function from a population of subjects at risk, suffering from severe atherosclerosis of the abdominal aorta.

PATIENTS AND METHODS

Since 1985 we have investigated pre-operative renal function in 60 consecutive patients suffering from occlusive and/or aneurismatic atherosclerosis of the abdominal aorta and/or of the iliac-femoral vessels. There were no diabetics and all were over fifty years old. Each patient was submitted to aortography with study of the renal arteries, to evaluation of creatinine clearance, proteinuria, urinary sediment and uroculture. In 9 patients, in the presence of atherosclerotic lesions of the renal arteries (7/9), abnormal urinary sediment

(9/9), reduction of creatinine clearance (7/9) and proteinuria (4/9) we performed a renal biopsy in the course of intervention on the abdominal aorta. In 3 cases with reduced pre-operative creatinine clearance and deceased due to post-operative non-renal complications, we examined the kidneys hystologically. In all the biopsy cases, immunofluorescence (anti IgG, IgA, IgM, Fibrinogen) and electronic microscopy were carried out, while the hystological examination was performed with hematoxiline-eosine, Masson's trichrome, PAS-PASM staining. No fragment contained less than 30 glomeruli. At the time of the study there were no embolic signs and renal function was stable.

RESULTS

On the 12 patients examined, the hystological examination revealed in 6 the presence of nephroangiosclerosis and in 6 cholesterol emboli affecting the renal vessels of various diameter in association with nephroangiosclerotic lesions. Immunofluorescence was negative in all the cases examined. On the basis of the hystological findings, we analysed the clinical characteristics of the patients and the pattern of renal function in the last three years. The 6 patients with nephroangiosclerosis (group A) were between 55 and 75 years of age. Creatinine clearance varied between 100 and 50 ml/m, blood pressure was high in 2/6 cases, ESR was normal and the urine test showed slight alterations in sediment and proteinuria not higher than 20 mg/dl. In all cases, anamnesis showed no deterioration in renal function in the last three years. Of the 6 cases with cholesterol emboli, in 3 (Group B1) the emboli affected only the interlobular and arcuate arteries and in the glomeruli either ischemic alterations or an increase in the mesangial matrix were present. In 3 cases (group B2) they were also present within the glomeruli in association with fibrinoid necrosis and/or segmental sclerosis, in the absence of extracapillary proliferation and fibrinoid necrosis of the arterioles. All 6 patients were hypertensive, between 59 and 77 years of age, with creatinine clearance ranging from 65 to 16 ml/m, but those in group B1 had normal ESR, slightly abnormal urinary sediment, proteinuria not higher than 20 mg/dl, normal serum complement, an absence of eosinophilia and absence of renal failure progression in the last three years. Those in group B2, on the other hand, had proteinuria higher than 50 mg/dl, frankly abnormal sediment, high ESR and renal failure progression over the last three years (in one case resulting in periodic dialysis treatment and in one case partial recovery of renal function after a brief period of hemodialysis.

DISCUSSION

Atheroembolic renal disease may be the cause of acute, chronic or rapidly progressive renal failure (2). Frequently elderly subjects, over 50 years of age, hypertensive and with severe aorto-iliac atherosclerosis both of the occlusive and aneurismatic type are affected (4). The emboli can affect vessels of different diameter, determining the various clinical pictures on the basis of the number and the diameter of the occluded vessels. If the most affected vessels are the interlobular and arcuate arteries, an extensive occlusion may give rise to multiple infarctions with acute renal failure and irreversible oligoanuria. If the entity of the embolic phenomenon is limited, the evolution of acute renal failure may be more favourable and lead to a moderate reduction in creatinine clearance. The glomerular and tubulo-interstitial lesions are usually aspecific (glomerular collapse and tubulo-interstitial atrophy) but they may also be the consequence of direct damaging action of microemboli affecting the pre-glomerular arterioles and the capillaries, as in the cases of rapidly progressive renal failure described by Goldman et al. and Remy and al. (5,6) with a histological picture of segmental fibrinoid glomerular necrosis and extracapillary proliferation associated with cholesterol microemboli with negative immunofluorescence. If the clinical history reveals nothing significant, atheroembolic nephropathy may present itself with a picture of chronic renal failure with arterial hypertension and be mistaken for nephroangiosclerosis, with the risk of further deteriorations provoked by angiography, angioplasty and surgery of the aorta. Our hystological study of 12 subjects with impaired renal function in a population of 60 atherosclerotic patients, showed up atheroembolic renal disease in 50% of cases. All the cases were spontaneous chronic forms, not clinically suspect due to the absence of causal events in the clinical history. The search for anatomo-clinical correlations led to the identification of two different types of evolution of renal failure corresponding to different hystopathological pictures. Only the patients with glomerular lesions such as necrosis and/or segmental sclerosis associated with cholesterol microemboli had shown a progression towards uraemia in the last three years and had the lowest creatinine clearance values. Eosinophilia was not present in any of the cases while it was pointed out several times in the acute phases of atheroembolic nephropathy (7). The glomerular lesions in our cases differed from those pointed out by Goldman and Remy because of the absence of extracapillary proliferation and the importance of the segmental sclerosis phenomena, within which cholesterol crystals were identified. In these patients, ESR was high and proteinuria more marked with respect to patients with atheroembolism limited to the interlobular and arcuate arterioles. The clinical characteristics and course of the latter patients were not distinguishable from that of patients with simple nephroangiosclerosis.

In conclusion, our study has confirmed the high frequency of spontaneous atheroembolic renal disease in atherosclerotic patients and the possibility to differentiate two types of evolution of chronic renal failure on the basis of hystological lesions.

For this reason, we believe that impairment of renal function, in a patient with generalised atherosclerosis must always lead to the clinical suspicion of atheroembolic nephropathy to assess the opportunity for renal biopsy.

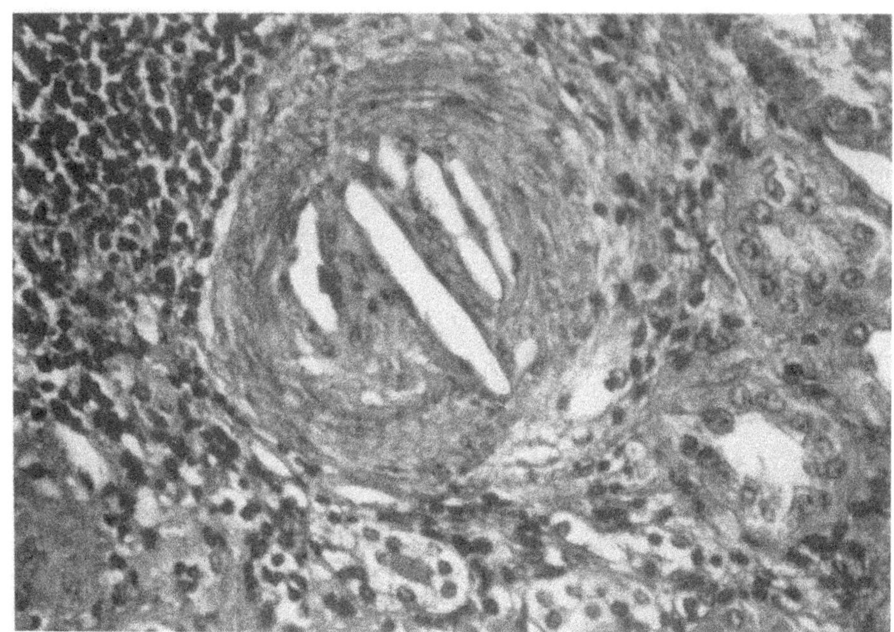

Fig. 1. Renal biopsy demonstrating an interlobular artery with the characteristic needle-shaped clefts of cholesterol embolization. Note the presence of a typical foreign-body inflammatory reaction to the emboli. (Masson's thrichrome stain, magnification x 250).

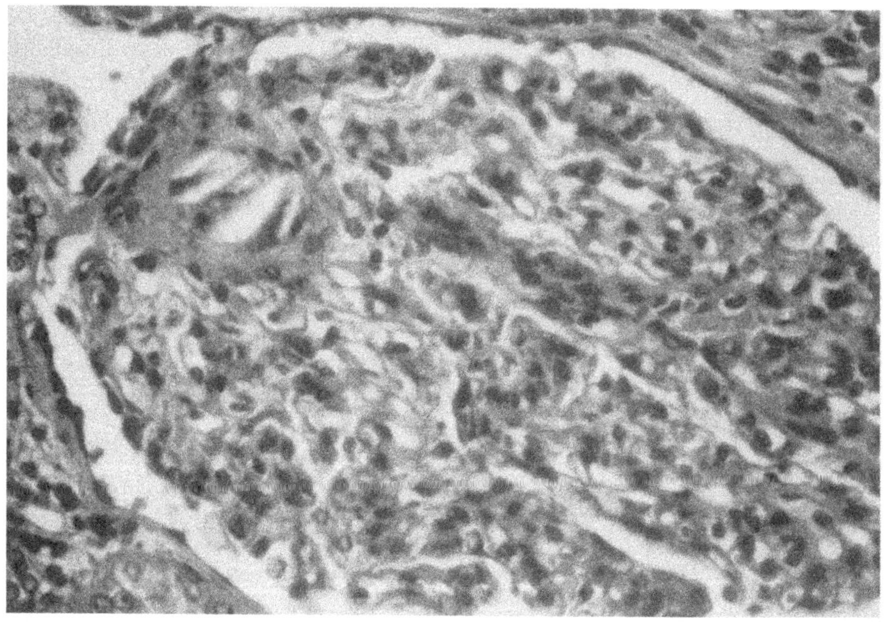

Fig. 2. Glomerulus with several cholesterol clefts in the afferent arteriole. Capillaries necrosis absence. (Masson's trichrome stain, magnification x 400).

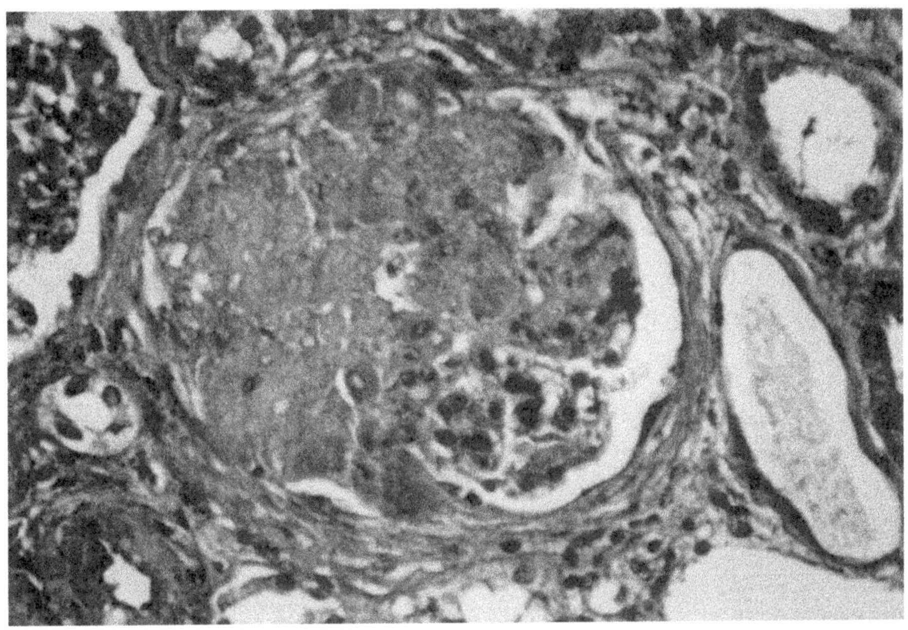

Fig. 3. Glomerulus showing segmental necrotizing lesions associated with extensive sclerosis (Masson's trichrome stain, magnification x 250).

ACKNOWLEDGMENT

We are indebted to Elena Gecchelin and Franco Cristofoli for their technical assistance.

REFERENCES

1) J.A. Carvajal, R. Anderson, L.Weiss, J.Grismer and R.Berman: Atheroembolism. An etiologic factor in renal insufficiency, gastrointestinal hemmorrhages, and peripheral vascular diseases. Arch.Int.Med. 119: 593-599 (1967.).
2) M.C. Smith, M.K. Ghose and A.R. Henry: The clinical spectrum of renal cholesterol embolisation. Am.J. of Med. 71: 174-180 (1981).
3) J.A. McGowan and A.Greenberg: Cholesterol atheroembolic renal disease. Report of 3 cases with emphasis on diagnosis by skin biopsy and extended survival. Am.J.Nephrol. 6: 135-139 (1986).
4) W.T. Thurlbeck and B.Castleman: Atheromatous emboli to the kidneys after aortic surgery. N.E.J.of Med. 257, 10: 442-447 (1957).
5) M.Goldman, Y. Thoua, M. Dhaene and C. Toussaint: Necrotising glomerulonephritis associated with cholesterol microemboli. Brit.Med.J. 290: 205-206 (1985).
6) P. Remy, C. Jacquot, C. Nochy, C. d'Auzac, P. Yéni and J. Bariéty: Cholesterol atheroembolic renal disease with necrotising glomerulonephritis. Am.J. of Nephrol. 7: 164-165 (1987).
7) B.S. Kasinath, H.L. Corwin, A.K. Bidani, S.M. Korbet, M.M. Schwartz and J.L. Lewis: Eosinophilia in the diagnosis of atheroembolic renal disease. Am.J. of Nephrol. 7: 173-177 (1987).

RENAL INVOLVEMENT IN TUBEROUS SCLEROSIS

F.Dossi*,A.M. Marconi**,P. Riegler***,M. Broggini****, and D.Donati*

* Dept. of Nephrology; ** Dept. of Urology; **** Dept. of Internal Medicine, General Hospital Varese - *** Dept. of Nephrology, General Hospital Bolzano - Italy

Tuberous Sclerosis (T.S.) is an autosomal dominant inherited disease with high penetrance but variable expressivity. According to recent studies the gene for T.S. is on the distal long arm of chromosome 9.[1] Criteria for diagnosis have been established and include clinical and radiological criteria.[2,3]
Clinical: adenoma sebaceum (60%-70%), seizures (80%), mental retardation (50%), hypomelanotic macules, shagreen patches, ungueal fibromas.
Radiological: X ray of skull: fibrotic plaques, X ray of hands and feet: cysts and periostal new bone formation, computed tomography of brain: periventricular calcifications and subependimal hamartromas, computed tomography of kidney: cysts and/or angiomyolipomas, ultrasound of hearth: rhabdomyoma.
Renal involvement in T.S. is frequent (80%)[4] and consists of: angiomyolipoma (40-80%), cysts (rare).[5,9] Recently glomerular lesions in form of focal and segmental hyalinosis have been described. This glomerulopathy would represent an example of glomerular lesion secondary to hyperfiltration.[6] Clinical expression of the renal involvement in T.S. is wide: palpable tumours, flank pain, hypertension, micro and/or macroscopic hematuria, proteinuria, chronic renal failure.[6,7]
Prognosis is rather poor since early deaths because of neurological complications occur in a high proportion of patients.[4,8]

MATERIAL AND METHODS

In the last few years four patients affected by T.S. and renal involvement came to our observation: two males aged 26 y.(n.1) and 44 y. (n.2) and two females aged 21 (n.3) and 11 (n.4).
Mean clinical and private data are listed in table 1.

Table 1. Private and clinical data of the patients

pt	sex	age	at d.[a]	syst.signes	r.funct.[b]	r.pathology	r.presenting sympt.
1	m	26	5	seizures adenomas	ESRD-RTX[c]	cysts hamartromas	uremia
2	m	44	birth	skin lesions seizures mental ret.	inc.CRF	hamartromas	incipient CRF
3	f	21	birth	seizures adenomas mental ret.	normal	hamartromas mycroscopic cysts	enuresis renal colic
4	f	11	5	adenomas mental ret.	normal	hamartromas	enuresis acute pyelonephritis

a. age at diagnosis of T.S.

b. actual renal funcion
renal pathology
renal presenting symptoms

c. renal transplantation

PATIENTS

Case report n.1

Male aged 26 years. Seizures since he was 1 year old. Skin lesions at the age of 5 years. At the age of 19 presented with End stage renal disease requiring replacement treatment (uremic pericarditis).
CT examination showed coesisting cysts and hamartromas (Fig.1 and Fig.2)
The patient underwent Continous ambulatory peritoneal dialysis. After a few months of treatment macroscopic hematuria occurred and after 2 further years the patient was moved to hemodialysis because of recurrent peritonitis.
A first unsuccessful cadaveric renal transplant was carried out (conventional immunosuppressive agents) then a second allograft was performed (figure 4).
The patient had been maintained on cyclosporine with a high daily dose regimen due to the concomitant assumption of anticonvulsivant drugs.
So far he his alive and well with his graft normally functioning; no apparent changes such as relapses of the basis disease are present.
Figure 3 shows the typical periventricular calcifications.

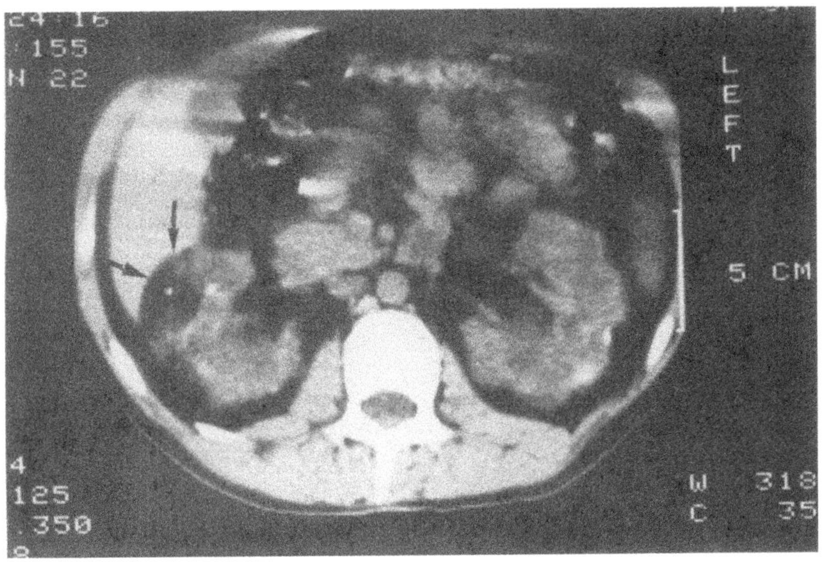

Figure 1. Renal hamartroma (arrows)

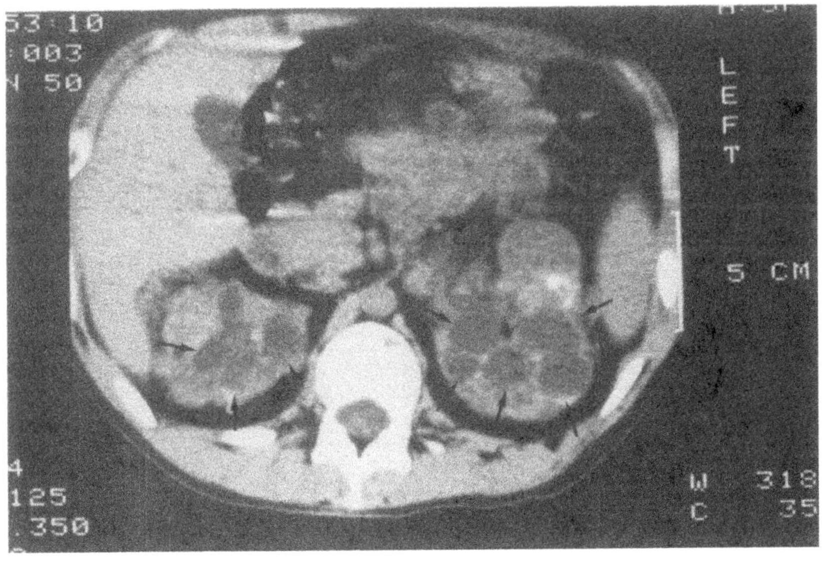

Figure 2. Renal cysts (arrows)

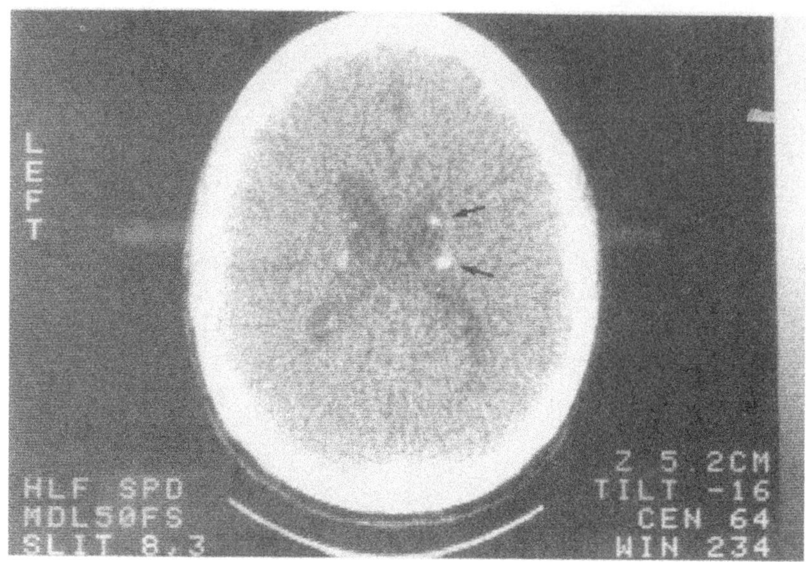

Fig.3 Periventricular calcifications

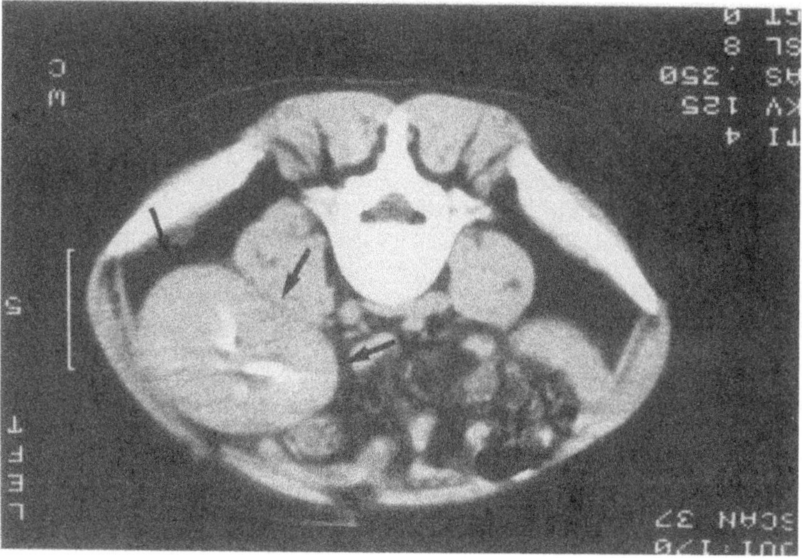

Fig.4 Successful renal transplantation. No relapses are present

Case report n.2

Male aged 44 years. Early diagnosis of T.S. was made because of adenoma sebaceum on his face, shagreen patches on lower abdomen, seizures, behaviour abnormalities and mental retardation.
At the age of 41 years he was admitted because of 1st degree coma which spontaneously recovered. Cardiac examination showed tachiarrythmia from atrial fibrillation.
On physical examination a palpable tumour on the right flank was observed. CT and US scans demonstrated enlargement of both kidneys which were massively devastated by angiomyolipomas of various size. This finding was confirmed by renal arteriography.
Serum creatinine was 1.6 mg/dl. Creatinine clearance was 68 ml/min.
Urinalysis showed microscopic hematuria and mild proteinuria.
Blood pressure was normal.
The patient was dismissed on anticonvulsivant and antiarrythmic drugs.
After 3 years, while in Psychiatric division, residual renal function is satisfactory: serum creatinine 1.8 mg/dl; creatinine clearance 59 ml/min.

Case report n.3

Female aged 25 years. Diagnosis of T.S. was made in infancy because of the classic triad. Maternal grandfather and an aunt were mentally retarded. At the age of 11 years she was admitted because of enuresis. Despite urographic and angiographic examinations demonstrated a right renal mass with the typical aspects of hamartromas, she was submitted to explorative lombotomy in suspition of malignancy. Right nephrectomy was carried out but hystologic examination confirmed the hamartromatous nature of the mass.
On revision, the microscopic speciment showed several cystic changes together with the angiomyolipoma which infiltrated the normal parenchima. The left kidney was preserved at that time but 9 years later she was admitted again because of left renal colic.
CT scan showed a 4.5 cm diameter mass on the left kidney.
Two further years later the mass was increased in size and extended outside the kidney in the retroperitoneal space.
Renal function is normal, so far.

Case report n.4

Female aged 11. Seizures were present since birth. Diagnosis of T.S. was made at 5 years of age because of adenoma sebaceum, hypomelanotic macules and mental retardation.
She had been suffering from pelvic pain for few years and used to micturate by abdominal compression.
At the age of 9 years she was submitted to urodinamic examination that showed depressed detrusorial activity during the emptying phase and increased uretral activity during the filling phase.
Urographic, cystographic and US investigations showed no abnormalities.

One and a half years later the child was admitted because of fever and urinary tract infection. Diagnosis of acute pyelonephritis was made. CT scanning demonstrated multyple small angiomyolipomas which were confirmed by arteriography.
At dismission urinalysis showed only mild microscopic hematuria.
Renal function is still normal.

DISCUSSION

Renal involvement in Tuberous Sclerosis is frequent[4] but chronic renal failure is rare.[6,7]
It has been stated that chronic renal failure is more likely to occur when cystic changes are present, with or without hamartromas.[7]
This can be explainated by the faster growth in size of the cysts, compaired with that of hamartromas, which replace and compress the normal parenchima.
On the other hand, expressivity is age-dependent then, as management of the neurological complications has become more effective and survival longer, C.R.F. could well develop also in those patients where angio-myolipomas are the only renal pathological finding. In our series of patients CRF developed in the patient with macroscopic cysts but also the oldest patient, whose kidneys were affected by angiomyolipomas without apparent cystic changes, suffered from incipient chronic renal insufficiency.
Moreover the girl whose removed kidney could be studied by hystological investigation showed microscopic cysts.
It can be hypotized that cystic pathology is more frequent than supposed and that this transformation begins early in the course of the disease.
Microscopic specimen was obtained only in one patient with normal renal function but urinalysis (of all patients) did not suggest an underlying glomerulopathy which has been regarded as a cause of CRF.[6]
Hypertension was not observed in any patient but in one case when clinical uremia occurred.
Sex-linkage of CRF can hardly be supported, reviewing literature, although in our experience it affected only male patients (but still older, when compaired with the female).
Clinical expression of nephropathy in T.S. is rather wide.
In the two females of our series the first symptom was enuresis which, in one case, reflected a condition of neurological bladder complicated by pyelonephritis. This pathological finding has often been described on autoptic specimens.
Although never reported before, neurological abnormalities of micturition could well occur in such a neurological disease as T.S.
Renal involvement in T.S. is often hardly distinguishible from polycystic disease when hamartromas are absent.[5,8]
A hyperplastic eosinophilic epithelial lining around the cysts of T.S. has been described[9] but the microscopic bioptic specimen are not routinarely obtained in these patients and the renal cysts alone are rather unusual in this disease.

It is the evidence of renal cystic disease associated with neurocutaneous abnormalitis that should drive the physician toward diagnosis of T.S. The possibility of T.S. should be evaluated when a child present with a cystic disease which appears to be the adult-type of polycystic disease. The hamartromatous tumours of the kidney may sometimes lead to a wrong diagnosis of malignancy.[10]
As a matter of fact, malignant transformation is very rare and although T.S. and cancer share some clinical, radiological and even hystologic signes the hamartromatous nature of the neoplasia should be carefully considered.
An eventual nephrectomy in such patients,whose renal disease comes from replacement of functioning parenchima, could have dreadful effects on prognosis.
As already asserted, survival is prolonging and probably renal failure is to become a more frequent presenting symptom.
In our one-case-experience both dialysis and transplantation can be successfully performed in these patients. As already reported[10], in spite of the multisystemic disorder, we consider patients affected by T.S. good candidates to any available renal replacement treatment.

REFERENCES

1. A.E. Fryer, J.M. Connor, S. Povery, J.R.W. Yates, A. Cholmers, I. Fraser, A.D. Yates, J.P. Osborne, Evidence that the gene for tuberous sclerosis is on chromosome 9, The Lancet i: 659-661(1987)
2. M.R. Gomez,"Tuberous sclerosis", Raven Press, New York (1979)
3. K. Simmons, Early diagnosis, genetic marker sought for tuberous sclerosis, JAMA 251: 3061-3063 (1984)
4. A.M. Chonko, J.M. Weiss, J.H. Stein, T.F. Ferris, Renal involvement in tuberous sclerosis, Am.J.Med. 56: 124-132 (1974)
5. J.S. Mitnick, M.A. Bosniak, S. Hilton, B. Nagesh Raghavendra, B.R. Subramanyam, N.B. Genieser, Cystic renal disease in tuberous sclerosis, Radiology 147: 85-87 (1983)
6. J.P. Herve, D. Chevet, J.Cledes, P. Le Pogamp, J.P. Leroy, A. Heyrier, Chronic renal failure in tuberous sclerosis (Bourneville disease), Kid. Int. 21: 899 (1982) Abstract
7. R.D. Okada, M.A. Platt, J.Fleishman, Chronic renal failure in patients with tuberous sclerosis. Association with renal cysts, Nephron 30: 85-88 (1982)
8. R.L. Scheing, P. Bornstein, Tuberous sclerosis in the adult. An unusual case without mental deficiency or epilepsy, Arch. Intern. Med. 108: 789-795 (1961)
9. F.B. Stapleton, D. Johnson, G.W. Kaplan, W. Griswold, The cystic renal lesion in tuberous sclerosis, J. Pediatr. 97: 574-579 (1980)
10. P.R. Jochimsen, P.M. Braunstein, J.S. Najarian, Renal allotransplantation for bilateral renal tumours, JAMA 210: 1721- 1724 (1969)

SEVERE RENAL INVOLVEMENT IN PRIMARY SJOGREN'S SYNDROME

A. Gentric*, J.P. Herve*, Y.L. Pennec**,
J.P. Leroy*** and J. Cledes*

* Service de Néphrologie
** Service de Médecine Interne HARVIER
*** Laboratoire d'Anatomo-Pathologie
C.H.U. Morvan 29285 Brest Cedex

Primary Sjögren's syndrome is a chronic inflammatory autoimmune disorder that is characterized by a mononuclear cell infiltration of the exocrine glands. Similar lymphocytic infiltrates may invade visceral organs, and this results in several extra glandular manifestations, including renal disease.

Various rare renal lesions have been reported, such as membranous and membranoproliferative nephrithis (7), necrotizing glomerulonephritis (13), renal lymphoma and pseudolymphoma (1).

The characteristic histological finding is a focal interstitial nephritis which occurs in about 50 percent of the patients. Its frequency may be underestimated. The interstitial nephritis results in latent or overt tubular defects : (table I) distal renal tubular acidosis type one (20 to 25 % of the patients) (13), with possible nephrocalcinosis (2), nephrogenic diabetes insipidus (reported in up to 50 percent of the patients) (13), rarely proximal renal tubular acidosis (13) and Fanconi syndrome. Aseptic leucocyturia (11), proteinuria (with levels below 0,5 g/day) and mild renal impairment (8) are quite common.

Three cases of rapidly evolutive and severe tubulo-interstitial nephritis (creatinine clearance below 30 ml/mn) are described in the literature. Tu and al in 1968 (10) and Gerhard and al in 1978 (5) Cobo Reinoso (4) reported the observations of three females who had a PSS and whose creatinine clearance were respectively 16, 20 and 23 ml/mn. No therapeutical trial was initiated.

We are going to report here 5 cases of PSS with marked deterioration in renal function.

5 females, mean age 55,2 years (range : 25 to 68 years) admitted for tiredness satisfied the criteria for the diagnosis of PSS (Homma's criteria), (table II).

- xerophtalmia
- abnormal Schirmer test : less than 5 mm of filter paper was moistened after 5 mn).
- keratoconjonctivitis sicca with Rose Bengal staining (11)
- xerostomia
- and a characteristic biopsy of the minor salivary glands : grade IV in the classification of Chisholm and Mason with more than one focus of lymphocytes for $4mm^2$ gland section (3).

Furthermore 4 patients had an elevated erythrocyte sedimentation rate. Hypergammaglobulinemia was present in three cases. Antibodies to SSA and to SSB were always negative. None of the patients met clinical or serological criteria for an additional auto-immune disease (rheumatoid arthritis, systemic lupus erythematosus, systemic sclerosis, polymyositis, polyarteritis nodosa). They didn't tacke any nephrotoxic drug. Three patients had other disease features Raynaud's phenomenon, arthritis, peripheral neuropathy, pulmonary fibrosis.

Laboratory and renal morphological data are summarized in table N°III.

Arterial blood pressure was normal. The mean creatinine clearance was 11,1 ml/mn (range 4 to 25 ml/mn), the mean urinary protein excretion was 980 mg/d (range : 500 to 1660 mg). Microscopic hematuria and aseptic leycocyturia were present in each case.

Two patients had distal renal tubular acidoses ; there was no impairment of proximal tubular function. The kidneys were normal in 3 cases, nephrocalcinosis was present in patient N°1, and small sized kidneys were seen in patient N°5.

All renal biopsy specimens revealed a dense mononuclear cell interstitial infiltrate, and fibrosis. The tubular pattern was destroyed by tubular dilatation and atrophy. Segmental glomerular sclerosis was seen in 3 patients. The glomeruli were normal in all other cases. Immunofluorescence was negative in cases 1,2 and 4, it revealed staining of the interstitium and the tubular basement membranes for IgM and C3 in cases 3 and 5.

None of the usual causes of interstitial nephritis could be retained : familial nephropathy, chronic pyelonephritis, drug, toxic, infection or metabolic induced interstitial nephropathy.

The treatment and the evolution are shown in table IV. Patient 5 was immediately stârted on chronic hemodialysis. A therapeutic trial of glucocorticoids (1 mg/kg/day), was initiated in the other patients. Renal function didn't improve in patient 3, hemodialysis was undertaken 1 month later. Clinical and laboratory improvements were observed in patients 1, 2, and 4. A corticodependance appeared in patient 4 who died from staphylococcal infection 7 months after starting corticotherapy. In patients 1 and 2, treatment was stopped after two years, creatinine clearances were respectively 40 ml/mn and 25 ml/mn.

The pathogenesis of the renal disease of PSS is not known. An immune complex deposition has been implicated. However, glomeruli are generally spared, immune deposits in tubular basement membranes are not always seen, interstitial nephritis is the most frequently observed renal lesion. So another hypothesis, suggests that the renal involvement might be attributed to a cell mediated immunological mechanism. A delayed type hypersensitivity may be suspected. As in salivary glands, the majority of infiltrating cells are T cells, most activated and belonging to the helper/inducer subset (OKT 4+). These cells might react against an unknown renal antigen. In many other forms of interstitial nephritis cytotoxic/suppressor T cells are the predominant identified cell types.

In conclusion we suggest that when the etiology of interstitial nephritis is obscure, associated auto-immune diseases, including PSS, should be considered. Interstitial nephritis of PSS may result in severe and rapidly evolutive renal impairment. Pathogenic immune mechanisms are suspected, so long terme glucocorticoid therapy may improve renal function but side effects must be considered.

TABLE I

RENAL MANIFESTATIONS IN P.S.S.

- NEPHROGENIC DIABETES INSIPIDUS (RENAL CONCENTRATING DEFECT)	:	50 %
- DISTAL RENAL TUBULAR ACIDOSIS	:	20 - 25 %
- NEPHROCALCINOSIS	:	6 - 8 %
- PROXIMAL RENAL TUBULAR ACIDOSIS	}	RARE
- FANCONI SYNDROME	}	RARE

TABLE II

PATIENT	1	2	3	4	5
AGE	25	68	59	64	60
XEROPHTALMIA SCHIRMER TEST	+	+	+	+	+
KERATOCONJONCTIVITIS SICCA	+	+	+	+	+
XEROSTOMIA	+	+	+	+	+
LABIAL SALIVARY GLAND BIOPSY	IV	IV	IV	IV	IV
ESR (Mn/H)	-	117	90	90	54
HYPERGAMMAGLOBULINEMIA	+	+	-	+	-
OTHER DISEASE FEATURES	Raynaud's phenomenon	-	. Peripheral nephropathy . Pulmonary fibrosis	-	Arthritis pulmonary fibrosis

TABLE III

PATIENT	1	2	3	4	5
CREATININE (clearance ml/mn)	25	10	6	10,8	4
PROTEINURIE (g/d)	0,5	0,75	1,40	0,60	1,66
LEUCOCYTURIA (WBC/mn)	32 000	100 000	52 000	12 400	36 000
HEMATURIA (RBC/mn)	10 000	33 000	46 000	30 000	36 000
TUBULAR ACIDOSIS	+	-	-	-	+
KIDNEY MORPHOLOGY	NEPHROCALCINOSE	N	N	N	Little sixed kidneys

TABLE IV

TREATMENT AND EVOLUTION

PATIENT	1	2	3	4	5
TREATMENT	PREDNISONE 1mg/kg/d	PREDNISONE 1mg/kg/d	PREDNISONE 1 mg/kg/d	PREDNISONE 1mg/kg/d	HD
TREATMENT DURATION	2 years	2 years	1 month	7 months	
EVOLUTION	Improvement → Creatinine clearance 40 ml/mn	Improvement → Creatinine Clearance 28 Ml/mn	HD	Death	

BIBLIOGRAPHIE

1 - ANDERSON L.G., TALAL N.
The spectrum of benign to malignant lymphoproliferation in Sjögren's syndrome
Clin. Exp. Immunol. 1971, 9, 199-221

2 - BUCKALEW VW, PURVIS ML, SCHUMAN MG et al.
Hereditary renal tubular acidosis : report of a 64 member-kindred with variable clinical expressions including idiopathic hypercalciuria.
Medecine, 1974, 53, 229-254

3 - CHISHOLM D.M., MASON D.K.
Labial salivary gland biopsy in Sjögren's syndrome.
J. Clin. Path. 1968, 21, 656.

4 - COBO REINOSO E., COLLAZOS GONZLEZ J., CHOCARRO A.
Linfoma immunoblastico y nefritis interstitial en un sindrome de Sjögren.
Med. Clin. 1984 ; 83, 420-423

5 - GERHARD RE, LOEBL DH, RAD RN.
Interstitial immunofluorescence nephritis of Sjögren syndrome.
Clin. Nephrol. 1968, 10, 201-207.

6 - HOMMA M., YAMMAGATA H.
Japan Sjögren's syndrome commitee
1977

7 - MOUTSOPOULOS HM, LAWLEY JT, BALOW E.J. et al
Immune complex glomerulonephritis and circulating immune complex in patients with sicca syndrome.
Arth. and Rheum, 1978, 2, 58.

8 - TALAL N, ZISMAN E, SCHUR P.H.
Renal tubular acidosis, glomerulonephritis and immunological factors in Sjögren's syndrome.
Arth. and Rheum 1968, II, 774

9 - TU W, H, SHEARN AM, LEE CJ et al.
Interstitial nephritis in Sjögren's syndrome
Ann. Intern. Med., 1968, 69, 1163-1170.

10 - TAKAYA M., ICHIKAWA Y., SCHIMIZU H et al.
T lymphocyte subsets of the infiltrations cells in the salivary gland and kidney of a patient with Sjögren's syndrome associated with interstitial nephritis.
Clin. Exp. Rheumatol., 1985, 3, 259.

11 - VAN BIJSTERVELD OP
Diagnostic tests in the sicca syndrome
Arch. Ophtalmo, 1969, 82, 10.

12 - LEBB J., VINCE J., WHALEY K et al.
Studies of renal function in Sjögren's syndrome and rheumatoid arthritis.
Rheumatism, 1975, V, 263-282.

13 - WINER L., ROBERT M.
Renal complications of Sjögren's syndrome.
Current therapy in nephrology and hypertension 1985, 167-171.

IgA NEPHROPATHY IN SYSTEMIC DISEASES

G Piccoli, R Coppo, D Roccatello, and A Amore
Instiute of Nephro-Urology, University of Turin
Nuova Astanteria Martini, Turin, Italy

In the last years growing interest has been focused on the pathogenesis of the glomerular diseases characterized by mesangial IgA deposits. Some pathogenetic mechanisms are common to all these nephropathies, either idiopatic or those associated to systemic disorders. Moreover, the analysis of individual diseases shows that their relative weight may be different, and this allows to consider at the same time at least a few of their pathogenetic mechanisms.

The granular pattern on immunofluorescence, together with the electron dense deposits on the electron microscopy examination, strongly suggest an immune complex pathogenesis (1,2).

IgA-containing immune complexes in renal deposits are thought to derive from the general circulation according to this hypothesis, high levels of IgA-containing circulating immune complexes (IgACIC) have been detected by several investigators, and by ourselves, with different techniques (3-8) in 35-70% of sera from patients with idiopathic IgA nephropathy (IgAGN), in about 80% of sera from patients with Schoenlein-Henoch syndrome and up to 100% in cases with alcoholic cirrhosis-associated glomerulonephritis. By using a specific solid-phase assay (3) we found mean values of IgACIC significantly higher than controls in patients affected by idiopathic IgAGN [0.91 OD values at 400 nm (range 0.10-3.00 OD) in patients, versus (vs) O.25 (0.17-0.61) OD in healthy subjects, $p< 0.01$] (9). We observed also very high mean IgACIC levels in Schoenlein-Henoch nephritis [1.05 (0.05-3.00) OD, $p< 0.01$] (9) and in chronic alcoholic liver cirrhosis [0.71 (0.33-1.62) OD, p<0.01] (10).

Opinions that deny any pathogenetic significance to these findings are also present (11). These IC are in effect intermittently present in the circulation and their levels were related to the extent of haematuria in same researches (3, 5, 7, 12), but not in others (11). These are however commonly found in IC diseases, where the cinetic behaviour of tissue deposits is never the same to that of the immune complexes in circle, and the impossibility to demonstrate CIC, at least in some phases of the disease, may be due, along to different moments of activity, also to a limited sensibility to methodics and to the speed of departure from the circle of the CIC themselves.

It is therefore our opinion that the lack of a regular correspondence between serical and tissue findings and clinical signs of disease activity reduces and may cancel the semeiotic significance in isolated controls of the CIC but that, at least in the actual state of knowledge, their significance in pathogenetic interpretation of disease has still to be considered acceptable.

The detection of relevant amount of IgACIC in sera from IgA nephropathy patients provided the stimulus for the examination of the mechanisms of regulation of IgA synthesis as well as the formation and the fate of IgACIC. More recently, some antigens, supposed to be able to trigger this sequence of events, have received increasing interest.

Information inferred from these studies, although non-unequivocably agreed, suggests a general design of pathogenesis of the diseases grouped under the heading of IgA mesangial nephropathy.

It is worthy to remind that an increased synthesis of serum IgA, especially polymeric, was reported by several Authors, in IgAGN idiopathic and related to systemic diseases (13-16). Moreover the levels of IgA antibodies to infectious and alimentary antigens in these patients were found to be higher than in the controls (17-21), and IgA response to subcutaneous injection of influenza haemoagglutinins seems increased as well (22). Finally IgA with rheumatoid or antiidiotypic activity were detected in these patients (23-24).

Abnormalities in the mechanisms of regulation of IgA synthesis are supposed to underlie a picture of immunological hyperreactivity which includes increase of IgA bearing lymphocytes (16), B cell hyperreactivity (20), unbalance of lymphocyte subsets with prevalent T helper cells (13).

From the clinical point of view, a mucosal immune system involvement is suggested by the well known observation of frequent relapses which parallel infections of upper respiratory tract, gut and urinary tract. In agreement with this hypothesis, is the remark that polymeric IgA, of prevalently mucosal origin, are probably mostly involved in the formation of circulating IC and immune deposits (25, 26). Moreover some reports detecting J-chains in mesangial deposits further support the relevance of the mucosal immune system in these nephropathies.

Although some Authors, using monoclonal antibodies, detected only IgA1 subclass in IgAIC from sera of IgAGN patients (25), Coppo et al in our group, by employing specific polyclonal antibodies prepared by Vaerman and Delacroix, documented, in circulating IC, the presence of IgA2 subclass together with IgA1 (9). By using a specific modified conglutinin solid-phase assay, mean levels of IgA1CIC were found to be significantly increased in primary IgAGN in comparison to controls [0.64 (0.17-2.05) OD, vs 0.25 (0.10-0.65) OD, $p<0.01$]. Similar data were found for IgA2CIC [0.43 (0.10-1.80) OD, $p<0.01$]. In the same studies high levels of IgACIC, constituted by both IgA1 and IgA2 subclasses, were detected in alchoolic cirrhosis - associated GN (10) [IgA1CIC: 0.91 (0.47-1.80) OD, $p<0.01$ and IgA2CIC: 1.13 (0.67-1.75) OD, $p<0.01$] and in Schoenlein-Henoch purpura nephritis (18) in which, however, a prevalence of IgA1 on IgA2 was found. [IgA1CIC : 0.84 (0.14-3.15) OD, $p<0.01$; IgA2CIC 0.41 (0.05-0.84, $p<0.01$].

As IgA of mucosal provenience are constituted of IgA from both subclasses, we had interpreted that these findings, inserted in a group of contrasting information, were an ulterior evidence that IgACIC in IgAGN have a mucosal origin; as we will discuss the actual state of knowledge, and in particular some data of sperimental pathology, seem to offer ulterior evidence in favour of this eventuality.

An experimental confirmation on the pathogenetical relevance of polymeric IgA derived from Rifai's mouse model of IgAGN (27). Renal IgA deposits could be produced by injecting mouse with polymeric IgA obtained from murine myeloma MOP 305 complexed with BSA-conjugated DNCB. Of interest, only injection with IC containing polymeric IgA results in glomerular deposition. Monomeric IgA, even if complexed with DNCP does not. More elements have been provided by Emacipator's model (28), that we will discuss later.

Other studies focused on the removal of IgA containing CIC in humans. Roccatello et al, from our group, assessed the clearance of IgG-sensitized erytrocytes in IgAGN patients. A defective IgG Fc-receptor function was found (29) [T1/2 values: 57.3 (22-180) min, vs 32.9 (27-46) min in controls, $p<0.005$] .The extent of the immune clearance defect can change over the time. It is generally greater in the patients with major urinary abnormalities and high levels of IgACIC. These results were confirmed by other Authors (30).

A small sample of volunteers affected by IgAGN was subsequently examined in our laboratories to study the hepatic clearance of human aggregated IgA (HAIgA). Also HAIgA removal from the circulation was found to be delayed in IgAGN patients compared to normals (31). This suggests a generalized defect of the mechanisms of clearance of immune material. Hence one can suppose that the delayed removal of circulating IC, by favouring their persistence in the blood stream, leads to an increased mesangial deposition. This hypothesis was demonstrated in experimental models, including IgAGN (32).

In the recent years the association of alcoholic cirrhosis with IgA GN stimulated the studies on nephritis occurring in experimentally-induced chronic liver disease. These models could be obtained in rats by chronic administration of CCl4 or by biliary duct-ligation (33).

It is currently accepted that in rat a transhepatocitic transport system of polymeric IgA via secretory tract receptors provides the uptake of polymeric IgA and IgA transport from sinusoidal circulation to bile (34). In humans (like mouse) these mechanisms are probably less important than in rats. It is likely that in humans Kuppfer cell system represents the most involved component of immune clearance. Sclerotic changes in alcoholic cyrrhosis could impair also Kuppfer cell function.

In other reports on liver alcoholic cirrhosis, a blockade of the monocyte-macrophage system was found (29). This blockade was supposed to be consonant with a saturation by circulating IC, formed in excess as a consequence of an increased gut permeability to alimentary antigens. These observations make even more complicated the interpretation of the immunological events leading to a glomerular deposition of IgA in alcoholic cyrrhosis.

Finally a defective complement-mediated IC solubilization activity was reported in patients with IgA GN (35).

A still open question regards the fact if IgAGN patients must be thought as "high responders" to whatever stimulation able to induce an IgA response or wether one or several antigens may trigger out, maintain or amplify the immunoregulatory disorder.

Of interest, injection of mouse with dextrans causes mesangial deposition of IgA, suggesting the possible involvement of bacterial or viral carbohidrates in the development of IgAGN (36). Based on these experimental data, Clarkson and coworkers assessed the reactivity of serum IgA from patients with IgAGN and detected high levels of IgA directed to capsular antigens of pneumococci (17).

Chronic viral infections, like lymphocytic corionmeningitis or aleutian mink disease, are associated to IgAGN in experimental animals (33).

The possible role of viral antigens in humans was further stated by Tomino et al, which demonstrated that eluats from renal tissue obtained from IgAGN patients bind the nuclear region of cultured cells infected with tonsillar extracts from the same patients (37).

On the other hand, Emancipator and coworkers were able to produce experimentally a deposition of IgA by administering in mouse bovine gammaglobulins, ovalbumin or horse splenic ferritin (28). This model stressed the possible role of alimentary antigens.

Based on this study our group extended the analysis to another well known alimentary antigen, gluten, and its antigenic potential. In a pilot clinical investigation (38) in a sample of 6 IgAGN patients with persistently high levels of IgACIC, major urinary abnormalities and jejunal biopsy excluding a subclinic coeliac disease, a remarkable decrease in IgACIC levels was observed after gluten-free diet. With short term dietetic regimens, the IgACIC levels were found to decrease only after gluten-free diet [from 1.10 (0.52-1.60) OD to 0.48 (0.30-0.95) OD, $p<0.02$] and not after egg-free or meat-free diet. The reintroduction of gluten in diet was associated after one month to a new increase in IgACIC [from 0.48 (0.25-0.80) OD to 0.71 (0.52-1.10) OD, $p<0.04$].

The relevance of these data is now under further investigation.

The effects of a gluten-free diet were up to now evaluated in 27 IgAGN patients (39). Five patients followed a gluten-free diet for 3 years, 7 for 1 year and 15 for 6 months. In unrestricted diet, the mean levels of IgACIC in these patients were higher than normal controls [0.64 (0.10-2.45) OD, $p<0.01$] with positive data (>0.50 OD) in 17 out of 27 cases. A significant decrease in mean levels of IgACIC was already observed after 6 months of gluten-free diet. In 64 per cent of patients with high basal values, IgAIC levels were normalized.

The patients with high basal values of IgACIC presented with elevated levels of IgA directed to alimentary antigens: bovine serum albumin, ovalbumin and various gluten antigens including bicarbonate-soluble gliadin, ethanol-soluble gliadin and the lectin fraction called glyc-gli.

After 1 year-diet a decrease in level of IgA anti-ethanol-soluble gliadin and glyc-gli has been observed as well as anti-ovalbumin.

Also in Shoenlein-Henoch patients significantly high levels of IgA anti-alimentary antigens were detected. They included carbonate buffer-soluble gliadin [1.11 (0.65-1.74) OD vs 0.35 (0.15-0.80) OD in controls, $p<0.00003$) and glyc-gli fraction [1.12 (0.75-1.63) OD vs 0.58 (0.25-1.14) OD, $p< 0.0001$].

Moreover, high levels of IgA directed to bovine albumin [0.57 (O.36-0.91) OD, vs 0.43 (0.18-1.11) OD, $p<0.004$], ovalbumin [0.50 (0.22-0.84) OD, vs 0.37 (0.11-0.64) OD, $p<0.005$] and glyc-gli fraction [0.69 (0.35-0.80), vs 0.58 (0.25-1.14) OD, $p<0.01$] were found in patients with alcoholic cirrhosis.

Experimentally, we could confirm in mice a relationship between gluten administration and development of IgA deposit in mesangium by following Emancipator's experimental design with other alimentary antigens (40).

Clinical and experimental data are therefore consistent with the possible role of gluten in the pathogenesis of IgAGN.

Other genetic informations are provided by the study of IgA GN associated to other diseases. In IgAGN associated with gluten enteropathy (i.e. coeliac disease and dermatitis herpetiformis) the main pathogenical mechanism probably consist in an abnormal permeability of gut mucosa. This may be due to an exaggerated response to the binding of gliadin to mannosyl-glycoprotidic radicals on the surface of intestinal epithelial cells in genetically predisposed individuals (41). This might trigger out cytotoxic reactions resulting both in epithelial damage with villous atrophy and an immune response with production of antigliadin IgA and CIC formation. The possible detection of numberless antibodies to other alimentary antigens could indicate an increased intestinal permeability (42).

Analogous mechanism might occur also in IgAGN: gluten, particulary gliadin, might increase intestinal permeability. This might also favour the absorbtion of other alimentary antigens and lead to an exaggerated production of polymeric IgA. Finally, these phenomena might trigger out, maintain or amplify the immunological events resulting in glomerular lesions.

Alcohol or even other alimentary substances might act on gastrointestinal tract with similar mechanism.

Finally, chronic infections of respiratory tract, by producing a tissue damage, could result in an increased permeability to macromolecules related or unrelated to the infectant microorganism (43). Again, this may be followed by the immunological events resulting in glomerular lesions.

These data, however, do not explain some differences among the various glomerulonephritis of the group, particularly they cannot explain the leucocytoclastic vasculitis characterizing Shoenlein-Henoch syndrome and absent in the histologically and immunologically related idiopathic form of IgAGN.

Recently Rifai indicated the antigen itself as a possible cause of the vascular damage (44). Conversely, renal tissue lesions would require antigen binding with IgA.

As regard to the less frequent IgAGN associated to non-renal disorders, some pathogenetic mechanisms, supposed to play a role in idiopathic disease, are probably involved in different ways.

In IgAGN associated to hepato-biliary disfunctions, it is likely that the most important pathogenetical mechanism is the reduction of IgA clearance combined with an increase intestinal permeability. In IgAGN occuring along the course of Ankylosing Spondylitis the high incidence of intestinal infections could result in persistently high IgA response (45).

On the other hand, the unfrequent association between monoclonal IgA dysgammaglobulinaemia and IgAGN agrees with Rifai's experimental data which demonstrate that monomeric IgA are relatively non-nephrotoxic as compared to polymeric IgA, particularly when complexed with antigen (27).

In Cyclic Neutropenia polymorphonuclear leukocytes were found to be defective as regard to their IgA clearance capacity (45).

In Mycosis Fungoides a remarkable increase in T helper and B cell activity, favouring an exaggerated IgA response, was demonstrated (45).

In IgAGN associated to Pulmunary Hemosiderosis, as well as those occuring during Primary Fibrosis or Obstructive Bronchiolitis, the involved mechanism seems to be related to IgA of respiratory secretions (43). It was postulated an activation of alveolar macrophages by IgAIC with subsequent production of toxic radicals of molecular oxigen. These oxidizing species could increase the permeability of respiratory mucosa.

In conclusion, these data, considered together, could delineate a pathogenetical hypothesis, common to different IgA nephropathies (45, 38, 29).

An exaggerated IgA response, prevalently of mucosal origin and of polymeric type, leads to the formation of high amounts of IC. IgACIC clearance is impaired mainly by a chronic overload of removal systems. Because of this chronic saturation new antigenic stimulations result in sudden increase in CIC levels leading to clinical relapse.

This increased IgA response in IgAGN, compared to healthy people, might be inherited or acquired. Substances able to increase the mucosal permeability -including gluten, at least in some patients- may trigger out, maintain or amplify this process. Except for some particular diseases, like coeliac and alcoholic enteropathies, the pathogenetical sequence resulting in glomerular damage is not so clear to lead a rational therapy.

Maybe this perspective is not far, but it remains a hope for the future.

BIBLIOGRAFIA

1. Berger, J., 1969, IgA glomerular deposits in renal disease. Transplant Proc 1: 939.
2. Emancipator, S.N., Gallo, G.R., Lamm, M.E., 1985, IgA nephropathy: perspectives on pathogenesis and classification. Clin Nephrol 24: 161.
3. Coppo, R., Basolo, B., Martina, G., Rollino, C., De Marchi, M., Giacchino, F., Mazzucco, G., Messina, M., Piccoli, G., 1982, Circulating immune complexes containing IgA, IgG and IgM in patients with primary IgA nephropathy

and with Henoch-Schoenlein nephritis: Correlation with clinic and histologic signs of activity. Clin Nephrol 18: 230.

4. Lesavre, P., Digeon, M., Bach, J.F., 1982, Analysis of circulating IgA and detection of immune complexes in primary IgA nephropathy. Clin Exp Immunol 48: 61.
5. Valentijn, R.M., Kauffmann, R.H., Brutel de la Riviere, G., Daha, M.R., Van Es, L.A., 1983, Presence of circulating macromolecular IgA in patients with hematuria due to primary IgA nephropathy. Am J Med 74: 375.
6. Hall, R.P., Stachura, I., Cason, J., Whiteside, T.L., Lawley, T.L., 1983, IgA-containing circulating immune complexes in patients with IgA nephropathy. Am J Med 74: 56.
7. Egido, J., Sancho, J., Rivera, F., Hernando, L., 1984, The role of IgA and IgG immune complexes in IgA nephropathy. Nephron 36: 52.
8. Coppo, R., Basolo, B., Roccatello, D., Piccoli, G., 1985, Circulating immune complexes in immunologically mediated glomerular diseases. Contr Nephrol 48: 137.
9. Coppo, R., Basolo, B., Piccoli, G., Mazzucco, G., Bulzomi, M.R., Roccatello, D., De Marchi, M., Carbonara, A.O., Barbiano di Belgioioso, G., 1984, IgA1 and IgA2 immune complexes in primary IgA nephropathy and Henoch-Schoenlein nephritis. Clin Exp Immunol 57: 583.
10. Coppo, R., Aricò, S., Piccoli, G., Basolo, B., Roccatello, D., Amore, A., Tabone, M., De La Pierre, M., Sessa, A., Delacroix, D., L., Verman, J.P., 1985, Presence and origin of IgA1- and IgA2-containing circulating immune complexes in chronic alcoholic liver diseases with and without glomerulonephritis. Clin Immunol Immunopathol 35: 1.
11. Breda Vriesman, P., Tiebosch, T., 1987, Idiopathic IgA nephropathy: a local immune complex disease? (Abs) XXIVth Congress of EDTA-European Renal Association, p 89.
12. Feehally, J., Beattie, T.J., Brenchley, P.E.C., Coupes, B.M., Mallick, N.P., Postlethwaite, R.J., 1986, Sequential study of the IgA system in relapsing IgA nephropathy. Kidney Int 30, 924.
13. Egido, J., Blasco, R., Sancho, J., Lozano, T., 1983, T cell dysfunctions in IgA nephropathy: specific abnormalities in the regulation of IgA synthesis. Clin Immunol Immunopathol 26: 201.
14. Lopez-Trascasa, M., Egido, J., Sancho, J., Hernando, L., 1980, IgA glomerulonephritis (Berger's disease): evidence of high serum levels of polymeric IgA. Clin Exp Immunol 42: 247.

15. Danielsen, H., Eriksen, E.F., Johansen, A., Solling, J., 1984, Serum immunoglobulin sedimentation patterns and circulating immune complexes in IgA nephropathy and Schoenlein-Henoch nephritis. Acta Med Scand 215: 435 .

16. Nomoto, Y., Sakai, H., Arimori, S., 1979, Increase of IgA bearing lymphocytes in peripheral blood from patients with IgA nephropathy. Am J Clin Path 71: 158 .

17. Drew, P.A., Nieuwhof, N., Clarkson, A.R., Woodroffe, A.J., 1987, Increased concentration of serum IgA antibody to Pneumococcal polisaccarides in patients with IgA nephropathy. Clin Exp Immunol 67: 124.

18. Nagy, J., Vj, M., Szucs, G., Trinn, C., 1984, Herper virus antigens and antibodies in kidney biopsies and sera of IgA glomerulonephritic patients. Clin Nephrol 21: 259.

19. Woodroffe, A.J., Gormly, A.A., McKenzie, P.E., Clarkson, A.R., 1980, Immunologic studies in IgA nephropathy. Kidney Int 18: 342.

20. Hale, G.M., McIntosh, S.L., Hiki, Y., Clarkson, A.R., Woodroffe, A.J., 1986, Evidence for IgA-specific B cell hyperreactivity in patients with IgA nephropathy. Kidney Int 29: 718.

21. Nagy, J., Scott, H., Brandtzaeg, P., 1987, Food antigens in the pathogenesis of IgA nephropathy. (Abs) XXIVth Congress of EDTA-European Renal Association, p 39.

22. Endoh, A., Suga, T., Miura, M., 1983, In vivo altaration of antibody production in patients with IgA nephropathy. Clin Exp Immunol 57: 564.

23. Nomoto, Y., Sakai, H., 1979, Cold reacting antinuclear factor in sera from patients with IgA nephropathy. J Lab Clin Med 94: 76.

24. Jackson, S., Montgomery, R.I., Julian, B.A., Galla, J.H., Czerninsky, C., 1987, Aberrant synthesis of antibodies directed at the Fab fragment of IgA in patients with IgA nephropathies. Clin Immunol Immunopathol 45: 208.

25. Valentijn, R.M., Radl, J., Haaijnon, J.J., 1984, Circulating and mesangial secretory component-binding IgA_1, in primary IgA nephropathy. Kidney Int 26: 760.

26. Komatsu, N., Nagura, H., Watanabe, K., Nomoto, Y., Kobayashi, K., 1983, Mesangial deposition of J chain-linked polymeric IgA in IgA nephropathy. Nephron 33: 61.

27. Rifai, A., Millard, K., 1985, Glomerular deposition of immune complexes

prepared with monomeric or polymeric IgA. Clin Exp Immunol 60: 363.

28. Emancipator, S.N., Gallo, G.R., Lamm, M.E., Experimental nephropathy induced by oral immunization. J Exp Med 157: 572.

29. Roccatello, D., Coppo, R., Piccoli, G., Cordonnier, D., Martina, G., Picciotto, G., Sena, L.M., Amoroso, A., 1985, Circulating Fc-receptor blocking factors in IgA nephropathies. Clin Nephrol 23: 159.

30. Nicholls, K., Kincaid-Smith, P., 1984, Defective in vivo Fc and C3b receptor function in IgA nephropathy. Am J Kidney Dis 4: 128.

31. Roccatello, D., Picciotto, G., Coppo, R., Piccoli, G., Molino, A., Cacace, G., Amore, A., Sena, L.M., 1987, Delayed clearance of IgA immune complexes-like material in IgA nephropathy patients. (Abs) XXIVth Congress of EDTA-European Renal Association, p 86.

32. Sato, M., Idema, T., Koshikawa, S., 1986, Experimental IgA nephropathy in mice. Lab Invest 54: 377.

33. Rifai, A., 1987, Experimental models for IgA-associated nephritis. Kidney Int 31: 1.

34. Orlans, E., Peppard, J., Fry, J.F., Hinton, R.H., Mullock , B.M., 1979, Secretory component as the receptor for polymeric IgA on rat hepatocytes. J Exp Med 150: 1577.

35. Schena, F.P., Pastore, A., Sinico, R.A., Ladisa, N., Montinaro, V., Fornasieri, A., 1987, Studies on the mechanisms producing solubilization of immune precipitates in serum of patients with primary IgA nephropathy. Sem Neprol 7: 336.

36. Isaacs, K.L., Miller, F., 1982, Role of antigen size and charge in immune complex glomerulonephritis. I. Active induction of disease with dextran and its derivatives. Lab Invest 47: 198.

37. Tomino, Y., Sakai, H., Endoh, M., Cross reactivity of IgA antibodies between renal mesangial areas and nuclei of tonsillar cells in patients with IgA nephropathy. Clin Exp Immunol 51: 605.

38. Coppo, R., Basolo, B., Rollino, C., Roccatello, D., Martina, G., Amore, A., Bongiorno, G., Piccoli, G., 1986, Mediterranean diet and primary IgA nephropathy. Clin Nephrol 26: 72.

39. Coppo, R., Roccatello, D., Amore, A., Quattrocchio, G., Molino, A., Maffei, S., Amoroso, A., Bajardi, P., Piccoli, G., Effects of gluten-free diet in primary IgA nephropathy (submitted for pubblication).

40. Coppo, R., Mazzucco, G., Martina, G., Sena, L.M., Roccatello, D., Amore, A., Novara,

R., Bargoni, A., Ragni, R., Piccoli, G., 1987, Experimental IgA nephropathy induced by gluten-rich diet. (Abs.) Xth International Congress of Nephrology, London p. 320.

41. Kottigen, E., Volk, B., Kluga, F., Gerok, W., 1982, Gluten, a lectin with oligomannosyl specificity and the causative agent of gluten-sensitive enteropathy. Biochem Biophys Res Commun 109: 168.

42. Scott, H., Fauza, O., EK, J., Brandtzaeg, P., 1984, Immune response patters in coeliac disease. Serum antibodies to dietary antigens measured by an enzyme-linked immunosorbent assay (ELISA). Clin Exp Immunol 57: 25.

43. Endo, Y., Hara, M., 1986, Glomerular IgA deposition in pulmonary diseases. Kidney Int 29: 557.

44. Rifai, A., Chen, A., Imai, H., 1987, Complement activation in expeerimental nephropathy: an antigen-mediated process. Kidney Int 32: 838.

45. Clarkson, A.R., Woodroffe, A.J., Aarons, I., Hiki, Y., Hale, G., 1987, IgA nephropathy. Am Rev Med 38: 157.

DIABETIC NEPHROPATHY: NEW PATHOGENETIC ASPECTS

August Heidland, Markus Teschner, and Roland Schaefer

Division of Nephrology, Department of Internal Medicine, University of Würzburg, Josef-Schneider-Str. 2, 8700 Würzburg, FRG

200 years ago the well-known italian physician Domenico Cotugno was the first to describe the appearance of protein in the urine of diabetics. He noted that urine of many diabetics coagulates when exposed to heat (1,2). In the past several years a better understanding of the mechanisms and consequences of proteinuria has been developed.

Stages And Course Of Diabetic Nephropathy

Nowadays 5 stages of diabetic nephropathy (DN) have been established.

Table 1

STAGES IN DIABETIC NEPHROPATHY

	Stage	Chronology	Characteristic Symptoms
I	Hyperfunction / Hypertrophy	Diagnosis of Diabetes	UAE (↑), GFR ↑↑, > Kidneys in Sonography
II	Histological kidney alterations clinically silent	2 – 5 years	UAE N, GFR ↑, > Kidneys, > BM, > Mesangium
III	Incipient Nephropathy	5–10 years	Microalbuminuria, GFR ↑, BP ↑, Retinopathy ↑
IV	Ouvert Nephropathy	10–25 years	Proteinuria (> 0.5 g/d), GFR → ↓, BP ↑ 60–70 %, > Retinopathy ↑ ↑
V	Renal Insufficiency	15–30 years	Proteinuria, GFR ↓ ↓, BP ↑ 90 %, Retinopathy ↑ ↑ ↑

In particular we differentiate between clinical silent and apparent forms. At the time of diagnosis of diabetes the first hint of renal involvement is an increased glomerular filtration rate (GFR) in the presence of enlarged kidneys (stage I). Occasionally, microalbuminuria can be detected, if the carbohydrate metabolism is badly controlled. 2 to 5 years after onset of diabetes histological alterations in form of thickening of basement membrane and expansion of the mesangium can be seen (stage II). Incipient nephropathy (stage III) is characterized by microalbuminuria, while GFR in these patients is still increased. 10 to 20 years after onset of diabetes (stage IV) the patients suffer from ouvert nephropathy as indicated by clinical proteinuria and a progressive decline of GFR. Within a few years these patients develop endstage renal failure (stage V).

As soon as clinical nephropathy develops proteinuria shows an exponential rise, while GFR decreases dramatically, averaging 13 ml/min/year. The individual variation, however, is great.

The incidence of DN in patients with type I diabetes mellitus averages about 40-50 % and 15 to 20 % in type II diabetes mellitus (4, 5).

Risk Factors of Diabetic Nephropathy

The question arises which diabetics are prone for nephropathy. Important risk factors are poor control of diabetes (6), hypertension (7-10), high initial GFR (11), early manifestation and long duration of the disease (11, 12), and heavy smoking (13, 14). Recently, it was shown that genetic disposition of hypertension is of tremendous importance. Having a parent with hypertension tripled the risk of nephropathy (15).

Microalbuminuria: Definition And Clinical Consequences

In the individual case we can detect those diabetics with the risk for developing nephropathy by demonstrating microalbuminuria (16, 17). As shown by Mogensen et al. (18) within 10 years 80 % of diabetics with microalbuminuria show clinical proteinuria with consecutive renal failure. On the other hand, patients without microalbuminuria remain stable over the whole decade concerning their renal function.

According to the Consensus Conference (19) microalbuminuria is defined as an increase of albumin excretion from 30 mg to 300 mg/24 hours. It must be found in 2 of 3 urine samples within half a year.

However, we must consider that a lot of non-diabetic factors, such as exercise, fever, urinary tract infection, essential hypertension and congestive heart failure also may induce proteinuria. Furthermore, non-diabetic renal diseases, such as membranous and membrano-proliferative glomerulonephritis as well as rapid progressive glomerulonephritis are frequently observed in diabetics (20-22). In particular in the presence of infectious problems, for instance osteomyelitis, immune complex nephritis may develop.

Microalbuminuria is not only indicative for the development of ouvert nephropathy. It also is associated with various other disturbances such as enhanced transcapillary leakage of albumin (23, 24), a mild rise of arterial blood pressure, proliferative retinopathy and neuropathy. In addition cardiovascular morbidity and mortality is enhanced (25, 26). All these disturbances indicate the prevalence of general vascular disease in patients with microalbuminuria.

Pathogenetic Mechanisms Of Diabetic Nephropathy

The pathogenesis of diabetic nephropathy is a synergistical effect of glomerular capillary hypertension and biochemical changes of glomerular components, induced by nonenzymatic glycation and enhanced polyol pathway. It is demonstrated that the synthesis of glomerular basement membrane collagen is increased (27-30), whereas its turnover is reduced (31-33). Furthermore, the decrement of proteoglycans, such as heparan sulfate (34) induce marked changes of anionic sites and charge selectivity, thereby promoting albuminuria (35).

Hemodynamic Factors

Early stages of diabetes mellitus are characterized by renal hyperperfusion and glomerular hyperfiltration in humans and animals (36-40). As shown in the pioneering experiments of Hostetter, Rennke and Brenner (1982) in diabetic rats, single nephron hyperfiltration results from elevations of the glomerular capillary plasma flow rate and hydraulic pressure, which are in turn associated with progressive morphologic injury.

Meanwhile lots of mechanims have been incriminated in the pathogenesis of hyperfiltration: First of all hyperglycemia results in a rise of GFR (41, 42), probably caused by an altered tubulo-glomerular feedback (43). Recently elevated levels of atrial natriuretic peptide concentration depending on the quality of blood glucose control have been demonstrated in man and rats (44-46). With the aid of specific antibodies of ANP glomerular hyperfiltration could be normalized in the diabetic rat (47). Underlying mechanism for increased ANP level is the well-known renal sodium retention with expansion of extracellular fluid volume in diabetes. In addition enhanced levels of sorbitol (48) and ketone bodies (49) induce a rise in GFR.

At the glomerular level prostaglandines seem to play a central role in mediating the hyperfiltration (50). However, short-term inhibition of prostaglandin synthesis had no effect on the elevated GFR levels of early insulin-dependent diabetics (51). Contrary results were shown by others (52). Glomerular hyperfiltration is not associated with elevated plasma levels of glucagon and growth hormone (53).

The altered glomerular hemodynamics are not only of functional importance, but also induce various structural lesions.

Increased capillary hydraulic pressure may induce disruption of endo- and epithelial surfaces, enhanced mesangial matrix production, thickening of basement membrane (due to stretch and tension) and deposition of macromolecules. However, recently the central role of increased glomerular pressure initiating diabetic nephropathy has been questioned (54).

Role Of Non-Enzymatic Glycosylation

The quality of diabetic control is related to non-enzymatic glycosylation of proteins which is a condension reaction between carbohydrate and the free amino groups at the NH_2 terminus or E-amino groups of lysine residues of proteins. The extent of glycosylation in vivo depends on the degree and duration of hyperglycemia, half life of the protein in the circulation or the tissue, permeability of tissue to free glucose, number of free amino groups, accessibility and pK of the amino groups within the structure of the proteins (Cohen, 1986). It is now clear, that practically all proteins may be involved. Consequently a multitude of functional changes may arise from non-enzymatic glycosylation such as enhanced oxygen affinity of hemoglobin (56), altered transendothelial albumin transport (57), impaired function of immunoglobulins (58), decreased uptake and degradation of low density lipoproteins (59, 60), decreased fibrinolysis (61) and reduced activity of antithrombin III (62).

Not only plasma but also structural proteins, particular those with long half-lifes are involved in the process of glycosylation. As a consequence of glycation of glomerular basement membrane collagen abnormal cross-links and enhanced trapping of proteins such as albumin, IgG and LDL may occur (63, 64).

Enhanced Polyol Pathway

Besides glycation of proteins elevated blood glucose levels lead to the formation of intracellular sorbitol due to stimulation of the aldose reductase reaction.

In epithelial cells of glomeruli of streptozotocin diabetic rats an enhanced polyol pathway is found, which results in increased sorbitol levels and a depletion of myoinositol, whereas sodium/potassium ATPase activity is reduced (65, 66). All these changes are prevented by the administration of the aldose reductase inhibitor sorbinil (67, 68).

Altered Proteinase Activity In Diabetic Glomeruli

Since in the initiating process of diabetic nephropathy the decreased degradation of glomerular basement proteins and an accumulation of macromolecules within the mesangium plays a central role (69, 70) we investigated the degradative capacity of proteins, that means the protease activity in isolated glomeruli of diabetic rats (Teschner et al., 71).

3 weeks after induction of diabetic nephropathy in rats by streptozotocin (STZ)-application the proteolytic activity in isolated glomeruli was assayed using azocasein as a substrate. The results showed a significant reduction of the proteolytic activity in the diabetic rats in comparison with normal controls. Insulin treatment, however, ameliorated the impaired proteolytic activity (Fig. 1).

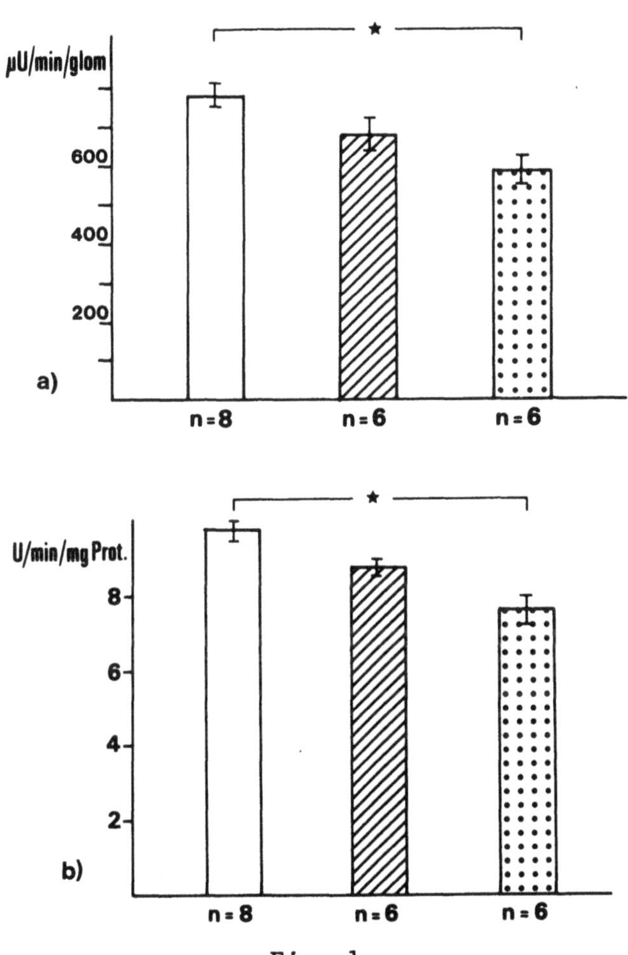

Fig. 1

Glomerular proteinase activity in diabetic rats, either well (hatched column) or poorly (dotted column) controlled and non-diabetic animals (white column), when enzyme activity is expressed as U/min/mg protein (Fig. 1 a) or µU/min/glomerulus (Fig. 1 b), respectively. The values are given as means $\pm$ SEM, * $p < 0.01$ for poorly controlled diabetic animals versus non diabetic controls.

We assume that the decreased activity of proteases is involved in the accumulation of proteins in the glomeruli representing an important pathogenetic factor in the development of intercapillary glomerulosclerosis.

Our results of an altered protease activity in glomeruli fits well with the findings of lowered activities of cathepsin D, cathepsin B and L in the tubules of rats with experimental diabetes (71, 72).

A hint that this might be true also for diabetic patients is the finding of an enhanced concentration of inactive plasma renin due to decreased conversion of active renin by cathepsin B and G (73).

At the present time we cannot decide whether decreased protease activity in the glomeruli is the consequence of glycosylation of the enzymes or of a functional lesion.

Protease Activity of Polymorphonuclear Leukocytes

Surprisingly, protease activity in the phagocytes show in the opposite direction. An increased content of elastase was observed in isolated polymorphonuclear leukocytes (74). Furthermore, the plasma concentration of granulocyte elastase is significantly increased in diabetics, particularly in patients with microangiopathy (75). Teschner et al. could show that stimulation of PMN leukocytes of diabetic patients by the calcium ionophore A 23187 resulted in an exaggerated response as compared to controls (unpublished). Investigations of Hörl and Heidland (76) proved that the hemodialysis induced rise of elastase alpha$_1$-proteinase inhibitor complex is markedly increased in diabetic patients as compared to non-diabtic uremic patients. Therefore, it has to be questioned, whether the increased release of granulocyte proteases due to various stimuli may contribute to endothelial damage of the vascular system in diabetes.

Conclusion

When summarizing the different mechanisms of diabetic nephropathy it seems to be that the diabetic milieu induces 3 fundamental alterations as there are renal hyperperfusion and glomerular hypertension, an altered chemical composition of glomerular components and furterhmore a decrease of glomerular protease activity. The central result of all these processes is the accumulation of glomerular and circulating proteins within the mesangium and glomerular basement membrane with consequent progressive glomerulosclerosis.

Literature

1. D. Contunnii, "De ischiade nervosa commentarius", Napoli (1764)
2. C. Haslacher and E. Ritz, Effect of control of diabetes mellitus on progression of renal failure, Kidney Int., 22: 853 (1987)
3. C.E. Mogensen, C.K. Christensen and E. Vittinghas, The stages in diabetic renal disease with emphasis on the stage of incipient nephropathy, Diabetologia 32: 64 (1983)
4. T. Deckert, J.E. Poulsen and M. Larsen, Prognosis of diabetes with diabetes onset before the age of thirty-one. I. Survival, causes of death, and complications. Diabetologia 14: 363 (1978)
5. T. Deckert, J.E. Poulsen and M. Larsen, Prognosis of diabetes with diabetes onset before the age of thirty-one. II. Factors influencing the prognosis, Diabetologia 14: 371 (1978)
6. A.S. Krolewski, J.H. Warram, A.R. Christlieb, E.J. Busieck and C.R. Kahn, The changing natural history of nephropathy in type I diabetes. Am. J. Med. 78 (S): 785 (1985)
7. C.E. Mogensen, High blood pressure as a factor in the progression of diabetic nephropathy. Acta Med. Scand. (Suppl.), 602: 29 (1976)
8. S.M. Mauer, W.M. Steffes, S. Azar, S.K. Sandberg and D.M. Brown, The effects of Goldblatt hypertension on development of the glomerular lesions of diabetes mellitus in the rat, Diabetes 27: 738 (1978)
9. A.M. Cohen and E. Rosenmann, Role of genetics, hypertension (Goldblatt Kidney) and carbohydrate metabolism disturbance on the development of diabetic nephropathy, Diab. Nephr., 4: 66 (1985)
10. C.H. Haslacher, W. Stech, P. Wahl and E. Ritz, Blood pressure and metabolic control as risk factors for nephropathy in type 1 diabetes, Diabetologia, 28: 6 (1985)
11. C.E. Mogensen, Early glomerular hyperfiltration in insulin-dependent diabetics and late nephropathy. Scand. J. Clin. Lab. Invest, 46: 201 (1986)
12. A. Kofoed-Enevoldsen, K. Borch-Johnsen, S. Kreiner, J. Nerup and T. Deckert, Declining incidence of persistent proteinuria in type I (insulin-dependent) diabetes, Diabetes, 36 (2): 205 (1987)
13. J.S. Christiansen, Cigarette smoking and prevalence of microangiopathy in juvenile onset insulin-dependent diabetes mellitus, Diabetes Care 1: 146 (1978)
14. I. Mühlhauser, P. Sawicki and M. Berger, Cigarette smoking as a risk factor for macroproteinuria and proliferative retinopathy in type 1 (insulin-dependent) diabetes. Diabetologia, 29: 500 (1986)
15. A.S.D. Krolewski, M.D. Canessa, J.H. Warram, L.M.B. Laffel, R.A. Christlieb, W. Knowler, L. Rand, Predisposition to hypertension and susceptibility to renal disease in insulin-dependent diabetes mellitus, N. Engl. J. Med., 318: 140 (1988)
16. H.H. Parving, B. Oxenboll, P.A. Svendsen and A.R. Andersen, Early detection of patients at risk developing diabetic nephropathy, Acta Endocr., 100: 500 (1982)

17. G.C. Viberti, R.D. Hill, R.J. Jarrett, A. Argyropoulos, U. Mahmud and H. Keen, Microalbuminuria as a predictor of clinical nephropathy in insulin-dependent diabetes mellitus. Lancet, 1: 1430 (1982)
18. C.E. Mogensen and C.K. Christensen, Predicting diabetic nephropathy in insulin-dependent patients, N. Engl. J. Med., 311: 89 (1984)
19. C.E. Mogensen, A. Chachati, C.K. Christensen, C.F. Close, T. Deckert, E. Hommel, J. Kastrup, P. Lefebvre, E.R. Mathiesen, B. Feldt-Rasmussen, A. Schmitz and G.C. Viberti, Microalbuminuria. An early marker of renal involvement in diabetes, Uremia Investigation, 9: 85 (1985)
20. S. Aziz, A.H. Cohen, R.L. Winer, F. Llach and S.G. Massry, Diabetes mellitus with immune complex glomerulonephritis, Nephron, 23: 32 (1979)
21. J. Olivero and W.N. Suki, Acute glomerulonephritis complicating diabetic nephropathy. Archs. Intern. Med., 137: 732 (1977)
22. T. Cavallo, J. Pinto and S. Rajaramon, Immune complex disease complicating diabetic glomerulosclerosis, Am. J. Nephrol., 4: 347 (1984)
23. B. Feldt-Rasmussen, Increased transcapillary escape rate of albumin in insulin-dependent diabetic patients with microalbuminuria, Diabetologia, 29: 282 (1986)
24. L. Bent-Hansen, B. Feldt-Rasmussen, A. Kverneland and T. Deckert, Transcapillary escape rate and relative metabolic clearance of glycated and non-glycated albumin in type 1 (insulin-dependent) diabetes mellitus, Diabetologia, 30: 2 (1987)
25. M. Wiseman, G. Viberti, D. Mackintosh, R.J. Jarrett and H. Keen, Glycemia, arterial pressure and microalbuminuria in type 1 (insulin-dependent) diabetes mellitus, Diabetologia, 26: 401 (1984)
26. H.H. Parving, E. Hommel, E. Mathiesen, P. Skott, B. Edsberg, M. Bahnsen, M. Lauritzen and P. Hougaard, Prevalence of microalbuminuria, arterial hypertension, retinopathy and neuropathy in patients with insulin-dependent diabetes, Br. Med. J., 296: 156 (1988)
27. M.P. Cohen and C. Vogt, Evidence for enhanced basement membrane synthesis and lysine hydroxylation in renal glomerulus in experimental diabetes, Biochem. Biophys. Res. Commun., 49: 1542 (1972)
28. M.E. Grant, R. Harwood and I.F. Williams, Increased synthesis of glomerular basement membrane collagen in streptozotocin diabetes, J. Physiol. (London), 257: 56P (1976)
29. M.P. Cohen and A. Khalifa, Effect of diabetes and insulin on rat glomerular protocollagen hydroxylase activities, Biochem. Biophys. Acta, 496: 88 (1977)
30. M.P. Cohen, Glomerular basement membrane synthesis in diabetes. In: Kefalides, N.A. (ed.) Biology and Chemistry of Basement Membranes. Academic Press, New York, San Francisco, London, 523 (1978)
31. W. Romen and R. Morath, Diffuse glomerulosclerosis - a dysfunction of the mesangium? Virchows Arch. (Cell Pathol.), 31: 205 (1979)

32. W. Romen, Zur Morphologie und Pathogenese der diabetischen Glomerulosklerose. Klin. Wochenschr., 58: 1013 (1980)
33. W. Romen and A. Takahashi, Autoradiographic studies of the proliferation of glomerular and tubular cells of the rat kidney in early diabetes, Virchows. Arch. (Cell Pathol.), 40: 339 (1982)
34. D.H. Rohrbach, C.W. Wagner, V.L. Star, G.R. Martin, K.S. Brown and I.W. Yoon, Reduced synthesis of basement membrane heparan sulfate proteoglycan in streptozotocin-induced diabetic mice, J. Biolog. Chem., 258: 11672 (1983)
35. T. Deckert, B. Feldt-Rasmussen, R. Djurup and M. Deckert, Glomerular size and charge selectivity in insulin-dependent diabetes mellitus, Kidney Int., 33: 100 (1988)
36. T.H. Hostetter, H.G. Rennke and B.M. Brenner, The case for intrarenal hypertension in the initiation and progression of diabetic and other glomerulopathies, Am. J. Med., 72: 375 (1982)
37. T.H. Hostetter, Diabetic nephropathy, N. Engl. J. Med., 312: 642 (1985)
38. R. Zatz, T.W. Meyer, H.G. Rennke and B.M. Brenner, Predominance of hemodynamic rather than metabolic factors in the pathogenesis of diabetic glomerulopathy, Proc. Natl. Acad. Sci., 82: 5963 (1985)
39. C.E. Mogensen, Glomerular filtration rate and renal plasma flow in short-term and long-term juvenile diabetes mellitus, Scand. J. Clin. Lab. Invest., 28: 91 (1971)
40. C.E. Mogensen and M.J.F. Andersen, Increased kidney size and glomerular filtration rate in early juvenile diabetes, Diabetes, 22: 706 (1973)
41. J.S. Christiansen, M. Frandsen and H.H. Parving, Effect of intravenous glucose infusion on renal function in normal and in insulin-dependent diabetics. Diabetologia 21: 368 (1981)
42. M.J. Wiseman, R. Mangili, M. Alberetto, H. Keen and G. Viberti, Glomerular response mechanisms to glycemic changes in insulin-dependent diabetics, Kidney Int., 31: 1012 (1987)
43. R.C. Blantz, O.W. Peterson, L. Gushwa, B.J. Tucker, Effect of modest hyperglycemia on tubuloglomerular feedback activity, Kidney Int., 22: 206 (1982)
44. C. Kinddermans, K. Laborde, B. Thiriet, L. Marchal, C. Sachs and M. Dechaux, Atrial natriuretic peptide (ANF) in type 1 diabetes: relationship with glomerular filtration rate, extracellular fluid volume and plasma renin activity, Kidney Int., 33: 270 A (1983)
45. S.L. Jones, N. Perico, A. Benigni, G. Remuzzi, G.C. Viberti, Glomerular filtration rate, extracellular fluid volume and atrial natriuretic factor in insulin dependent diabetes, Kidney Int., 33: 268 A (1988)
46. G.M. Bell, R.K. Bernstein, S.A. Atlas, G.D. James, M.S. Pecker, J.E. Sealey and J.H. Laragh, Increased plasma atrial natriuretic factor in early controlled diabetes mellitus, Kidney Int., 33: 254 A (1988)
47. F.V. Ortola, B.J. Ballermann, S. Anderson and B.M. Brenner, A role for atrial natriuretic peptide in mediating glomerular hyperfiltration in diabetic rats. 10th Int. Cong. of Nephrology, London, 205 (1987)

48. S.A. Goldfarb, D.A. Simmons, and E. Kern, Amelioration of glomerular hyperfiltration in acute experimental diabetes by dietary myo-inositol and by an aldose reductase inhibitor, Clin. Res., 34: 725 A (1986)
49. R. Trevisan, R. Nosadini, P. Fioretto, A. Avogaro, E. Duner, E. Jori, A. Valerio, A. Doria and G. Crepaldi, Ketone bodies increase glomerular filtration rate in normal man and in patients with type 1 (insulin-dependent) diabetes mellitus. Diabetologia, 30: 214 (1987)
50. M. Schambelan, S. Blake, J. Sraer, M. Bens, M.P. Nivez and F. Wahbe, Increased prostaglandin production by glomeruli isolated from rats with streptozotocin-induced diabetes mellitus, J. Clin. Invest., 75: 404 (1985)
51. J.S. Christiansen, B. Feldt-Rasmussen and H.-H. Parving, Short-term inhibition of prostaglandin synthesis has no effect on the elevated glomerular filtration rate of early insulin-dependent diabetes, Diabet. Med., 2: 17 (1985)
52. E. Hommel, E. Mathiesen, S. Arnold-Larsen, B. Edsberg, U. B. Olsen and H.-H. Parving, Effects of indomethacin on kidney function in type 1 (insulin-dependent) diabetic patients with nephropathy, Diabetologia, 30: 78 (1987)
53. M.J. Wiseman, G.C. Viberti, S. Redmond and H. Keen, The glomerular hyperfiltration of diabetes is not associated with elevated plasma levels of glucagon and growth hormone, Diabetologia, 28: 718 (1985)
54. N. Bank, R. Klose, H.S. Aynedjian, D. Nguyen and L.B. Sablay, Evidence against increased glomerular pressure indicating diabetic nephropathy, Kidney Int., 31: 898 (1987)
55. M.P. Cohen, Diabetes and Protein Glycosylation. Measurement and Biologic Relevance. Springer-Verlag, New York-Berlin-Heidelberg-Tokyo, 1 - 142 (1986)
56. J. Ditzel, Changes in red cell oxygen release capacity in diabetes mellitus, Fed. Proc., 38: 2484 (1977)
57. S.K. Williams and N.J. Solenski, Enhanced vesicular ingestion of non-enzymatically glucosylated proteins by capillary endothelium, Microvasc. Res., 28: 311 (1984)
58. M.A. Cohenford, J.C. Urbanowski, D.C. Shepard, et al., Nonenzymatic glycosylation of human IgG: In vitro preparation, Immunol. Commun., 12: 189 (1983)
59. J.L. Witztum, E.M. Mahoney, M.J. Branks, et al., Nonenzymatic glucosylation of low-density lipoproteins alters its biologic activity, Diabetes, 31: 283 (1982)
60. H.J. Kim and I.V. Kurup, Decreased catabolism of glycosylated low density lipoprotein in diabetic rats, Diabetes, 26: 218 (1984)
61. M. Brownlee, H. Vlassara and A. Cerami, Nonenzymatic glycosylation reduces the susceptibility of fibrin to degradation by plasmin, Diabetes, 32: 680 (1983)
62. R.N. Banerjee, A.L. Sahni and V. Kumar: Antithrombin 3 deficiency in maturity onset diabetes mellitus and atherosclerosis, Thromb. Diath. Haemorrh., 31: 339 (1974)
63. M.P. Cohen, E. Urdanivia, M. Surma and V.Y. Wu, Nonenzymatic glycosylation of basement membrane. In vitro studies, Diabetes, 30, 367 (1981)

64. M. Bronlee, H. Vlassara and A. Cerami, Nonenzymatic glycosylation and the pathogenesis of diabetic complications, Ann. Int. Med., 101: 527 (1984)
65. C.N. Cordes, J.M. Braughles and P.A. Culp, Quantitative histochemistry of the sorbitol pathway in glomeruli and small arteries of the human diabetic kidney, Folia Histochem. Cytochem., 17: 137 (1979)
66. M.P. Cohen, A. Sasmahapatra and E. Shapiro, Reduced glomerular sodium potassium adenosine triphosphatase activity in acute streptozotocin diabetes, Diabetes, 34: 1071 (1985)
67. A. Beyer-Mears, L. Ku. and M.P. Cohen, Glomerular polyol accumulation in diabetes and its prevention by oral sorbinil. Diabetes, 33: 604 (1984)
68. A. Beyer-Mears, E. Varagiannis and E. Cruz, Effect of sorbinil on reversal of proteinuria. Diabetes, 35 (Suppl. 1): 101A (1985)
69. E.N. Wardle, Mesangial cell dysfunction detected by accumulation of aggregated protein in rats with streptozotocin induced diabetes. Biomed., 23: 299 (1975)
70. S.M. Mauer, M.S. Steffes, M. Chern and D. Brown, Mesangial uptake and processing of macromolecules in rats with diabetes mellitus. Lab. Invest., 41: 401 (1979)
71. M. Teschner, R.M. Schaefer, U. Heidland, A. Svarnas and A. Heidland, Proteinase activity in isolated glomeruli of diabetic and non-diabetic rats. Kidn. Int., 1989, in press
72. B. Greisinger, C.J. Olbricht and K.M. Koch, Decreased activity of intralysosomal proteolytic enzymes as possibly relevant factor for tubular hypertrophy in the early diabetic kidney. Kidn. Int., 33: 376, Abstract (1988)
73. M.A. Nerurker, J.G. Satar and S.S. Katyare, Insulin dependent changes in lysosomal cathepsin D-activity in rat liver, kidney, brain and heart. Diabetologica, 31: 119 (1988)
74. J.A. Luetscher, F.B. Kraemer, D.M. Wilson, H.C. Schwartz and M.B. Bryer-Ash, Increased plasma inactive renin in diabetes mellitus. N. Engl. J. Med., 312 (1985)
75. G- Öberg, R. Hällgren, L. Moberg and P. Venge, Bacterial proteins and neutral proteases in diabetes neutrophils. Diabetologia, 29: 426 (1986)
76. A. Collier, M. Jackson, D. Bell, A.W. Patrick, D.M. Matthews, R.J. Young, B.F. Clarke and J. Dawes, Increased neutrophil elastase activity in Type 1 (insulin-dependent) diabetic patients. Diabetologia, 30: 509 (1987)
77. W.H. Hörl and A. Heidland, Evidence for the participation of granulocyte proteinases on intradialytic catabolism. Clin. Nephrol., 21: 314 (1984)

URIC ACID AND KIDNEY

Giorgio Fuiano, Stefano Federico, Giuseppe Conte, and Vittorio E. Andreucci

Department of Nephrology
Second Faculty of Medicine
University of Naples, Naples, Italy

Uric Acid Metabolism

Uric acid is the end product of purine metabolism in humans. In animals other than mammals uric acid undergoes further degradation because of the activity of enzymes such as uricase, allantoinase and allantoicase; in some species the urea that is formed is further hydrolyzed to ammonia and CO2 by the urease of intestinal bacteria (1).

Uric acid derives from endogenous purines (normally at a constant rate) and from dietary purines. Variations in uric acid production rate derives mainly from variations of dietary intake of purines (purine-rich foods include poultry, meat, liver and fish). As much as 50% of uric acid derived from dietary purines may be recovered in the urine (2). One quarter of the uric acid produced daily is excreted through intestinal secretions undergoing uricolysis by intestinal bacteria (3, 4); a very small amount of the remaining three quarters is excreted through the skin (5), the nails (6), the saliva and the hair (1), while the remnant appears in the urine; in chronic renal failure the extrarenal elimination is increased as a compensatory phenomenon (1).

In the blood, at pH 7.4, uric acid is almost entirely as monovalent anion; since its protein binding is minimal, more than 95% of plasma urate is freely filtered by glomeruli.

About 90% of the filtered urate undergoes proximal tubular reabsorption; but after this reabsorption, uric acid secretion at a similar rate (i.e. 90% of the filtered load) occurs, presumably in the proximal tubule. It has been demonstrated that a further postsecretory reabsorption takes place, which also approximates 90% of the filtered load and is believed to be the major determinant of final urinary excretion of uric acid which amounts to about 10% of the filtered urate.

Factors that may influence urinary urate excretion are: plasma urate concentration, urine flow rate and effective blood volume. Thus, extracellular volume expansion by saline increases urate clearance causing hypouricemia; by contrast, volume contraction decreases urate clearance causing hyperuricemia (1).

Table 1 - Conditions favouring uric acid stone formation

A. HYPERURICOSURIA
   I. Secondary to hyperuricemia
      (a) Gout (20% form uric acid stones)
      (b) Rare enzymatic disorders
      (c) Secondary uric acid overproduction (Myeloproliferative disorders, Leukemia, Lymphomas, Multiple myeloma, Neoplasia, Hemolytic Anemia)
   II. Without hyperuricemia
      (A) Uricosuric drugs (only acutely) (Probenecid, Salicylates in high doses, Contrast media)
      (B) Tubular disorders
      (C) High dietary intake of purine-rich foods (meat, liver, poultry, fish) (it causes also low urine pH)
      (D) Gout (with acid urine pH)

B. LOW URINE VOLUME AND/OR LOW URINE pH WITHOUT HYPERURICOSURIA
   1. Gastrointestinal disorders (by dehydration and bicarbonate loss) (e.g. Ulcerative colitis, Regional enteritis, Ileostomy)
   2. Dehydration
   3. Physical exercise
   4. "Idiopathic uric acid lithiasis" (low urine pH)

Hyperuricosuria may cause renal injury by three different mechanisms (7): (a) uric acid nephrolithiasis or calcium oxalate nephrolithiasis; (b) deposition of sodium urate crystals in the renal interstitium thereby causing chronic urate nephropathy (the so-called "gouty kidney"); (c) deposition of uric acid in collecting ducts (8, 9) with the consequent intrarenal obstructive nephropathy known as acute Uric Acid Nephropathy (UAN)(10, 11).

Uric Acid and Stone Formation

The first proton of uric acid has a pK (dissociation constant) of 5.4 in urine at 37°C (12). When pH of urine exceeds pK (e.g. 6.5 or more), the urate anion (product of uric acid dissociation) forms salts mainly with sodium (monosodium urate); thus, under such circumstances, more than 90% of uric acid is in form of urate. When pH of urine is lower than pK (e.g. 5.0 or less), uric acid remains mainly (about 90%) undissociated. But the undissociated uric acid is soluble in urine only up to the concentration of about 95 mg/litre at 37°C (13). Oversaturation of urine at pH of 5.0 or less with undissociated uric acid leads to uric acid stone formation. Oversaturation of urine at pH of 6.0 or more with monosodium urate will lead to calcium oxalate stone formation.

Uric Acid Nephrolithiasis

The incidence of uric acid nephrolithiasis in the general population is very low (about 0.01%). It becomes high in patients with primary gout, reaching 20%. The disorders frequently associated with uric acid stones are summarized in Table 1. Gouty population usually exhibits increased urinary excretion of uric acid which is further increased by high intake of purine-rich foods; 50% of patients with uric acid excretrion rate greater than 1000 mg/day form uric acid stones (1). High urine acidity greatly contributes to uric acid stone formation in gouty patients. As a matter of fact these patients may form uric acid stones even in the absence of hyperuricosuria. The pathogenesis of the high urine acidity of gouty patients is not known; urinary excretion of titratable acid is increased, while ammonia excretion is decreased (1).

Myeloproliferative disorders (50% of these patients form uric acid stones), leukemia, lymphomas, multiple myeloma, neoplasia and hemolytic anemia may cause uric acid nephrolithiasis because of increased rate of nucleoprotein metabolism. This occurs through a severe hyperuricemia and the consequent hyperuricosuria and is made more severe and more frequent during therapy (7).

Hyperuricosuria occurs acutely, without hyperuricemia, after administration of uricosuric drugs, such as probenecid, salicylates, contrast media, by inhibition of tubular reabsorption of uric acid; with chronic administration of the same drugs, however, uric acid excretion returns to normal.

Hyperuricosuria may also occur, even without hyperuricemia, in subjects under high dietary intake of purine-rich foods; these subjects have also a low urinary pH (14).

There is finally the possibility of uric acid nephrolithiasis without hyperuricosuria. It occurs in some gastrointestinal diseases, such as regional enteritis or ulcerative colitis, and following ileostomy; under such conditions, uric acid renal stone formation is presumably secondary to dehydration and enteric loss of bicarbonate with the consequent high concentration and increased acidity of urine (1). Obviously dehydration by itself may account for the high incidence of uric acid nephrolithiasis in some arid countries (e.g. 40% of population in Israel) and in subjects performing physical exercise (in addition to a low urine pH)(15). The so-called "Idiopathic uric acid lithiasis" is the uric acid nephrolithiasis occurring without hyperuricemia and without hyperuricosuria in subjects who exhibit only persistently very acid urine (5).

Hyperuricosuric Calcium Oxalate Nephrolithiasis
(HyperUricosuric Calcium Urolithiasis or HUCU)

Hyperuricosuria is frequently associated with calcium nephrolithiasis. This association has been called HyperUricosuric Calcium Urolithiasis (HUCU) (2). Typical feature of HUCU is the association of (a) hyperuricosuria (urinary excretion of uric acid greater than 600 mg daily in at least two out of three 24-hour urine collections), (b) calcium oxalate (mainly) and/or calcium phosphate stones, (c) urinary pH greater than 5.5, in the absence of hypercalciuria, hyperoxaluria or hypocitraturia (1).

The hyperuricosuria of patients with HUCU is usually due to abitudinal high dietary intake of purine-rich foods (16, 17); only in 30% of the patients it is due to uric acid overproduction (1).

Urine of patients with HUCU are supersaturated with respect to monosodium urate, having a pH greater than 5.5 (18). There is evidence that monosodium urate participates in calcium stone formation either by inducing crystallization of calcium stones by heterogeneous nucleation (19, 20) or by binding inhibitors of calcium oxalate crystallization (21).

Thus, when, in patients with HUCU undergoing purine-restricted diet, urinary excretion of uric acid was increased by oral purine load

(3 grams of ribonucleic acid), urine specimens became more supersaturated with respect to monosodium urate. The urinary Activity Product Ratio (APR) of monosodium urate and uric acid (i.e. the ratio activity products before and after incubation of urine samples with 5 mg monosodium urate/ml; a ratio of 1 indicates saturation, less than 1 undersaturation, more than 1 supersaturation), in fact, increased with the increase of urinary uric acid (16). This rise of APR Na urate was associated with a decrease in the Formation Product Ratio (FPR) of calcium oxalate (i.e. the minimum APR at which a spontaneous precipitation of calcium oxalate occurs 3 hours after the addition of a solution of sodium oxalate) (16). These observations demonstrate that increase of urinary excretion of uric acid facilitates the spontaneous nucleation of calcium oxalate. After a two to four month-pretreatment with allopurinol (300 mg daily) urinary excretion of uric acid was reduced during both the purine-restricted diet and the purine load, thereby leading to a decrease of the urinary APR of monosodium urate with the consequent increase in urinary FPR of calcium oxalate (16). These observations indicate that allopurinol therapy decreases the saturation of urine with respect to monosodium urate thereby preventing calcium oxalate formation (16).

Clinical conditions associated with hyperuricemia

As already mentioned, severe hyperuricemia usually occurs in patients with malignancies, mainly leukemia, lymphomas and, less frequently, multiple myeloma and large solid tumors. In these conditions the hyperuricemia is due to the massive destruction of tumor cells; cell destruction will cause the release of great amounts of nucleoproteins and their metabolites and the consequent formation of unusually large amounts of uric acid. Since cell destruction is even more marked during chemotherapy and radiation therapy, the most severe hyperuricemia typically occurs during aggressive cytolytic treatment of these neoplastic disorders. Values of hyperuricemia as high as 90 mg/dl have been reported, causing acute renal failure (22).

Other disorders associated with increased production of uric acid (bacause of accelerated breakdown of tissue nucleotides) include primary gout, hypercatabolic states and conditions of severe tissue hypoxia, such as acute myocardial infarction, cardiomyopathy, cardiogenic shock, hemorrhagic shock, rhabdomyolysis (23).

Hyperuricemia may also result from impaired urinary escretion of uric acid. This typically occurs as a consequence of chronic renal failure or organic acute renal failure (Acute Tubular Necrosis, ATN) (7). Renal failure induces the retention of waste products of nitrogen metabolism including uric acid; the resulting hyperuricemia, however, is blunted by the increase of uric acid clearance per residual nephron (the ratio uric acid clearance to creatinine clearance is, in fact, increased).

A hyperuricemia out of proportion to the degree of renal failure typically occurs in prerenal ARF, as result of proximal tubular overreabsoption which takes place in the attempt to correct ECV depletion.

Hyperuricemia may also occur following long-term treatment with diuretics, particularly thiazides; it is due to impaired excretion of uric acid (increase in tubular reabsorption and presumably decrease in secretion because of an interference of diuretics with organic acid secretory mechanism) and is not harmful to the kidney (7). Finally a retention hyperuricemia due to increase in tubular reabsorption of uric acid may occur in congestive heart failure and in cirrhosis.

Gouty kidney

The pathogenesis and even the existence of a chronic gouty nephropathy is still matter of controversy (24). That uric acid precipitates may be present both in the lumina of tubules and in the

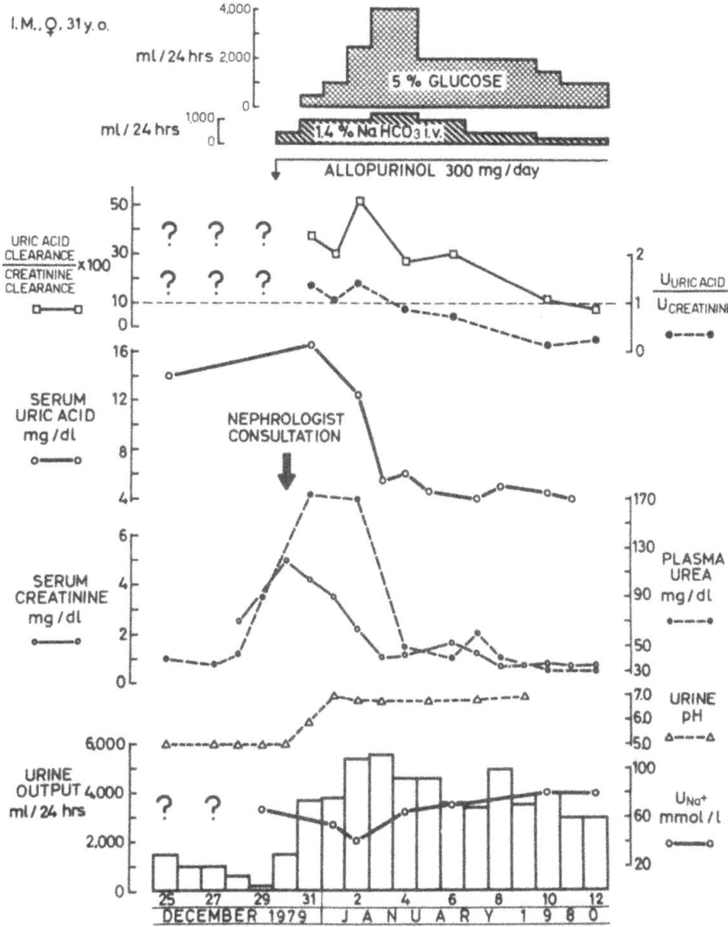

Figure 1. Acute renal failure due to Acute Uric Acid Nephropathy. A pregnant woman (28th week of gestation) was admitted to the hospital because of lumbar pain. She had a hystory of stones in the right kidney. Oligo-anuria occurred with urine pH of 5.0. No renal stones were detected by ultrasonography. Serum uric acid reached values greater than 16 mg/dl; the ratio between uric acid clearance and creatinine clearance was greater than 0.30; the ratio between urinary uric acid and urinary creatinine was greater than 1. Treatment with sodium bicarbonate i.v., glucose sol. i.v. and allopurinol per os normalized urine output, serum uric acid and renal function in a few day. A healthy girl was born two months later. After delivery, i.v. pyelography did not show any renal stone. (Reprinted with permission from V.E.Andreucci and A.Dal Canton, Proc. EDTA, 17: 123,1980)

surrounding interstitium has been suggested by Charcot in 1881 (25). But whether cortical microtophi are the cause or the consequence of interstitial fibrosis is still unknown (26). On the other hand microtophi have been observed also in the absence of gout or hyperuricemia; furthermore in many patients with gout no microtophi have been found in the kidney. Thus, it is believed that interstitial nephritis occurring in gouty patients may be the result of several mechanisms, such as ureteral obstruction, intratubular crystal deposition, pyelonephritis and possibly the nephrotoxicity of hyperuricemia (26). Even the progressive evolution to renal failure of "Gouty kidney" has been challanged (27, 28). Berger and Yu (29, 30) systematically studied 600 gouty men, carrying out PAH and inulin clearances in each individual patient at intervals of 7 and 12 years; they concluded that gout and hyperuricemia alone did not cause renal insufficiency.

Recent studies have suggested that some patients with chronic hyperuricemia and renal dysfunction have chronic lead nephropathy. The hyperuricemia and the renal urate deposition in these patients is the result rather than the cause of renal impairment (23).

Acute uric acid nephropathy (UAN)

Acute uric acid nephropathy (UAN) is an oliguric acute renal failure (ARF) (Figure 1) which is attributed to massive intratubular crystallization of uric acid; this takes place mainly in the collecting ducts (8), where the tubular fluid becomes very concentrated and uric acid solubility is decreased because of the acidic pH (10). The resulting widespread tubular obstruction by uric acid crystals will increase the intratubular pressure in proximal and distal tubules, thereby leading to a fall in GFR (8). The demonstrated associated impairment of renal blood flow (10) has been attributed to simultaneous obstruction of the distal renal vasculature because of the urate deposits in deep cortical and medullary vessels or because of compression of these vessels secondary to the increase in tubular and interstitial pressure (8). Although this reduction in renal blood flow may represent also a pathogenetic factor, undoubtedly it is the tubular obstruction the primary cause of renal function impairment (7). Even the hyperuricosuria that follows the use of urographic or cholecystographic agents (due to enhanced tubular secretion of uric acid) has been suggested as playing a pathogenetic role in contrast-induced ARF (7).

Sometimes hyperuricosuria may cause ARF of postrenal type, through the obstruction of the urinary tract by uric acid stones (Figure 2) or calcium oxalate stones. In these cases the symptoms of acute obstructive uropathy may occur (e.g. colicky pain, back pain, hematuria, etc) (7). It has been suggested that the ARF of postrenal type occurs predominantly following a gradual onset of hyperuricemia (with the consequent hyperuricosuria) while the acute uric acid nephropathy occurs after a sharp rise in serum uric acid (22). The diagnosis of this type of ARF is based on ultrasonography, high-dose i.v. pyelography, gamma camera renography or computed tomography (Figure 2). It is also possible that acute uric acid nephropathy and acute obstructive uropathy coexist in the same patients, both contributing to the renal shutdown (7).

UAN is readily reversible with early adequate therapy. This makes early diagnosis absolutely necessary. Urinary excretion of uric acid is reduced with the fall of GFR, but less than expected from the impairment of renal function. Thus, the ratio uric acid

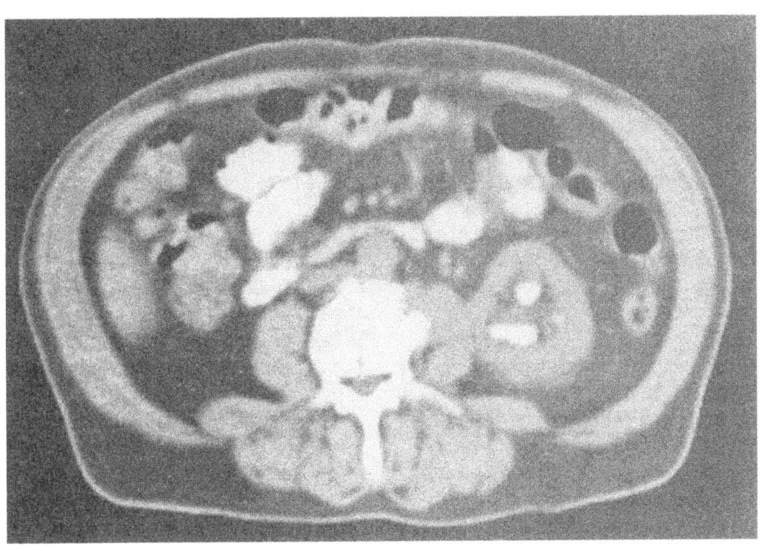

Figure 2. Computed tomography (CT) in a 69-year-old one-kidney patient with postrenal ARF due to uric acid stone. This patient had for several years a serum creatinine around 1.5 mg/dl. A progressive decrease of urine output (until 100 ml/24 hours) led to the evaluation of renal function: serum creatinine had reached 13 mg/dl. Plain film tomogram did not show renal stones. CT demonstrated the absence of the right kidney and a renal stone (arrows) in the left renal pyelocalyceal system that was clearly dilated. A retrograde pyelography confirmed a non-radiopaque obstructing stone (uric acid stone) in the pelvis. Ureteral catheterization up to the pelvis allowed resumption of urine output; the catheter was left in place for a couple of weeks. Treatment with allopurinol per os and sodium bicarbonate i.v. led to dissolution of the uric acid stone (as shown by the tomogram after injection of contrast material through the catheter) and resumption of renal function (serum creatinine returning to basal values of 1.5 mg/dl).(Reprinted with permission from V.E. Andreucci, "Acute Renal Failure", Martinus Nijhoff Publishing, Boston, 1984)

clearance/creatinine clearance, usually about 0.10 when GFR is normal, raises to 0.26 when GFR is between 4 and 20 ml/min (31). In UAN this ratio may easily exceed 0.26, reflecting a striking hyperuricosuria (Figure 1). It has also been suggested that the urinary uric acid/urinary creatinine ratio is a useful test in order to differentiate UAN (in which the ratio is greater than 1) from other forms of ARF (in which the ratio is less than 1) (Figure 1) (7). A mean ratio of 1.68 (0.63 SD) has been reported in 5 patients with UAN, while the ratio was 0.43 (0.19 SD) in 27 patients with other forms of ARF (11).It is better to measure this ratio in 24-hour urine specimens rather than in spot samples (32).

Treatment of hyperuricemia and/or hyperuricosuria

Treatment of hyperuricosuria is very important in preventing renal stone formation. It is based on three points:

(a) Dietary restriction of proteins, calcium and sodium

Since dietary animal proteins represent a purine load, leading to increase in urinary uric acid, decrease in urine pH and citrate, and increase in urinary calcium, high protein diets (more than 1.7 gm per kg b.w. per day) must be avoided. A moderate limitation of the ingestion of meat, poultry, liver and fish may be helpful, by omitting, for instance, animal proteins in one meal every day; a pure vegetarian diet has not been found protective against stone formation and may be even dangerous by increasing oxalate excretion (33). Excessive intake of calcium (greater than 1 gm per day), should be avoided even when intestinal calcium absorption is normal; this is obtained by limiting dairy products and dark green vegetables (33). A moderate sodium restriction (by avoiding obviously salty foods) is also indicated since high sodium intake increases urinary calcium excretion meanwhile reducing citrate excretion (33).

(b) Increase in fluid intake

Stone formers usually do not drink much, thereby having low urine output (less than 1 liter per day). They should be advised to increase fluid intake in order to have a urine output of at least 2 liters per day; this will greatly reduce the urinary saturation of stone-forming salts (34).

(c) Treatment with allopurinol and potassium citrate

Allopurinol, at a daily dosage of 300 mg, reduces uric acid synthesis and consequently uric acid excretion. It is therefore very useful not only in patients with uric acid overproduction, but also in those used to high dietary purine intake (33).

Potassium citrate has been introduced in 1985 for preventing stone formation, since it lowers ionic calcium concentration (by complexing calcium) and inhibits heterogeneous nucleation of calcium oxalate by monosodium urate (35). Given at the dosage of 60 mEq per day, it can increase citrate excretion to the normal values of about 600 mg per day (33). Thus the increase in citraturia can prevent not only urinary saturation of calcium oxalate but also urate-induced crystallization of calcium oxalate (33).

The ideal conditions for preventing recurrent renal stone formation in patients at risk are summarized in Table 2.

Table 2. Ideal urinary conditions for preventing recurrent renal stone formation in patients at risk.

Urine output:	more than 2 litres/day
Urinary calcium:	less than 250 mg/day
Urinary oxalate:	less than 45 mg/day
Urinary citrate:	more than 300 mg/day
Urinary uric acid:	less than 600 mg/day
Urinary pH:	more than 5.5 but less than 7.0

As mentioned, even the oliguric ARF due to UAN may be reversed with adequate conservative therapy. This is based on the following procedures (7):

(A) To induce a high urinary flow rate (with the purpose to flush out obstructing uric acid crystals) we may use either high-dose furosemide or i.v. infusion of saline and/or glucose solutions, or both. Solute and water diuresis will prevent further uric acid deposition within the collecting ducts by diluting uric acid in the tubular fluid, thereby enhancing its solubility. In volume-expanded patients saline infusion may be hazardous and furosemide alone should be preferred.

(B) To alkalinize the urine (with the purpose to increase the solubility of uric acid in the urine) the i.v. drip infusion of sodium bicarbonate is indicated (lactate is contraindicated, inhibiting uric acid secretion). Sodium bicarbonate may also be given per os in frequent divided doses in order to maintain the urinary pH between 6.5 and 7.0.

(C) Acetazolamide may be combined with sodium bicarbonate to alkalinize the urine by reducing tubular reabsorption of bicarbonate (11). Acetazolamide should be used alone in volume-expanded patients in whom bicarbonate infusion may be hazardous (22).

(D) Allopurinol is given at high dosage, between 300 and 900 mg daily. In patients treated with 6-mercaptopurine, azathioprine or cyclophosphamide, the dosage of these drugs should be reduced since allopurinol potentiates their action and toxicity.

(E) In some cases of UAN due to extensive cell destruction (e.g. leukemia, malignancies), the hyperuricemia that follows the antineoplastic therapy may be associated with hyperphosphatemia due to release of intracellular phosphorus. These patients should be given aluminum hydroxide in order to prevent metastatic calcification and acute nephrocalcinosis (22).

(F) Severe hyperkalemia should be treated immediately.

(G) Should dialysis become necessary, hemodialysis is preferable. If hyperphosphatemia is present, dialysate calcium should be decreased in order to prevent metastatic calcification (22).

(H) Should the patient respond to conservative therapy with increase of urine output, hydration, alkalinization and administration of allopurinol should be continued until normalization of renal function (7).

In patients with malignancy, prevention of UAN is based on hydration, alkalinization and administration of allopurinol which must be started several days before chemotherapy and continued throughout the treatment (7).

References

1. N.A. Breslau and K. Sakhaee, Pathophysiology of nonhypercalciuric causes of stones, in : "Renal Stone Disease", C.Y.C. Pak, ed., Martinus Nijhoff Publishing, Boston (1987), pp. 47-84.
2. E.W. Holmes, Uric acid nephrolithiasis, in :"Nephrolithiasis", F.L. Coe, ed., Churchill Livingstone, New York (1972), pp. 325-336.
3. L.B. Sorensen, Role of the intestinal tract in the elimination of uric acid, Arth. Rheum., 8: 994 (1965).
4. L.B. Sorensen, Extrarenal disposal of uric acid, in : "Uric acid", W.N. Kelley and I.N. Weiner, eds., Springer-Verlag, New York (1978), pp. 325-336.

5. A. Atsmon, A. DeVries and M. Frank, "Uric Acid Lithiasis", Elsevier, Amsterdam (1963).
6. A. Bollinger and R. Gross, Ammonia, urea and uric acid content of toe nails in renal insufficiency and gout, Aust. Exp. Biol. Med. Sci., 31: 385 (1953).
7. V.E. Andreucci, "Acute Renal Failure", Martinus Nijhoff Publishing, Boston (1984).
8. J.D. Conger, S.A. Falk, S.J. Guggenheim and T.J. Burke, A micropuncture study of the early phase of acute urate nephropathy, J. Clin. Invest., 58: 681 (1976).
9. J.D. Conger and S.A. Falk, Intrarenal dynamics in the pathogenesis and prevention of acute urate nephropathy, J. Clin. Invest., 59: 786 (1977).
10. R.E. Rieselbach, C.J. Benzel, E. Cotlove, E. Frei and E.J. Freireich, Uric acid excretion and renal function in the acute hyperuricemia of leukemia, Am. J. Med., 37: 872 (1964).
11. J. Kelton, W.N. Kelley and E.W. Holmes, A rapid method for the diagnosis of acute uric acid nephropathy, Arch. Intern. Med., 138: 612 (1978).
12. B. Finlayson and A. Smith, Stability of first dissociable proton of uric acid, J. Chem. Eng. Data, 19: 94 (1974).
13. F.L. Coe, A.L. Stauss, V. Tembe and M.S.L. Dunn, Uric acid saturation in calcium nephrolithiasis, Kidney Int., 17: 661 (1980).
14. C.Y.C. Pak, N.A. Breslau and J.A. Harvey, Nutrition and metabolic bone disease, in : "Nutritional Diseases: Research Directors in Comparative Pathobiology", D.G. Scarpelli and G. Migaki, eds., Alan R. Liss, New York (1986) pp 115-140.
15. C.Y.C. Pak, "Renal Stone Disease", Martinus Nijhoff Publishing, Boston (1987).
16. C.Y.C. Pak, D.E. Barilla, K. Holt, L. Brinkley, R. Tolentino and J.E. Zerwekh, Effect of oral purine load and allopurinol on the crystallization of calcium salts in urine of patients with hyperuricosuric calcium urolithiasis. Am. J. Med., 65: 593 (1978).
17. F.L. Coe and A.G. Kavalach, Hypercalciuria and hyperuricosuria in patients with calcium nephrolithiasis, N. Eng. J. Med., 291: 1344 (1974).
18. C.Y.C. Pak, O. Waters, L. Arnold, K. Holt, C. Cox and D.E. Barilla, Mechanism of calcium urolithiasis among patients with hyperuricosuria: supersaturation of urine with respect to monosodium urate, J. Clin. Invest., 59: 426 (1977).
19. C.Y.C. Pak and L. Arnold, Heterogeneous nucleation of calcium oxalate by seeds of monosodium urate, Proc. Soc. Exp. Biol. Med., 149: 930 (1975).
20. F.L. Coe, R.L. Lawton, R.B. Goldstein and V. Tembe, Sodium urate accelerates precipitation of calcium oxalate in vitro, Proc. Soc. Exp. Biol. Med., 149: 926 (1975).
21. C.Y.C. Pak, K. Holt and J.E. Zerwekh, Attenuation by monosodium urate of the inhinitory effect of mucopolysaccharide on calcium oxalate nucleation, Invest. Urol., 17: 138 (1979).
22. C.M. Kjellstrand, D.C.H. Campbell, B. von Hartitzsch and T.J. Buslmeier, Hyperuricemic acute renal failure, Arch. Intern. Med., 133: 349 (1974).
23. J.O. Woolliscroft, H. Colfer and I.H. Fox, Hyperuricemia in acute illness: a poor prognostic sign, Am. J. Med., 72: 58 (1982).
24. L.H. Beck, Requiem for gouty nephropathy, Kidney Int. , 30: 280 (1986).
25. J.M. Charcot, Clinical lectures on senile and chronic diseases. Translated by W.S. Tuke, The New Sydenham Society, London (1881).
26. R.P. Wedeen and V. Batuman, Tubulo-interstitial nephritis induced

by heavy metals and metabolic disturbances, in : "Tubulo-interstitial nephropathies", R.S. Cotran, ed., Churchill Livingstone, New York (1983) pp. 211-241.
27. W.J. Fessel, Renal outcomes of gout and hyperuricemia, Am. J. Med., 67: 74 (1979).
28. T.F. Yu, T.L. Berger, D.J. Dorph and H. Smith, Renal function in gout. V. Factors influencing the renal hemodynamics, Am. J. Med., 67: 766 (1979).
29. T.F. Yu and T.L. Berger, Renal disease in primary gout: a study of 259 gout patients with proteinuria, Semin. Arthritis Rheum., 4: 293 (1975).
30. T.L. Berger and T.F. Yu, Renal function in gout. IV. An analysis of 524 gouty subjects including long-term follow-up studies, Am. J. Med., 59: 605 (1975).
31. T.F. Yu and T.L. Berger, "The kidney in gout and hyperuricemia", Futura Publishing, Mount Kisco, NY (1982).
32. R.L. Wortmann and I.H. Fox, Limited value of uric acid to creatinine ratios in estimating uric acid excretion, Ann. Intern. Med., 93: 822 (1980).
33. C.Y.C. Pak, Prevention of recurrent nephrolithiasis, in : "Renal Stone Disease", C.Y.C. Pak, ed., Martinus Nijhoff Publishing, Boston (1987).
34. N.A. Breslau, K. Sakhaee, C. Crowther and L. Brinkley, Evidence justifying a high fluid intake in treatment of nephrolithiasis, Ann. Intern. Med., 93: 36 (1981).
35. C.Y.C. Pak and R. Peterson, Successful treatment of hyperuricosuric calcium oxalate nephrolithiasis with potassium citrate, Arch. Intern. Med., 146: 863 (1986).

PRE-ECLAMPSIA AS A MULTI-SYSTEM DISEASE

John M Davison

Medical Research Council Human Reproduction Group
Princess Mary Maternity Hospital
Newcastle upon Tyne
NE2 3BD, England

INTRODUCTION

Hypertension complicates 1 in 10 pregnancies. Approximately 50-60% of these women have pre-eclampsia, which occurs primarily in first pregnancies, usually after the twentieth gestational week and most often near term. Of the various systemic changes in pre-eclampsia, hypertension, oedema and proteinuria have been given significant status for the purpose of definition.[1] Indeed, other clinical labels include pregnancy-induced hypertension(PIH), hypertension peculiar to pregnancy and pregnancy associated hypertension, perhaps mistakenly reflecting the exclusive importance of raised blood pressure(BP). Hypertension, oedema and proteinuria are merely conveniently accessible clinical signs which are not specific or characteristic of the disorder but secondary features of whatever comprises the primary pathology. Furthermore, in clinical terms, there is difficulty distinguishing between pre-eclampsia, essential or secondary hypertension, renal disease or combinations of these entities.[2]

This review will assess the relevance of the clinical signs used in pre-eclampsia and will consider the primary pathology, the multi-system pathophysiology and the many and variable clinical sequelae of this disorder.

RELEVANCE OF CLINICAL SIGNS IN PRE-ECLAMPSIA

An appropriate definition of hypertension requires cognizance of BP changes in normal pregnancy so that the criteria decided on will truly establish a dividing line between normal and abnormal levels. In fact, mean BP decreases early in pregnancy, reaching a nadir by midtrimester when diastolic levels are often 10 to 15 mmHg below values measured postpartum. BP then increases gradually, approaching nonpregnant values near term. Since cardiac output rises quickly during the first trimester (to 140 to 160% of nonpregnant values) and remains relatively constant thereafter until term, the decrease in BP is due to a marked decrement in peripheral vascular resistance.[3] This is greatest in the uterine vasculature, which becomes a large "low resistance shunt," but vasodilatation does occur in other organ systems including the kidney and skin. The return of mean BP from a midtrimester nadir toward nonpregnant values near term is of interest because it demonstrates that increasing vasoconstrictor tone is a feature of late normal pregnancy.

Given these above normal alterations in pregnancy, what constitutes high BP? Categorisation is by either an absolute threshold or by an increment from a baseline in early pregnancy. Although many thresholds have been advocated the conventional dividing line is 140/90.[4] If, however, hypertension is only identified above a certain threshold in late pregnancy it might not be possible to distinguish a permanently raised BP from a transient gestationally-induced state. Thus BP increments from a early baseline have been defined.

Despite both these approaches there is still confusion and categorisation can be erroneous. For instance, although the American College of Obstetricians and Gynecologists[4] specifies systolic and diastolic changes of +30 and +15mmHg respectively, the diastolic increment is probably too low because the average for all women is about 10-12mmHg[5] and others therefore recommend that the increase should be 20 or 25mmHg[6]. Furthermore, the American College´s definition of hypertension is based on "either/or" conditions: a systolic pressure of >140mmHg or an increment of >30mmHg or a diastolic of >90mmHg or an increment of >15mmHg. In effect it incorporates two alternative absolute thresholds, which if not reached, can be replaced by limits based on increments. British definitions specify that a threshold of 90mmHg after midpregnancy is diagostic of pre-eclampsia,[7] provided there was no previous reading at or above this level. Thus a woman whose pressures rise from a baseline diastolic of 88mmHg (mild chronic hypertension for example) are grouped with women with a parallel rise from a baseline diastolic of 70mmHg or less. Consequently hypertension is an artificial concept: it depends on a variable which is difficult to measure accurately, it has large sampling errors, definitions vary and it is not the primary cardiovascular anomaly in the pathogenesis of pre-eclampsia.

Considering the other clinical signs: oedema is commonplace in normal pregnancy, its assessment is subjective and although it can be present in pre-eclampsia the so-called "dry" variant can occur. Proteinuria usually occurs as a late sign in pre-eclampsia but it is not a necessary component. All in all, pre-eclampsia cannot be defined precisely by its signs.

LEVELS OF PATHOLOGY IN PRE-ECLAMPSIA

The primary pathology is unknown but must be localised within the pregnant uterus because pre-eclampsia always resolves after delivery. Although the presence of trophoblast is necessary, the fetus is not, because pre-eclampsia can develop with hydatidiform mole. The primary change of pre-eclampsia must therefore be either an abnormality of the trophoblast itself or of the maternal adaptation to the presence of trophoblast. Two lesions involving the uterine spiral arteries, supplying the intervillous space have been identified. There is a relative lack of physiological dilatation of the arterial walls induced by the endovascular trophoblast[8] as well as acute atherosis - aggregates of fibrin, platelets and lipid-loaded macrophages which partially or completely block the arteries.[9] Neither change, however,

TABLE 1

MATERNAL TARGET SYSTEMS : MULTI-SYSTEM INVOLVEMENT

ARTERIAL	INCREASES IN SENSITIVITY TO AII, IN TPR & IN BP
RENAL	DECREASED RENAL HAEMODYNAMICS & $C_{uric\ acid}$, PROTEINURIA
COAGULATION	DECREASED PLATELETS & INCREASED FIBRINOGEN-FIBRIN TURNOVER
HEPATIC	ELEVATED ENZYMES & JAUNDICE

TABLE 2

MATERNAL TARGET SYSTEMS : ADDITIONAL SEQUELAE

ARTERIAL	PULMONARY OEDEMA
RENAL	ATN, ACN
COAGULATION	DIC
HEPATIC	RUPTURE
CNS	CONVULSIONS, HAEMORRHAGE, OEDEMA, RETINAL DETACHMENT

is specific to pre-eclampsia and can also occur with intrauterine growth retardation without maternal sequela.[10] This means that either the spiral artery changes are an associated but not primary feature of pre-eclampsia or that pre-eclampsia is a broader disorder than previously considered. If the latter, then the primary problem is an impaired uteroplacental circulation, to which the maternal system may not respond. The secondary pathology of pre-eclampsia is the actual maternal adaptation to the abnormal relationship between uterus and trophoblast. As normal pregnancy imposes changes on maternal physiology, probably due to humoral factors which enter the maternal circulation from the placenta, a disturbed uteroplacental relationship could be mediated in the same way, possibly by the same factors. The secondary or end-organ pathology (Table 1) includes the defining signs of pre-eclampsia and other peripheral disturbances (to be described later), which may become so severe that they themselves initate tertiary pathology (Table 2).

AETIOLOGY OF PRE-ECLAMPSIA

Pre-eclampsia can still justifiably be called the disease of theories,[11] not all of which can be considered here.

Decreased uteroplacental perfusion

Proponents of this theory hypothesize that decrements in uteroplacental perfusion trigger hypertensive mechanisms, possibly by increasing uterine venous efflux of vasopressor substances or decreasing the outflow of vasodilator hormones.[12] Animal experiments indicate that acute reductions in uteroplacental flow are accompanied by decreased amounts of prostaglandin(PG)-like material in the uterine veins and pregnancy hypertension can be produced by decreasing blood flow to uterus. There are no comparable human data, but the healthy human placenta must obviously function normally over a range of perfusing pressures, including the 15% decrease in mean arterial pressure that occurs at night during sleep. Interestingly, there is an observation in humans that high altitude increases the incidence of preeclampsia.[13]

Immunologic mechanisms

There is evidence to suggest that severe pre-eclampsia may have an immunological basis.[14,15] Circulating immune complexes, which have been found in preeclampsia in higher concentrations than in normal pregnancy, could trigger the disseminated intravascular coagulation (DIC) that has been found in pre-eclampsia by some investigators. High levels of IgG and IgM antibodies to laminin, a glycoprotein present in both trophoblast and glomerular basement membrane, have been detected in sera from pre-eclamptic women.[16] Immune complexes have been found in pre-eclamptic vascular lesions of the placental bed and the kidney the density of renal immunoglobulin deposits correlating with the severity of the disease.

At first consideration it would seem unlikely that severe pre-eclampsia has an immunological basis because it is most common in first pregnancies, in contrast to the best-documented immunological condition in pregnancy, rhesus isoimmunization. However, pre-eclampsia may be the result not of an excessive immune response but of an inadequate response, the protective immune response possibly being less efficient in first than in later pregnancies.[15] Evidence for an impaired immune response in pre-eclampsia compared with normal pregnancy comes from studies of lymphocyte DNA synthesis, lymphocyte response to phytohemagglutinin and lymphocytotoxic antibody titres.[17] Pregnancy always suppresses a mother's immune response to some extent, since rejection of an antigenically foreign fetus needs to be prevented, but this physiologic immunosuppression may be greater than usual in pre-eclampsia. This could account for the increased evidence of the disorder in conditions such as twin pregnancy and molar pregnancy, in which there are high plasma concentrations of human chorionic gonadotropin(hCG), a likely immunosuppressive agent.

Why should women with pre-eclampsia have a defective immune response? It is interesting that no particular maternal HLA antigen is associated with pre-eclampsia, nor is there excessive maternal-fetal HLA incompatibility.[18] However, what is apparent in some investigations is that pre-eclamptic gravidas have increased homozygosity for human leukocyte (HLA) antigens: Those who are homozygous for HLA-A and HLA-B antigens are more likely to have severe pre-eclampsia. This would account for the apparently increased HLA compatibility between mothers and fetuses, and also the decreased immune response. HLA genes are thought to be closely linked to immune-response genes at adjacent loci, and Redman and colleagues[18] have suggested that homozygosity of HLA genes in a given patient therefore would imply that the adjacent immune-response genes are almost certainly homozygous as well, suggesting the operation of a recessive gene in pre-eclampsia.

Genetic factors

One hypothesis is that there is homozygosity for recessive maternal immune-response genes linked to HLA and that genetic control of severe pre-eclampsia may depend on mendelian inheritance of a single recessive gene.[19] Because pre-eclampsia is manifest only in pregnancy the two obvious possibilities for the determining factor are the genotype of either the mother or the fetus.[20] If there is recessive inheritance, these two possibilities will not be distinguished by study of mother-daughter pairs. Instead, it is necessary to know the incidence of pre-eclampsia in sisters of affected women (higher than expected incidence if maternal genotype hypothesis is correct) or in the husband's female relatives (higher than expected incidence if the fetal hypothesis is correct). Cooper and Liston[20] re-analyzed the family data collected by Chesley[1] and found that the incidence of toxaemia in the sisters, the daughters, and the sisters-in-law of eclamptic women fitted closely with the notion of maternal homozygosity for a recessive gene. However, when they extended their analysis to two further sets of their own data, evidence for the fetal-genotype hypothesis was apparent, thus, as to be expected, there was a significant deficit of toxaemic illness in sisters of affected women. Thus a final decision on this matter was deferred.

Any hypothesis on the aetiology of pre-eclampsia has to account for first-pregnancy preponderance. If pre-eclampsia depended on the fetal gene, the influence of parity would be extremely difficult to explain. It is easier to accept the Chesley data and the re-analysis with the suggestion that the evidence in favour of the fetal-genotype hypothesis may be biased by problems of underascertainment. Parous women who conceive for the first time by a new partner seem to have an increased risk of pre-eclampsia, thus behaving as primigravidas.[21] This leads to the concept that pre-eclampsia results from an absent or deficient maternal immune response to the fetus, which is necessary for normal pregnancy and is more likely to be imperfectly developed in first exposure to fetal antigens.[15,21] Thus the first pregnancy preponderance of pre-eclampsia, its familial occurrence, and the HLA data can be gathered together by one genetic hypothesis; the putative gene and its function have not been identified, but circumstantial evidence suggests that it may be an immune-response gene.

PATHOPHYSIOLOGY OF PRE-ECLAMPSIA

Although cardiac output may decrease in pre-eclampsia,, it usually remains at or above nongravid levels. Therefore hypertension in pre-eclamptic women is essentially the result of an increment in peripheral resistance. The hypertension is characterized by its lability, a reflection of the intense vascular sensitivity these women have to their own endogenous pressor peptides and amines.

Vascular reactivity

Renin-angiotensin system. Healthy pregnant women are quite resistant to the pressor effects of infused angiotensin II but those destined to develop pre-eclampsia manifest increased pressor responsiveness to this peptide many weeks prior to the hypertension.[22] Inevitably, this has led to the suggestion that the renin-angiotensin system may be involved in the altered vascular reactivity. Most investigators note that renin concentration, renin activity and angiotensin II are decreased in pre-eclampsia when compared to measurements during normal pregnancy.[11,23] However, some have noted increments in both plasma renin activity and angiotensin II levels, the latter correlating with the degree of maternal hypertension.[24] Even if concentrations do decrease, these pressor substances may still have a pathogenic role, especially when the exquisite sensitivity to the vasculature is condiered.[22] When overt pre-eclampsia does occur the vasculature is more sensitive to angiotensin than it is in the non-pregnant, yet these gravidas usually have concentrations of angiotensin II that are as great as or greater than those of nonpregnant women.[25]

Prostaglandins. Pre-eclamptics display several aberrations in eicosanoid metabolism, which has led to the suggestion that pre-eclampsia is due to a relative or absolute PG deficiency.[2,4,28] The belief is that an imbalance occurs between the vasodilatory PG's and vasoconstrictor influences of angiotensin and/or thromboxane(TX). According to one hypothesis, increased PG production is required during normal pregnancy to counteract the vasoconstrictor actions of the elevated angiotensin II levels. In keeping with this view are several observations: (a)Ingestion of aspirin or indomethacin, both cyclo-oxygenase inhibitors, decreases the vascular resistance of normal gravidas to infused angiotensin II to the levels observed and in both nongravid subjects and women with pre-eclampsia[29] (b)Infusion of PG in pregnancy blunts vasopressor responses to coinfusion of angiotensin II (c)PG inhibition increases BP in pregnant animals and (d)Dietary restriction of the essential fatty acid precursors of PGs in pregnant animals leads to increased sensitivity to angiotensin II.

Evidence that circulating PG levels decrease in preeclampsia is equivocal. The strongest data, however, come from studies of PG metabolism in the products of conception and in fetal or maternal blood vessels.[30-32] The level or production of vasodiltory PG's are decreased in the placenta, decidua, chorion and amnion in women with pre-eclampsia, and there is reduced prostacyclin generation in the maternal and fetal vessels of such patients. The decrement in umbilical PGI generation is greater than that in the maternal vasculature, and this has been interpreted as evidence that fetomaternal blood flow is more impaired than maternal uteroplacental flow. Of interest also is the presence of increased levels of PGI-stimulating activity in plasma from pre-eclamptics in comparison with those having a normal pregnancy. This too, has been interpreted as a compensatory mechanism in response to subnormal PGI synthesis in pre-eclampsia. Data concerning the metabolism of TX during pregnancy are fragmentary and contradictory. However, if TX levels are stable or increase while PG synthesis decreases, both hypertension and blood clotting abnormalities might occur.

There are some aberrations in fatty acid metabolism that could relate to the alterations in PG described in pre-eclampsia. For instance decrements in placental and fetal arachidonic acid levels as well as increases in the maternal concentrations of this fatty acid have been reported in pre-eclampsia.[33]

Last, free radical oxidation products, which may be related to the synthesis of some PG's and their vasoactive derivatives, are increased during pregnancy.[34]

Other hormonal and metabolic factors. It was suggested that production of progesterone, a vasodilator hormone with natriuretic action, may be decreased in pre-eclampsia. This suggestion was based on measurement of urinary metabolites, but more recently plasma progesterone levels have been reported to be unaltered in pre-eclampsia. Infusions of the progesterone metabolite 5-hydroxyprogesterone into women with pre-eclampsia apparently abolished their increased sensitivity to angiotensin II.[35]

Prolactin is purported to antagonize the effect of circulating pressor substances, but levels of this hormone in pre-eclampsia vary and have been reported as decreased, normal and elevated.[12]

Urinary and uterine tissue norepinephrine and the pressor effects of this catecholomine increase in pre-eclampsia, but data concerning plasma norepinephrine and epinephrine levels are fragmentary and conflict. Urinary dopamine excretion appears unaltered.[11,12]

There is a considerable literature (in non-pregnant hypertensives) describing membrane transport abnormalities characterized by increased intracellular calcium in smooth muscle, which sensitizes it to constrictor stimuli.[36] It has been suggested that pre-eclampsia occurs in gravidas who manifest a temporary defect in their calcium transport system. In this formulation, pregnancy is an anabolic state, in which some women fail to produce sufficient calcium-transporting protein. Reports nothing that there are decrements in sodium-potassium adenosinetriphosphatase (Na-K-ATPase are of interest, because of a defect in the sodium pump has been postulated in the pathogenesis of the cellular calcium transport effect described above. There are also intriguing reports linking hypertension in pregnancy to inadequate calcium and/or vitamin E in the diet, all of which require further investigation.[12]

Unknown humoral substances and Infection: The literature abounds with reference to "unknown humoral substances" because plasma obtained from pre-eclamptics has been shown to have vasoconstrictor properties in nonpregnant subjects. Many of these reports await confirmation and further clarification.

There is an infection theory of pre-eclampsia, and recently one group of workers claims to have identified various forms of a parasitic helminth in the blood of pre-eclamptic patients and women with trophoblastic disease. The parasite was also identified in the placentas and cord blood of the offspring of patients and pre-eclampsia-eclampsia and in trophoblastic tumour tissue. It was also claimed that inoculates of this organism, Hydatoxi lualba, induced in toxaemia-like syndrome in pregnant beagles and that intrauterine transmission of the parasite occurred, explaining the higher incidence of pre-eclampsia in the daughters of mothers who have had the disease. Recent work, however, has revealed that the suggested organisms are artefacts created by cotton and other cellulose fibers and glove talc, introduced during the preparation of the microscope slides.[38-39]

Volume homeostasis and sodium retention

Pre-eclamptic patients usually have an impaired ability to excrete sodium, but pre-eclampsia can occur in the absence of fluid retention, and even when oedema is present, plasma volume (when compared with that of a normal pregnant woman) is usually decreased.[12] The cause of sodium retention in preclampsia is obscure. Glomerular filtration rate(GFR) decreases, but the decrement seems insufficient to explain the positive salt balance. Aldosterone levels in early or midpregnancy in gravidas destined to develop hypertension in the third trimester are similar to those in women who remain normotensive, and concentrations actually decrease in frank pre-eclampsia. Deoxycorticosterone (DOC) levels increase in normal pregnancy and are not suppressible by physiologic manoeuvres such as sodium loading, suggesting that this mineralocorticoid could play a role in maintaining oedema in preeclampsia.[12]

The decrement in plasma volume in pre-eclampsia is the basis of a major controversy in the management of the disease.[40] Some investigators believe that decreased intravascular volume is the primary event in pre-eclampsia that may be responsible for the rise in blood pressure (i.e. placental hypoperfusion may induce release of a pressor substance from the uterus, or relative hypovolaemia may result in excessive instead of compensatory secretion of catecholamines). This naturally leads to the recommendation of volume expansion therapy for pre-eclampsia, an approach rejected by traditional hypertension experts who believe that decrements in volume are secondary to vasoconstriction as well as to the effect of the hypertension on renal sodium excretion.

Platelets and coagulation abnormalities

During normal pregnancy, profound changes occur in both the coagulation and the fibrinolytic systems. Several clotting factors, including factors VII, VIII, X, and fibrinogen increase and reach peak values in the third trimester.[11,41] At the same time, fibrinolytic activity, as measured by circulating plasminogen levels, is depressed. This combination of changes suggests that the pregnant woman is particularly susceptible to the development of intravascular coagulation; indeed, some suggest that normal pregnancy is a chronic state of intravascular fibrin formation, which is exaggerated in pre-eclampsia.

There is controversy concerning the incidence and significance of coagulation abnormalities in pre-eclampsia.[42] Some have claimed that a decrement in platelet count and often a defect in platelet function (collagen-induced synthesis of TXB_2) is the earliest sign of pre-eclampsia and can occur weeks before clinical signs are evident. Indeed, there are reports of the unwary clinician mistakenly diagnosing idiopathic thrombocytopenic purpura.[43]

The possibility that coagulation problems and deficient PG production may be linked in this disease has also been suggested, because the appropriate balance between vascular PGI and platelet TX synthesis is considered important for normal clotting.[41] It has been suggested that even when the diagnosis of pre-eclampsia is a remote consideration an immediate platelet count is mandatory because severe thrombocytopenia may remain undiagnosed.[44] Furthermore, there is a defined subgroup of such patients to which the acronym HELLP syndrome (H, hemolysis; EL, elevated liver enzymes; and LP, low platelet counts) has been given.[45] Such patients may have extremely high (>1,000 units) transaminase levels, and their platelet counts may decrease rapidly to values below 40×10^3 $/mm^3$.

Contrasting with these views are studies that do not ascribe a primary role to coagulation abnormalities in the pathogenesis of pre-eclampsia. Pritchard and colleagues performed a battery of five tests (platelet count, plasma fibrinogen and its degradation products, fibrin monomer and thrombin time) and found evidence of disordered coagulation in only a minority of their eclamptic patients.[46] It was suggested that the thromobytopenia that occasionally accompanies pre-eclampsia could be due to platelet adherence at sites of disrupted vascular endothelium. Decrements in the level of clotting factors in pre-eclampsia could also be related to liver involvement in this disease.

Finally, in the renal biopsy series of Fisher et al fibrin-like material was evident on immunofluorescence in only 20 of 45 specimens with ultrastructural evidence of pre-eclampsia and in only 8 instances did its intensity exceed 1+.[22,47] Glomerular fluorescence for antihaemophilic globulin was present in 5 of 10 biopsy specimens, but it was greater than 1+ in only one case. These findings do not support a role for fibrin or other clotting factors in the genesis of the renal lesion.

CLINICAL SEQUELAE OF PRE-ECLAMPSIA

The kidneys

Renal haemodynamics decrease by approximately 25% compared with normal pregnancy. Since renal haemodynamics increase 30-50% in normal pregnancy, values in pre-eclamptic women often remain above prepregnancy values.[1,2] Occasionally, functional impairement is quite severe and pre-eclampsia can cause both tubular and cortical necrosis.

Uric acid clearance, which also increases during normal pregnancy, decreases markedly in pre-eclampsia.[3] The decrement is earlier and greater than that of GFR (although there is disagreement about this conclusion) and elevated serum uric acid levels may be one of the first indicators of the disorder with serum values >350umol/l (>5.9mg/dl) during pregnancy being abnormal and associated with a poor fetal outcome. The hyperuricaemia and decreased uric acid clearance in pre-eclampsia are due primarily to altered renal handling of uric acid, with increased net tubular reasborption.

Abnormal proteinuria that is moderately unselective is a hallmark of pre-eclampsia.[4,8] The increments in urinary protein excretion may be minimal to large. Pre-eclampsia is the most common cause of nephrotic syndrome in pregnancy.

Pre-eclampsia is accompanied by a characteristic renal lesion termed glomerular capillary endotheliosis. The glomerular swelling is due to a characteristic hypertrophy of the intracapillary cells involving mainly the endothelial and less commonly the mesangial cells. These swollen cells, which contain a variety of vacuoles and lipid clusters, encroach on the capillay lumen, thus creating the appearance of a bloodless glomerulus. Occasionally small endothelial deposits (thought to represent accumulation of protein) and tactoids of fibrin or a fibrinlike material may be seen. Such images may be due in part to the accumulation of several basement membrane proteins including laminin,type IV collagen, fibronectin and a proteoglycan in the glomeruli of pre-eclamptics.

The tubules are usually intact.

The liver

Pre-eclampsia may affect the liver, but this involvement is usually mild.[4,9] An exception is the variant called HELLP syndrome, already alluded to, marked by signs of severe liver dysfunction combined with coagulation changes.[4,5] Whether there is a characteristic liver lesion for pre-eclampsia is debated but fibrin deposition has been noted in liver biopsies. Subcapsular haematomas and rupture into the abdomen is a dangerous complication of pre-eclampsia.

The placenta

In women destined to develop pre-eclampsia there is inhibition of the secondary endovascular trophoblastic migration in the second trimester, so that myometrial segments of the uteroplacental arteries remain narrowed and responsive.[10] In addition, a necrotizing arteriopathy or "acute atherosis" may affect the small muscular arteries in the placental bed. Placental blood flow, as determined by the placental clearance or accumulation of various injected radiolabels, is reduced, with a concomitant decrement in intervillous blood oxygen saturation.

The central nervous system

Eclampsia is the convulsive phase of pre-eclampsia and may occur at any time prior to, during, or after delivery. As many as one-third of the reported cases present on the first postpartum day. Hypertension and convulsions have also been reported days to weeks into the puerperium and have been termed late postpartum eclampsia, but whether or not these patients in fact had pre-eclampsia is controversial.[40]

Cerebral haemorrhage is the major cause of maternal death from pre-eclampsia or eclampsia. As well as large haemorrhages, diffusely scattered infarcts, cortical petechiae, smaller subcortical haemorrhages, and necrotic arterioles (some containing fibrin thrombi) are found. The large hemorrhages are like those found in hypertension in nonpregnant individuals, and the other changes are like the autopsy findings seen in hypertensive encephalopathy.[50] To equate eclampsia with hypertensive encephalopathy, however, is not strictly correct because although eclampsia usually correlates with the severity of the hypertension, it may also arise when blood pressure elevations are mild.[12] Another possible cause of the convulsion is brain edema, but whereas some authors have offered selective evidence of such pathology - usually by computerized tomography (CT) scanning - many women who convulse have normal CT scans.

In summary, the pathogenesis of the eclamptic convulsion is poorly understood. Advocates of hypertensive encephalopathy invoke acute pressure-induced injury of the cerebral arterioles, which, on losing their ability to remain in protective spasm and participate in autoregulatory control, then expose the more peripheral vessels to high-pressure hyperfiltration and permeability changes affecting the blood-brain barrier. Others attribute convulsions to DIC characterized by platelet-fibrin clots that obstruct the cerebral microcirculation.[51]

REMOTE PROGNOSIS AFTER PRE-ECLAMPSIA

The remote cardiovascular prognosis of pre-eclampsia is disputed.[12] Some authors claimed that pre-eclampsia increased the incidence of chronic hypertension and cardiovascular deaths later in life, while others suggested that pre-eclampsia per se had no influence on these events. The signal study in this area seems to be that of Chesley, who has periodically re-examined 267 and 270 women who survived eclampsia during the years 1931 to 1951. The last report included 1974 in that some of these patients have been observed for over 40 years.[11] A special feature of this study is that it included only women with eclampsia; in the absence of renal biopsy, a convulsion strongly suggests that the patient had pure or superimposed pre-eclampsia. Caucasian women convulsing as nulliparas had a remote mortality rate and blood pressure profile similar to that of age-matched unselected women. However, in those who convulsed as multiparas, the remote mortality was substantially increased and these women had higher blood pressures than age-matched subjects in several large epidemiological studies. In addition, the prevalence of hypertension was greater in eclamptic primiparas if any of their subsequent gestations was complicated by hypertension. Chesley concluded that eclampsia was not a predictive sign nor a cause of remote hypertension, and that hypertensive pregnancies in multiparas were probably predictive, but not the cause of future essential hypertension. Similar conclusions were reached by the Chicago group who investigated black women with renal biopsy evidence of pre-eclampsia.[2,47]

SUMMARY

Pre-eclampsia cannot be defined precisely by clinical signs which are just readily detectable secondary features of the primary abnormality within the uterus. The multisystem sequelae could be thought of as a secondary maternal adaptation, with the large variation in clinical presentation reflecting variable susceptibility of maternal target organs. The changes may be characteristic of pre-eclampsia but are not specific and therefore reflect a process rather than a discrete disease entity. Because the pathogenesis is so controversial it is not surprising that views on management differ so much.

REFERENCES

1. Redman, C. W. G., 1987, The definition of pre-eclampsia."Hypertension in Pregnancy", F. Sharp & E. M. Symonds (Eds), Perinatology Press, N.Y., 3.
2. Fisher, K. A., Ahuja, S., Luger, A., et al., 1977, Nephrotic proteinuria with preeclampsia, Amer. J Obst Gynec. 129:643.
3. Dunlop, W. and Davison, J. M., 1987, Renal haemodynamics and tubular function in human pregnancy, Clin Obstet Gynae, 1:269.
4. Hughes, E. C., 1972, In: Obstetric-Gynecologic Terminology, Davis, Philadelphia, 422.
5. MacGillivray, I., Rose, G. A. and Rowe, B., 1969, Blood pressure survey in pregnancy, Clin Sci, 37:395.
6. Redman, C. W. G., and Jefferies, M., 1988, Revised definition of preeclampsia, Lancet 1:809.
7. Nelson, T. R., 1955, A clinical study of preeclampsia, J Obs Gynae, Br.Emp. 62:48.
8. Brosens, I. A., Robertson, W. B. and Dixon, H.G., 1972, The role of the spiral arteries in the pathogenesis of preeclampsia. In: Obstetrics and Gynecology Annual. Ed.R. M. Wynn, Appleton-Century-Crofts, New York, 177.
9. Robertson, W. B., Brosens, I. and Dixon H.G., 1967, The pathological response of the vessels of the placental bed to hypertensive pregnancy, J Path Bact, 93:581.
10. Fox, H., 1987, Histopathology of pre-eclampsia and eclampsia, In: "Hypertension in Pregnancy" F. Sharp & E. M. Symonds (Eds), Perinatology Press, N.Y. 119.
11. Chesley, L. C., 1978, Hypertensive Disorders in Pregnancy, New York: Appleton-Century-Crofts.
12. Lindheimer, M. D., and Katz, A. I., 1986, The Kidney in Pregnancy.In B. M. Brenner and R. O. Rector, Jr., (eds.), The Kidney (3rd ed.). Philadelphia: Saunders, 1986.

13. Moore, L. G., Hersye, D. W., Jahnigen, D. et al, 1982, The incidence of pregnancy-induced hypertension is increased among Colorado residents at high altitude. Am.J.Obstet Gynecol, 144:423.
14. Editorial, 1980, Genetic control of pre-eclampsia. Lancet 1:34.
15. Birkeland, S. A., and Kristofferson, K., 1979, Preeclampsia: A state of mother-fetus immune imbalance, Lancet 2:720.
16.Froidart, J. M., Hunt, J., Lapiere, C. M., et al, 1986, Kidney Int. Antibodies to laminin in preeclampsia, 29;1050.
17. Beer, A. E., 1978, Possible immunologic basis of pre-eclampsia/eclampsia, Semin.Perinatol, 2:39.
18. Redman, C. W. G., Bodner, J. G., Bodner, W. F., et al, 1978, HLA antigens in severe pre-eclampsia, Lancet 2:397.
19. Chesley, L. G., and Cooper, D. W., 1986, Genetics of hypertension in pregnancy: Possible single gene control of pre-eclampsia and eclampsia in the descendants of eclamptic women, Br J Obstet Gynaecol 93:898.
20. Cooper, D. W., and Liston, W. A., 1979, Genetic control of preeclampsia, J Med Genet 16:409.
21. Scott, J. S., Jenkins, E. M., and Need, J.A. 1978, Immunology of pre-eclampsia, Lancet 1:704.
22. Gant, N. F., Daley, G. L., Chand, S., et al, 1973, A study of angiotensin II pressor respone throughout primigravid pregnancy, J Clin Invest, 52:2682.
23. Weir, R. J., Doig, A., Fraser, R., et al, 1976, Studies of the Renin-Angiotensin-Aldosterone Sstem, Cortisol, DOC and ADH in Normal and Hypertensive Pregnancy. In M. D. Lindheimer, A. I. Katz, and F. P. Zuspan (eds), Hypertension in Pregnancy. New York, Wiley.
24. Broughton-Pipkin, F., Craven, D. J., and Symonds, E. M., 1981, The uteroplacental renin-angiotensin system in normal and hypertensive pregnancy, Contrib Nephrol 25:49.
25. Gant, N. F., and Pritchard, J. A., 1984, Pregnancy-induced hypertension, Semin Nephrol 4:260.
26. Demers, J. M., and Gabbe, S. G., 1976, Placental prostaglandin levels in pre-eclampsia, Am J Obstet Gynecol 126: 137.
27.Editorial, 1982, Pregnancy and the arachidonic acid cascade, Lancet 1:997.
28. Lamming, G. D., Broughton-Pipkin, F., and Symonds, E. M., 1980, Comparison of the alpha and beta blocking drug, labetalol, and methldopa in the treatment of moderate and severe pregnancy-induced hypertension. Clin Exp Hypertens 2:865.
29. Wallenburg, H. C. S., Dekker, G. A., Makovitz, J. W., et al, 1986, Low-dose aspirin prevents pregnancy-induced hypertension and pre-eclampsia in angiotensin-sensitive primigravidae, Lancet 1:3.
30. Makila, U. M., Joupilla, P., Kirkinen, P., et al, 1983, Relation between umbilical prostacyclin production and blood flow on the fetus, Lancet 1:728.
31. Moodley, J., Norman, R. J., and Reddi, K, 1984, Central venous concentrations of immunoreactive prostaglandins E, F, and 6-keto-prostaglandin Fla in eclampsia, Br Med J,, 288:1487.
32. Walsh, S. W., 1985, Preeclampsia: An imbalance in placental prostacyclin and thromboxane production, Am J Obstet Gynecol, 152:335.
33. Ongari, M. A., Ritter, J.M., Orchard, M. A., et al, 1984, Correlation of prostacyclin synthesis by human umbilical artery with status of essential fatty acids, Am J Obstet Gynecol, 149:455.
34. Wickens, D., Wilkins, M. H., Lunec, J., et al, 1981, Free-radical oxidation (peroxidation) products in plasma in normal and abnormal pregnancy, Ann Clin Biochem, 18:158.
35. Gant, N. F., and Pritchard J. A., 1984, A pregnancy-induced hypertension, Semin Nephrol, 4:260.

36. Spitz, B., Deckmyn, H., Van Bree, R., et al, 1985, Influence of a vitamin-E-deficient diet on prostcyclin production by mesometrial triangles and aortic rings from non diabetic and diabetic pregnant rats, Am J Obstet Gynecol, 151:116.
37. Aladjem, S., Lueck, J., and Brewer, J. I., 1983, Experimental induction of a toxemia-like syndrome in the pregnant bragle, Am J Obstet Gynecol, 145:27.
38. Long , E. G., Tsin, T., Reinarz, J. A., et al 1984, "Hydatoxoi lualba" identified, Am J Obstet Gynecol 16:274.
39. Gau, G. S., Bhundia, J. P., Napier, K. A., et al, 1984, Observations on an organism reported to be associated with gestational pathology, J Obstet Gynaecol, 4:209.
40. Davison, J. M., and Lindheimer, M. D., 1987, Hypertension and Prengancy In: "Diseases of the Kidney" R W Schrier & C W Gottschalk Eds. Little Brown & Co. Boston 1653.
41. Naumann, R. O., and Weinstein, L., 1985, Disseminated intravascular coagulation - The clinican´s dilemma, Obstet Gynecol Surv, 40:487.
42. Kelton, J. G., Hunter, D. J. S., and Neasme, P. B., 1985, A platelet function defect in preeclampsia, Obstet Gynecol 65:107.
43. Goldenberg, R. L., Huddleston, J. F., Davis, R. O., et al, 1983, Toxaemia of pregnancy masquerading as idiopathic thrombocytopenic purpura, Obstet Gynecol, 62:32S.
44. Schwartz, M. L., and Brenner, W. E., 1983, Pregnancy-induced hypertensin presenting with life-threatening thrombocytopenis, Am J Obstet Gynecol, 146:757.
45. Weinstein, L., 1985, Preeclampsia/eclampsia with hemolysis, elevated liver enzymes and thrombocytopenia, Obstet Gynecol, 66:657.
46. Pritchard, J. A., 1980, Management of pre-eclampsia and eclampsia, Kidney Int, 18-259.
47. Fisher, K. A., Luger, A., Sparto, B. H., et al, 1981, Hypertnesion in pregnancy: Clinical pathological correlations and late prognosis, Medicine 60:267.
48. Gaber, L. W., Spargo, B. M., Lindheimer, M. D., 1987, Renal pathology in preeclampsia, Clin Obstet Gynae 1:971.
49. De Swiet, M, 1985, Some rare medical complications of pregnancy, Br Med J, 290:2.
50. Redman, C. W. G., 1984, The management of hypertension in pregnancy, Semin Nephrol, 4:270.
51. McKay, G. G., 1981, Chronic intravascular coagulation in normal pregnancy and pre-eclampsia, Contrib Nephrol, 25:108.

ELECTROLYTE DISTURBANCES AND THE KIDNEY

ELECTROLYTE ABNORMALITIES IN CANCER

Manuel Martínez-Maldonado, and
Julio E. Benabe

Renal Section, Medical Service, Veterans Administration Medical Center and Departments of Medicine & Physiology, University of Puerto Rico School of Medicine

INTRODUCTION

This review will briefly discuss various electrolyte disturbances that occur in patients suffering from cancer. We will highlight those alterations in plasma composition that are directly due to the presence of tumor. Indeed, substances produced by tumors may be responsible for the production of various alterations in plasma composition including changes in the concentration of sodium, potassium, calcium and phosphate.

Fictitious Electrolyte Disorders

Baffling clinical problems may arise from fictitious changes in electrolyte composition. Table 1 lists four potentially confusing situations in the clinical assesment of electrolyte disturbances. Pseudo or fictitious states of lack or excess of certain ions, can be induced by changes in plasma protein concentration that lead to alterations in the physicochemical properties of plasma. A reduction in the percent of water content of a plasma sample that results from the presence of excess protein concentration, as in multiple myeloma or Waldenstrom's macroglobulinemia, will lead to an apparent decrease of plasma sodium concentration.(1)

Myeloma may also be responsible for the induction of fictitious hypercalcemia and hyperphosphatemia.(2) Great rises in plasma globulin concentration can increase protein bound calcium without any variation from normal in the fraction of ionized calcium. The importance of identifying this innocous phenomenon can not be overstressed, lest it lead to inappropriate therapy for non-existent hypercalcemia. Clearly, some of the therapeutic modalities recommended for the true hypercalcemia of myeloma, such as mithramycin and steroids are not free of potential danger. Adler et al (3) first reported the occurence of hyperphosphatemia in the presence of normal renal function in subjects with myeloma. It was subsequently shown that this phenomenon is the result of interference of abnormal plasma proteins with automated methods of phosphate determination.(4)

TABLE 1 ELECTROLYTE ABNORMALITIES IN CANCER FICTITIOUS (PSEUDO)

1. HYPONATREMIA

↑Serum Globulins or Total Proteins
Myeloma

Macroglobulins (Waldenstrom's)

2. HYPERCALCEMIA

↑Total Calcium - ionized no Δ
Myeloma

3. HYPERPHOSPHATEMIA

Abnormal Globulins interfere with automated measurements

4. HYPERKALEMIA
↑Pk - Lysis of leukocytes ($>5\times10^5/mm^3$)
or Platelets ($>10^6/mm^3$)

Equally troublesome is the lysis of blood cells such as leukocytes or platelets during or after the blood sample has been obtained.(5) This process may result in release of potassium in the sample and to the erroneous diagnosis and treatment of false hyperkalemia. Conditions characterized by high counts of leukocytes and platelets --chronic myelogenous leukemia, for example-- are common causes.

Hypo- and Hypernatremia

Hypo and hypernatremia are frequently seen in patients with cancer. The syndrome of inappropriate secretion of ADH, which leads to increased permeability of the collecting duct to water, volume expansion with natriuresis, and hyponatremia has been the subject of extensive review (6), and will not be covered here.

Hypernatremia may occur when hypercalcemia is present. Under these circumstances polyuria or the excretion of poorly concentrated urine, may result from decreased distal solute delivery secondary to reduced renal plasma flow and glomerular filtration rate, combined with diminished sodium reabsorption in the thick ascending limb of Henle and the nephrogenic diabetes insipidus syndrome induced by hypercalcemia.(7) These conditions can lead to hypernatremia.

Not infrequently hypercalcemia and increased ADH secretion may coexist and lead to the unusual circumstance of SIADH with an urine osmolality hypotonic to plasma. Clearly, when required because of symptomatology, therapy is directed at eliminating the underlying cause of the disturbance.

Hypo- and hyperkalemia

Significant and symptomatic alterations in plasma sodium and potassium have other origins. Metastatic disease leading to adrenal destruction, will result in hypoadrenalism. Reduced secretion of cortisol and aldosterone, leads to the characteristic findings of hyponatremia and hyperkalemia.

Tumors may also secrete polypeptides, such as ACTH and renin, and stimulate secretion of both mineralo and glucocorticoids.(8) Hypokalemia and a tendency to hypernatremia will ensue. Adrenal carcinoma may result in primary hyperaldosteronism, a condition that, as in the case of ectopic ACTH or renin secretion, is characterized by hypokalemia, hypernatremia and saline resistant metabolic alkalosis.(9) Also, myelomonocytic and monocytic leukemia can be associated with increased urinary excretion of lysozyme, a substance known to produce kaliuresis, a factor that may contribute to hypokalemia.(10)

In addition to adrenal metastases, lysis of tumor cells, as a result of chemotherapy or from spontaneous tumor necrosis, may lead to hyperkalemia, particularly in the presence of mild or moderate renal impairment, or on the background of conditions that induce inability to handle potassium loads.

Hypo- and Hyperphosphatemia

Severe hypophosphatemia can occur because of cell lysis (11) or uptake of the ion by large cell masses. Moreover, the cachexia of cancer can be accompanied by respiratory alkalosis. Furthermore, these patients are frequently treated by hyperalimentation and/or the frequent administration of glucose solution, all stimulants of phosphate uptake and sequestration in cells.(12)

Hypophosphatemia can also be the result of the Fanconi Syndrome induced by tumoral substances.(13) Various tumors and multiple myeloma can produce inhibitors of proximal tubular function and lead to the Fanconi Syndrome (hypophosphatemia and hypokalemia, bicarbonaturia and diminished plasma bicarbonate, uricosuria and hypouricemia, glucosuria, despite normal blood glucose, and aminoaciduria).(13) In the case of multiple myeloma, those with high k-chain excretion are the ones mostly associated with the syndrome. Crystalline inclusions in the proximal tubule cells, presumed to be light chains, have been frequently found in these cases.

Oat-cell carcinomas of the lung and hemangiopericytomas may induce so-called oncogenic hypophosphatemic osteomalacia, of which proximal tubule dysfunction (Fanconi Syndrome) is also a prominent component. It is thought that a substance produced by the tumor is responsible for the functional and anatomical changes since regression of the syndrome occurs upon excision or successful therapy of the tumor.(14,15) The substance is presumed to diminish proximal tubular reabsorption of phosphate and diminish activity of 1-alpha hydroxylase. Furthermore, in some cases, proximal tubule anatomical changes have been observed.(16) The proximal tubular lesions and the reduced phosphate availability, which reduces oxygen consumption, may impair reabsorptive processes at this site, leading to loss of various substances in the urine. Also, diminished 1,25 dihydroxycholecalciferol with reduced intestinal reabsorption of calcium and phosphate, can increase PTH secretion. The resulting fall in proximal reabsorption of phosphate contributes to the Fanconi Syndrome. The hypophosphatemia and the diminished $1,25(OH)_2D_3$

result in osteomalacia.(17) This part of the syndrome has also been shown to regress upon successful therapy.

Acid-Base Disturbances

As shown in Table 2, in addition to proximal tubular acidosis, other acid-base disturbances can occur in cancer. Distal RTA may be seen in myeloma and lymphomas and in other lymphoproliferative disturbances.(18,19) Both of these, proximal and distal RTA, are non-anion gap acidoses when they are clearly clinically present. Usually, distal RTA is of the "incomplete" type. Rarely, distal RTA in cancer is associated with metabolic acidosis severe enough to lead to buffering of bone salts, bone dissolution and hypercalciuria. Under these circumstances, there is also decreased urinary citrate and relatively alkaline urine, that may cause calcium precipitation, nephrocalcinosis and renal lithiasis.(8) The mechanism of distal RTA is unclear, but cell products of either plasma cells or lymphocytes may lead to local immunogenic disorders that impair hydrogen ion secretion.

TABLE 2 ELECTROLYTE ABNORMALITIES IN CANCER ACID-BASE

1. ACIDOSIS
   - PROXIMAL RTA (FANCONI)
   - DISTAL RTA
     myeloma, lymphoma, etc.
   - HYPERCHLOREMIC
     Apudoma's (VIP)
   - LACTIC ACIDOSIS
     leukemias, lymphomas
   - KETOACIDOSIS
     steroid therapy, pancreatic CA
2. ALKALOSIS
   - ECTOPIC ACTH $\bar{c}$ ↑glucocortidoids
   - ECTOPIC RENIN
   - EXCESS ALDOSTERONE

Hyperchloremic metabolic acidosis may also occur as a result of secretions by APUDoma tumors. The severity of the diarrhea is the most important determinant of the clinical syndrome.

Neoplastic cell invasion of organs or clogging-up of vessels with cells, as can be seen in disseminated lymphomas and high cell count leukemias, may lead to poor oxygenation and acute lactic acid acidosis. Also, it is conceivable that massive number of white cells can produce sufficient lactate to contribute to the clinical picture. Nevertheless, chronic lactic acid acidosis may be seen in some patients with acute leukemia in whom a clear-cut cause for the acidosis cannot be identified.(20) It has also been shown that tumors themselves may produce lactic acid. In most cases of non-hematological solid tumors, massive tumoral infiltration of the liver has been present, suggesting a decreased ability of hepatic lactate extraction. It is of interest that some neoplastic cells fail to show inhibition of glycolysis when exposed to oxygen (the Pasteur effect). Clearly this could also contribute to continued lactate excess under some circumstances. Be that as it may, reduction in cell mass as a result of therapy will revert the abnormality in most cases.(21)

There have been rare reports of ketoacidosis (another anion-gap acidosis) in patients with cancer as a result of steroid therapy and in patients with carcinoma of the pancreas.

Saline responsive metabolic alkalosis as a result of vomiting in patients with cancer is common. It is also a frequent complication of the hypokalemia and volume contraction (from diarrhea) that accompanies villous adenoma of the colon. Resistant metabolic alkalosis as a consequence of excess glucocorticoid or aldosterone from ectopic production of ACTH or renin, or from aldosterone elaboration by an adrenal tumor, may also occur. In these cases extracellular volume contraction, hypokalemia and an inappropriately acid urine contribute to the alkalosis.

Tumor Lysis Syndrome (Acute renal failure, hypocalcemia, hyperphosphatemia and hyperkalemia)

One of the most dramatic events in the treatment of cancer is the development of the acute tumor lysis syndrome with acute renal failure. The usual setting for the syndrome is in the patient with a poorly differentiated, high cell turnover-rate tumor, such as Burkitt's lymphoma, or in leukemias, such as lymphosarcoma cell and acute lymphoblastic leukemia.(22,24) Clinically, there is usually marrow invasion and large abdominal masses in these patients. Plasma lactic dehydrogenase activity is very high as a result of malignant cell glycolytic activity. Therapy undertaken without the proper precautions leads to massive rises in serum uric acid, phosphate, and potassium, and hypocalcemia. Moreover, precipitation of calcium phophate crystals and uric acid in the renal parenchyma induces severe acute renal failure, clinically characterized by exceedingly high serum creatinine concentration.

Prevention is the key to success and includes adequate hydration, and the administration of intravenous bicarbonate prior to therapy make urine pH exceed or equal 7.0 to avoid uric acid precipitation. Intravenous or oral allopurinol administered in doses of 300 to 500 mg per meter square 24 to 48 hours prior to chemo or radiotherapy, also decreases uric acid precipitation. Oral phosphate binders will reduce the tendency to hyperphosphatemia. If the WBC count exceeds 100,000/cubic millimeter, continous flow leukopheresis will reduce the risks of developing renal failure. If renal insufficiency is present before therapy hemodialysis should be considered, particularly if plasma creatinine concentration exceeds 2 mg/dl. If acute renal failure has developed, hemodialysis must be continued throughout the period of treatment. Normalization of uric acid level should prompt discontinuation of alkalinization to prevent the added danger of calcium phosphate precipitation. Treatment should also be watchful of the development of hypocalcemia, which merits immediate attention if symptomatic.

Hypocalcemia

The hyperphosphatemia of tumor lysis syndrome is probably the commonest cause of hypocalcemia associated with cancer. In one of the largest series reported so far 100% of the patients who developed acute renal failure with tumor lysis syndrome had hypocalcemia.(23) The hypocalcemia, particularly in patients harboring large cellular mass tumors, correlates directly with the degree of hyperphosphatemia.

It should be pointed out that some cancer patients have hypomagnesemia as the underlying cause for hypocalcemia. Also, therapy with cis-platin or gentamycin (and other aminoglycosides) may induce hypomagnesemia and, ultimately, hypocalcemia.

Hypercalcemia

One of the most exciting areas of recent investigation relates to the mechanisms of the hypercalcemia seen in patients with malignant disease. Because of space constraints, we will not be able to provide more than a schematic view of the novel findings in this area.

Clearly, the problem of hypercalcemia is serious: it has been estimated that cancer is responsible for 150 new cases of hypercalcemia per million population per year.(24) The general incidence is between 10% and 20%. It should be pointed out that hematologic malignant neoplasms are responsible for twice as many cases of hypercalcemia than solid tumors.

Mundy has best summarized the patterns of abnormalities in calcium homeostasis seen in the commonest malignancies that cause hypercalcemia.(25) Under normal circumstances, net gut reabsorption equals net calcium excretion, and bone resorption does not differ from bone formation. In multiple myeloma, there is increased bone resorption and decreased bone formation. Despite a diminution in gut calcium reabsorption, the reduction in its filtered load, because of impaired glomerular filtration, leads to hypercalcemia. In lung cancer, is a model of a solid tumor where bone metastases may or may not be present; bone formation and gut reabsorption, however, are similar to those in multiple myeloma. Yet, renal calcium reabsorption and, frequently, nephrogenous cyclic AMP are increased, suggesting the action of a substance capable of stimulating adenyl cyclase and causing increased calcium reabsorption as is the case with PTH. The situation in breast cancer is similar to that in lung cancer except that these patients usually have bone metastases and no increment in nephrogenous cyclic AMP. Finally, there is the unusual group of patients with various lymphomas and other malignancies whose hypercalcemia results from increased 1,25-dihydroxyvitamin D_3 concentration associated with increased bone resorption.

While hypercalcemia is more common in multiple myeloma than in other hematological disorders, it is present in almost all patients with human T-cell lymphotropic virus, type-1 adult T-cell lymphoma. Some of these patients have increased serum concentration of 1,25 dihydroxyvitamin D and increased calcium reabsorption from the gut, in clear contrast to most other forms of hypercalcemia of malignancy, in which both gut reabsorption and vitamin D levels are diminished.(26) Moreover, Mundy's group has shown that lymphoid cells infected with this virus can convert 25 hydroxyvitamin D_3 to 1,25 dihydroxyvitamin D_3.(27)

Metastases to bone are the commonest cause of hypercalcemia in cancer (28), but will not be discussed here so that we may concentrate on some of the recent developments in our understanding of humoral hypercalcemia.

As knowledge of the mechanisms of bone resorption in malignancy has expanded, it is clear that some substances play a major role in the hypercalcemia of malignancy. Some controversy exists among the experts in the field as to their nature and their relative importance, but we will attempt to give a general view of the most important factors involved. Six factors have been so far described as mediators of humorally-induced hypercalcemia.

Some of the characteristics of transforming growth factor alpha (TGF alpha) are listed in Table 3. We will not discuss TGF beta because less is known about its effects on bone. Many of the solid tumors associated with hypercalcemia produce TGF alpha. The human and murine polypeptide have been purified and the genes have been cloned. TGF is a 5000 dalton polypeptide with a sequence of 50 amino acids. The precursor molecule has a relatively unique structure without a leader sequence and an amino acid configuration suggesting that it is a transmembrane protein. Epidermal growth factor (EGF) receptor binds TGF alpha and all its effects are mediated through this receptor. Despite an homology of less than 40% with EGF, TGF alpha causes all the known biological effects of EGF. As in the case of EFG, TGF alpha stimulates osteoclastic bone resorption. Mundy and his collaborators have also found that TGF alpha stimulates formation of cells with osteoclastic characteristics by increasing proliferation of mononuclear cells.(29) Moreover, Tashjian et al (30) have demonstrated that EGF and recombinant human TGF alpha induce hypercalcemia when injected into intact mice. The hypercalcemia is independent of dietary calcium. These studies provide further evidence of the possibility that these and other related growth factors are potential mediators of tumor-induced hypercalcemia.

Recently it has become apparent that a PTH-like substance may be involved in tumoral hypercalcemia as well. Table 4 indicates some of the characteristics of the substance produced by tumors. About two thirds of the first amino acids of the factor are the same as those of the parathyroid hormone. In addition, it resembles PTH in its ability to stimulate adenylate cyclase in cultures of bone or kidney cells, resulting in increased levels of cyclic AMP. Moreover, a synthetic peptide from human tumor hypercalcemic factor was shown to be partially homologous to PTH in the aminoterminal 1-34 region. It interacted in vitro with PTH receptors and, in some systems, was more potent than PTH.(31) It also enhances bone resorption in vitro and causes calcium retention in isolated perfused rat kidneys.(32) Merendino et al (33) have suggested that the substance is similar to that produced by keratinocytes. These are skin cells that are the normal cellular counterparts of the squamous epithelial cells that form the kinds of tumors more likely to make the PTH-like peptide.

TABLE 3

TRANSFORMING GROWTH FACTOR

1) TGF ALPHA

- *PRODUCED BY TUMORS INCLUDING SOLID TUMORS COMMONLY ASSOCIATED WITH HYPERCALCEMIA
- *RAT AND HUMAN GENES HAVE BEEN CLONED
- *5000 DALTON / 50 AMINOACID SEQUENCE
- *EPIDERMAL GROWTH FACTOR RECEPTOR BINDS TGF ALPHA
- *AA HOMOLOGY <40% WITH EGF
- *STIMULATES OSTEOCLASTIC BONE RESORPTION (AS DOES EGF)

TABLE 4

PARATHYROID HORMONE-LIKE FACTORS

- *STRUCTURE SIMILAR TO THE PTH MOLECULE 2/3 OF THE FIRST 15 AMINO ACIDS ARE THE SAME AS THOSE OF PTH
- *STIMULATES ADENYLATE CYCLASE IN CULTURES OF BONE OR KIDNEY CELLS (↑ CAMP)
- *APPEARS TO ENHANCE BONE RESORPTION IN VITRO
- *MAY BE SIMILAR TO IF NOT IDENTICAL WITH A FACTOR PRODUCED BY KERATINOCYTES (THE NORMAL CELLULAR COUNTERPARTS OF THE SQUAMOUS EPITHELIAL CELLS THAT FORM THE KINDS OF TUMORS MOST LIKELY TO MAKE THE PTH-LIKE PEPTIDE)

Prostaglandins of the E series can produce bone resorption in vitro and lead to hypercalcemia when present in large concentrations. However, most patients do not respond to indomethacin or related drugs and it is difficult, if not impossible, at present to assign a role for prostaglandins in the humoral hypercalalcemia.

Cytokines of various kinds are produced by malignant cells. Bone resorbing activity, known as osteoclastic activating factor or OAF, is released by myeloma cells and by malignant lymphoid cell lines. It is now clearly apparent that a number of cytokines resorb bone and thus are potential members of the OAF family. These include interleukin-1, both alpha and beta molecules, lymphotoxin, and tumor necrosis factor. Possibly, many hematological malignancies involving monocytic cells may release interleukin-1 or tumor necrosis factor as the mediators of bone destruction.(25)

Space constraints forbid a detailed analysis of the remaining two factors: 1,25 dihydroxyvitamin D and colony-stimulating factor. In a small group of patients these two have been found to be potential mediators of hypercalcemia. A few patients with hypercalcemia and lymphoid malignancies have been described that exhibited elevated circulating concentrations of 1,25- dihydroxycholecalciferol. This, as already mentioned, contrasts with the majority of patients with the hypercalcemia of malignant disease, in whom 1,25-(OH)$_2$D$_3$ and gut calcium resorption are reduced.(34,35) Further studies, particularly of the possible role of vitamin D metabolites in some cases of adult T-cell lymphoma and Hodgkin's disease, will be necessary. Yet, the possibility that 1,25-(OH)$_2$D$_3$ mediates bone resorption is strengthened by the recent report that it may stimulate osteoblastic cells to release a soluble factor that increases osteoclastic bone resorption.(36)

The hypercalcemia of malignancy has also been reported in patients with marked leukocytosis. Inoculation of nude mice with these tumors has resulted in hypercalcemia and leukocytosis. The tumor extracts have contained colony-stimulating factors of the granulocyte-macrophage type. The nature of these factors, their appearance in patients from specific geographic areas (common in Japan, uncommon in United States), and other characteristics remain to be elucidated.(25,36,37)

It is amply clear that the mechanisms for increased bone resorption and hypercalcemia in malignancy are complex and heterogenous. Elucidation of these mechanisms may lead to the development of specific therapies of hypercalcemia according to their origin.

REFERENCES

1. M. Martínez-Maldonado, and L. Báez-Díaz, Renal Involvement in Multiple Myeloma, in: Nephrology, Vol. II, Proceedings of the IXth International Congress of Nephrology, R.R. Robinson, ed., Springer-Verlag, New York (1984).
2. J.P. Jaffe, and D.F. Mosher, Calcium binding by myeloma proteins, Am J Med 67:343-346 (1979).
3. S.G. Adler, S.A. Laidlaw, M.M. Lubran, Hyperglobulinemia may spuriously elevate measured inorganic phosphate, abstracted. Kidney Int 25:157 (1984).
4. J.C. Busse, M.A. Gelbard, J.J. Byrnes, R. Hellman, C.A. Vaamonde, Pseudohyperphosphatemia and dysproeinemia. Arch Intern Med 147:2045-2046 (1987).
5. W.R. Bronson, V.T. Devita, P.P. Carboneand E. Cotlove, Pseudohyperkalemia due to release of potassium from white blood cells during clotting, N Engl J Med 274:369-373 (1966).
6. M. Martínez-Maldonado, Idiopathic syndrome of inappropriate antidiuretic hormone secretion, Kidney Int 17(4):126-140 (1980).
7. J.E. Benabe, and M. Martínez-Maldonado, Hypercalcemic nephropathy, Arch Intern Med 138:777-779 (1978).
8. M. Fichman, and J. Bethune, Effects of neoplasms on renal electrolyte function, Ann NY Acad Sci 230:448-471 (1974).
9. D. Farge, G. Chatellier, J.Y. Pagny, X Jeunemaitre, P.F. Plouin, P. Corval, Isolated clinical syndrome of primary aldosteronism in four patients with adrenocortical carcinoma, Am J Med 83:635-640 (1987).
10. F.M. Muggia, H.O. Heinemann, M. Farhangi, and E.F. Osserman, Lysozymuria and renal tubular dysfunction in monocytic and myelomonocytic leukemia, Am J Med 47:351-366 (1969).
11. G.C. Tsokos, J.E. Balow, R.J. Spiegel, and I.T. Magrath, Renal and metabolic complications of undifferentiated and lymphoblastic lymphomas, Medicine 60:218-229 (1981).
12. J.P. Knochel, The pathophysiology and clinical characteristics of severe hypophosphatemia, Arch

Intern Med 137:203-220 (1977).
13. M. Martínez-Maldonado, J. Yium, W. Suki, and G.E. Eknoyan, Renal complications in multiple myeloma: Pathophysiology and some aspects of clinical management, J Chronic Dis 24:221-237 (1971).
14. D.J. Leehey, T.S. Ing, and J.T. Daugirdas, Fanconi syndrome associated with a non-ossifying fibroma of bone, Am J Med 78:708-710 (1985).
15. E.A. Ryan, and E. Reiss, Oncogenous osteomalacia: Review of the world literature of 42 cases and report of two new cases, Am J Med 77:501-512 (1984).
16. F. Lustman, R. Parmentier, and P. Dustin, Oncogenic osteomalacia and renal adenoid dysplasia, Ann Intern Med 102:869-870 (1985).
17. M.K. Drezner, and M.N. Feinglos, Osteomalacia due to 1 α,25 dihydroxycholecalciferol deficiency: Association with giant cell tumor of bone, J Clin Invest 60:1046-1053 (1977).
18. G.S. Lazar, and D.I. Feinstein, Distal renal tubular acidosis in multiple myeloma, Arch Intern Med 141:655-657 (1981).
19. R.C. Morris, Jr, and H.H. Fudenberg, Impaired renal acidification in patients with hypergammaglobulinemia, Medicine 46:57-62 (1967).
20. G.J. Roth, and D. Porte, Jr, Chronic lactic acidosis and acute leukemia, Arch Intern Med 125:317-321 (1970).
21. K. Rice, and S.H. Schwartz, Lactic acidosis with small cell carcinoma: Rapid response to chemotherapy, Am J Med 79:501-503 (1985).
22. J. Zusman, D.M. Brown, and M.E. Nesbit, Hyperphosphatemia, hyperphosphaturia and hypocalcemia in acute lymphoblastic leukemia, N Engl J Med 289:1335-1340 (1973).
23. L.F. Cohen, J.E. Balow, I.T. Magrath, D.G. Poplack, and J.L. Ziegler, Acute tumor lysis syndrome: A review of 37 patients with Burkitt's lymphoma, Am J Med 68:486-491 (1980).
24. G.R. Mundy, K.J. Ibbotson, S.M. D'Souza, E.L. Simpson, J.W. Jacobs, and T.J. Martin, The hypercalcemia of cancer: Clinical implications and pathogenic mechanisms, N Engl J Med 310:1718-1726 (1984).
25. G.R. Mundy, The hypercalcemia of malignancy, Kidney Int 31:142-155 (1987).
26. N.A. Breslau, J.L. McGuire, J.E. Zerwekh, E.P. Frenkel and C.Y.Z. Pak, Hypercalcemia associated with increased serum calcitriol levels in three patients with lymphoma, N Engl J Med 100:1-7 (1984).
27. D.A. Fetchick, D.R. Bertolini, P. Sarin, G.R. Mundy, and J.F. Dunn, Metabolism of 25-hydroxyvitamin D by human T cell lymphotrophic virus-transformed cord blood lymphocytes, J Bone Miner Res 1:323 (1986).
28. H.I. Scher, and A. Yagoda, Bone metastases: Pathogenesis, treatment and rationale for use of resorption inhibitors, Am J Med 82(Suppl 2A):6-28 (1987).
29. J. Hon, G.R. Mundy, R. Derynck, and G.D. Roodman, Recombinant human transforming growth factor (TGF-α) stimulates the formation of osteoclast (OCL)-like cells in long term human marrow cultures, J Bone Miner Res 1:68 (1986).
30. A.H. Tashjian, Jr, E.F. Voelkel, W. Lloyd, R. Derynck, M.E. Winkler and L. Levine, Actions of growth factors

on plasma calcium, J Clin Invest 78:1405-1409 (1986).
31. N. Horiuchi, M.P. Caulfield, J.E. Fisher, M.E. Goldman, R.L. McKee, J.E. Reagan, J.J. Levy, R.F. Nutt, S.B. Rodan, T.L. Schofield, T.L. Clemens, M. Rosenblatt, Similarity of synthetic peptide from human tumor to parathyroid hormone in vivo and in vitro, Science 238:1566-1568 (1987).
32. B.E. Kemp, J.M. Moseley, C.P. Rodda, P.R. Ebeling, R.E.H. Wettenhall, D. Stapleton, H. Diffenbach-Jagger, F. Ure, V.P. Michelangeli, H.A. Simmons, L.G. Raisz, T.J. Martin, Parathyroid hormone-related protein of malignancy: Active synthetic fragments, Science 238:1568-1570 (1987).
33. J.J. Merendino, Jr, K.L. Insogna, L.M. Milstone, A.E. Broadus, and A.F. Stewart, A parathyroid hormone-like protein from cultured human keratinocytes, Science 231:388-390 (1986).
34. K.J. Ibbotson, D.R. Twardzik, S.M. D'Souza, W.R. Hargreaves, G.J. Todaro, G.R. Mundy, Stimulation of bone resorption in vitro by synthetic transforming growth factor-alpha, Science 228:1007-1009 (1985).
35. K.J. Ibbotson, J. Harrod, M. Gowen, Effects of human transforming growth factor (TGF) alpha on bone resorption and formation in vitro, Proc Natl Acad Sci USA 83:2228-2232 (1986).
36. P.M.J. McSheehy, and T.J. Chambers, 1,25-Dihydroxyvitamin D_3 stimulates rat osteoblastic cells to release a soluble factor that increases osteoclastic bone resorption, J Clin Invest 80:425-429 (1987).
37. K. Sato, H. Mimura, D.C. Han, T. Kakiuchi, Y. Ueyama, H. Ohkawa, T. Okabe, Y. Kondo, N. Ohsawa, T. Tsushima, K. Shizume, Production of bone resorbing activity and colony stimulating activity in vivo and in vitro by a human squamous cell carcinoma associated with hypercalcemia and leukocytosis, J Clin Invest 78:145-154, 1986.

HYPERCALCEMIA AND THE KIDNEY

Wadi N. Suki

Baylor College of Medicine
Renal Section - 6565 Fannin
Houston, Texas 77030

Infrequently, the kidney may be involved in the etiology of hypercalcemia as might occur in diuretic-induced hypercalcemia (1) or the hypercalcemia of adrenal insufficiency (2), in which hypocalciuria and sodium and water diuresis may play a role. In these circumstances, the kidney may be considered the culprit in hypercalcemia. More often, however, the kidney is the victim of hypercalcemia suffering a number of derangements in hemodynamics and tubular function. The focus of this review shall be on the derangements in the structure and function of the kidney in hypercalcemic states. The spectrum of disorders of renal function and structure in hypercalcemia is summarized in Table 1. It is evident that a wide-range of renal derangements is observed in hypercalcemia. Consequently, only a few of these derangements will be the subject of a more detailed discussion.

Renal Hemodynamics

Acute hypercalcemia usually results in a decline in renal plasma flow and in the glomerular filtration rate. The decline in renal plasma flow is due to renal vasoconstriction induced by hypercalcemia (3). The decline in renal plasma flow will in turn cause a reduction in the glomerular filtration rate. It has been demonstrated, in addition, that hypercalcemia in the presence of parathyroid hormones can cause a reduction in the glomerular filtration coefficient (4), K_f, which is a function of both the filtering surfacing area, A, and the hydraulic permeability of the membrane, L_p,. Whether the reduction in K_f is the result of a diminution in the surface area, as might result from mesangial cell contraction, or from an impairment in the hydraulic permeability is not clear. When the hypercalcemia is persistent, renal function may deteriorate to the point of causing renal failure.

TABLE 1. Derangements in renal function and structure in hypercalcemia

A.	Renal Hemodynamics:	Decreased RBF Decreased GFR Renal Failure
B.	Monovalent Cation Excretion:	Sodium diuresis Kaliuresis
C.	Mineral Metabolism:	Hypercalciuria Hypermagnesuria Decreased/Increased Phosphate Excretion
D.	Acid-Base Balance:	Metabolic Alkalosis Metabolic Acidosis
E.	Urine Concentration:	Impaired Concentration
F.	Renal Structure:	Nephrocalcinosis Nephrolithiasis

Cation Excretion

The excretion of both sodium and potassium is increased by hypercalcemia (5). The sodium diuresis induced by hypercalcemia appears to be due to inhibition of sodium absorption in the proximal tubule (6,7), the thick ascending limb of Henle's loop (8,9), and in the distal tubule (10). Although the mechanism of these alterations is not fully known, it is possible that hypercalcemia increases the concentration of cytoplasmic calcium and that, in turn, exerts a negative effect on transport processes involved in the transepithelial translocation of sodium. Compounds which activate the calcium and phospholipid-sensitive protein kinase-C have recently been shown to inhibit proximal tubular transport (11). In addition, calcium is known to inhibit Na, K-ATPase (12). The urinary excretion of potassium is also increased in hypercalcemic states (5). This may result in clinical hypokalemia (13). The increased potassium excretion may be a consequence of the increased presentation of sodium to the distal nephron, coupled with activation of renin (14) and aldosterone caused by the hypercalcemia, sodium diuresis and intravascular volume depletion.

Mineral Metabolism

Hypercalcemia results in increased excretion of calcium and magnesium (15,16). The inhibition of the transport of these two cations appears to be localized to the proximal convoluted tubule (6) and the thick ascending limb of Henle's loop (17). The increased excretion of magnesium in hypercalcemic states may account for the hypomagnesemia encountered not infrequently in these disorders (16).

Elevation of the serum calcium may have divergent effects on the renal handling of phosphate. The acute elevation of serum calcium will often result in enhanced tubular absorption of phosphate (18). This has been shown to be a direct effect on proximal tubular phosphate transport exerted from the luminal surface presumably on sodium phosphate cotransport (19). The more chronic administration of calcium, however, results in depressed renal tubular absorption of phosphate (20). The exact mechanism of this latter effect is not known but may be due to increases in cytosolic calcium and activation of calcium-dependent pathways which may in turn inhibit the transepithelial translocation of phosphate.

Acid-Base Disorders

Both metabolic alkalosis (21) and metabolic acidosis (22) have been observed in hypercalcemic states. The acute administration of calcium and elevation of the serum calcium has been shown to raise the renal threshold for bicarbonate absorption (23). By contrast, the acute administration of parathyroid hormone has been shown to lower the renal threshold for bicarbonate (23). These effects of calcium and of PTH on HCO_3 transport have been reproduced in the isolated renal tubule microperfused in vitro (24,25). It would have been possible to extrapolate from these findings, therefore, that hypercalcemia resulting from disorders associated with suppressed parathyroid hormone would result in metabolic alkalosis while hypercalcemia resulting from elevated parathyroid hormone levels would result in metabolic acidosis. However, studies in which hypercalcemia was produced chronically by the administration of 1,25-dihydroxy cholecalciferol on the one-hand, or parathyroid hormone on the other have demonstrated the development of metabolic alkalosis under both circumstances (26). The source of the alkalosis appears to have been of non-renal origin, most likely buffer generated from bone dissolution, while the maintenance of the metabolic alkalosis must have been of renal origin since net acid excretion was not appropriately depressed. The augmented renal alkali absorption may have been due to the increased levels of 1,25 dihydroxycholecalciferol generated by exogenous administration in the former model, while in the latter model stimulated by the exogenous PTH administration. Hypercalcemia induced by exogenous calcium, however, resulted in metabolic acidosis (26). This may be due to the consumption of buffer which occurs when calcium salts are deposited in bone or in tissues. Another cause for the acidosis, which may be observed in hypercalcemic states may be the suppression of ammonia production which has been observed to occur with hypercalcemia per se (27), but which also may follow the loss of nephron mass when hypercalcemia has been severe and protracted resulting in nephrocalcinosis and renal insufficiency.

Urine Concentration

One of the commonest disorders in hypercalcemic states is that of polydipsia and polyuria accompanied by impairment in the renal concentrating ability (28). At least five factors may be responsible for the impaired urinary concentration: a) polydipsia resulting in polyuria and impaired concentration: In studies in rats, pair watered hypercalcemic rats exhibited improved urine concentration when compared to hypercalcemic rats allowed water ad lib (29); b) inhibition of sodium transport in the loop of Henle and impairment in the generation of hypertonic renal medulla (8,9): this effect may be in part a direct consequence of hypercalcemia, but in part may be due to increased prostaglandin production (30). Prostaglandins have been shown to inhibit sodium chloride transport in the medullary thick ascending limb (31). In at least one study, inhibition of prostaglandin production has been shown to ameliorate the concentrating defect of hypercalcemia in experimental animals (30). Conflicting results exist on this point, however, and other studies of the maximum urinary osmolality have shown that a brief exposure to indomethacin does not rectify the impairment in concentrating ability (29); c) impaired responsiveness of the collecting duct to vasopressin, due either directly to hypercalcemia per se, or secondarily to stimulation of prostaglandin production. Prostaglandin has been shown to inhibit the hydroosmotic effect of ADH on the cortical collecting tubule (32). The effects of calcium on collecting duct function have been conflicting. While an increase in calcium in the bathing medium did not impair the response of collecting tubules to ADH (33), studies in which intracellular calcium was increased have demonstrated an impairment in the responsiveness to ADH (34-36). Furthermore, activation of calcium and phospholipid-sensitive protein kinase-C with phorbol esters has also been shown to impair the effect of ADH on the collecting tubule (37). It is possible, therefore, that when hypercalcemia is sustained and cytoplasmic calcium concentration becomes elevated, concentrating function in the kidney will become impaired as a result of disordered collecting tubule function. Increased renal production of prostaglandins may play a contributing role. However, a recent study has demonstrated the important role of tubular transport of calcium rather than hypercalcemia per se (38). When animals made hypercalcemic were also phosphate restricted, so that tubular transport of calcium was reduced, the concentrating defect was totally prevented. It is possible, therefore, that the transcellular movement of calcium and, consequently, the elevation in cytoplasmic calcium may play a pivotal role in the development of impaired urinary concentration. Other factors contributing to the impaired concentrating ability are: d) increased medullary blood flow (39), and e) inhibition by hypercalcemia of ADH-dependent cAMP generation in the renal medulla (40) and in the thick ascending limb (41).

Renal Structure

In persistent hypercalcemia, nephrolithiasis and nephrocalcinosis occur (42,43). In this disorder calcium is deposited in the tubular lumina, tubular cells and in the interstitium leading to interstitial fibrosis and scarring (44).

It is clear from the foregoing that calcium elevation in the blood may have profound effects on a wide spectrum of renal function. While the mechanisms responsible for these derangements have been elucidated considerably in the last two decades, a great deal more remains to be done to more fully understand the physiologic and biochemical basis for these derangements.

REFERENCES

1. W.N. Suki, Effects of diuretics on calcium metabolism, Min. Elect. Metab., 2:125 (1979).
2. M. Walser, B.H. B. Robinson, and J.W. Duckett, Jr., The hypercalcemia of adrenal insufficiency, J. Clin. Invest., 42:456 (1963).
3. C.A. Edvall, Renal function in hyperparathyroidism. A clinical study of 30 cases with special reference to selective renal clearance and renal vein catheterization, Acta Chir. Scand., 229(Suppl):1 (1958).
4. H.D. Humes, I. Ichikawa, J.L. Troy, and B.M. Brenner, Evidence for a parathyroid hormone-dependent influence of calcium on the glomerular filtration, J. Clin. Invest., 61:32 (1978).
5. G. Fulgraff, G. Heinz, E. Sparwald, and O. Heidenreich, Die Wirkung von Calcium auf die Renale Ausscheidung von Kalium und Wasser und auf den renalen Solutengradienten beim Hund, Naunyn-Schmiedebergs, Arch, Pharmak. u. exp. Path., 261:299 (1968).
6. B.R. Edwards, R.A.L. Sutton, and J.H. Dirks, Effect of calcium infusion on renal tubular reabsorption in the dog, Am. J. Physiol. 227:13 (1974).
7. G.F. DiBona, Effect of hypercalcemia on renal tubular sodium handling in the rat, Am. J. Physiol. 220:49, 1971.
8. W.N. Suki, G. Eknoyan, F.C. Rector, Jr., and D.W. Seldin, The renal diluting and concentrating mechanism in hypercalcemia, Nephron, 6:50 (1969).
9. J-P. Guignard, N.F. Jones, and M.A. Barraclough, Effect of brief hypercalcaemia on free water reabsorption during solute diuresis: Evidence for impairment of sodium transport in Henle's loop, Clin. Sci., 39:337 (1970).
10. V. Guttman, and C.W. Gottschalk, Micropuncture study of the effect of calcium on sodium transport in the rat kidney, Israel J. Med. Sci., 2:243 (1966).
11. M. Baum, and S.R. Hayes, Phorbol myristate acetate and dioctanoylglycerol inhibit transport in rabbit proximal convoluted tubule, Am. J. Physiol., 254:F9 (1988).
12. F.H. Epstein, and R. Whitham, The mode of inhibition by calcium of cell-membrane adenosine-triphosphatase activity, Biochem. J., 99:232 (1966).
13. J.F. Zilva, and J.P. Nicholson, Plasma phosphate and potassium levels in the hypercalcemia of malignant disease, J. Clin. Endocrinol. Metab., 36:1019 (1973).
14. G.S. Brinton, W. Jubiz, L.D. Lagerqiust, Hypertension in primary hyperparathyroidism: The role of the renin-angiotensin system, J. Clin. Endocrinol. Metab., 41:1025 (1975).

15. R.A.L. Sutton, Disorders of renal calcium excretion, Kidney Int., 23:665 (1983).
16. R.A.L. Sutton, Plasma magnesium concentration in primary hyperparathyroidism, Brit. Med. J., 1:529 (1970).
17. G.A. Quamme, Effect of hypercalcemia on renal tubular handling of calcium and magnesium, Can. J. Physiol. Pharmacol., 60:1275 (1982).
18. A.R. Lavender, and T.N. Pullman, Changes in inorganic phosphate excretion induced by renal arterial infusion of calcium, Am. J. Physiol., 205:1025 (1963).
19. D. Rouse, and W.N. Suki, Modulation of phosphate absorption by calcium in the rabbit proximal convoluted tubule, J. Clin. Invest., 76:630 (1986).
20. E. Eisenberg, Effect of serum calcium level and parathyroid extracts on phosphate and calcium excretion in hypoparathyroid pateints, J. Clin. Invest., 44:942 (1965).
21. H.O. Heinemann, Metabolic alkalosis in patients with hypercalcemia, Metab. (Clin. Exp.), 14:1137 (1965).
22. A.A. Siddiqui, and D.R. Wilson, Primary hyperparathyroidism and proximal renal tubular acidosis: Report of two cases, Can. Med. Assoc. J. 106:654 (1972).
23. C.K. Crumb, M. Martinez-Maldonado, G. Eknoyan, and W.N. Suki, Effects of volume expansion, purified parathyroid extract, and calcium on renal bicarbonate absorption in the dog, J. Clin. Invest., 54:1287 (1974).
24. T.D. McKinney, and P. Myers, Effect of calcium and phosphate on bicarbonate and fluid transport by proximal tubules in vitro, Kidney Int., 21:433 (1982).
25. T.D. McKinney, and P. Myers, PTH inhibition of bicarbonate transport by proximal convoluted tubules, Am. J. Physiol., 39:F127 (1980).
26. H.N. Hulter, A. Sebastian, R.D. Toto, E.L. Bonner, Jr., and L.P. Ilnicki, Renal and systemic acid-base effects of the chronic administration of hypercalcemia-producing agents: Calcitriol, PTH, and intravenous calcium, Kidney Int., 21:445 (1982).
27. H.O. Heinemann, Reversible defect in renal ammonium excretion in patients with hypercalcemia, Metab., 12:792 (1963).
28. S.L. Cohen, M.C. Fitzgerald, P. Fourman, W.J. Griffith, and H.E. de Wardener, Polyuria in hyperparathyroidism, Quart. J. Med., 26:423 (1957).
29. M. Levi, L. Peterson, and T. Berl, Mechanism of concentrating defect in hypercalcemia. Role of polydipsia and prostaglandins, Kidney Int., 23:489 (1983).
30. E.R. Serros, and M.A. Kirschenbaum, Prostaglandin-dependent polyuria in hypercalcemia, Am. J. Physiol., 241:F224 (1981).

31. J.B. Stokes, Effect of prostaglandin E_2 on chloride transport across the rabbit thick ascending limb of Henle: Selective inhibition of the medullary portion, J. Clin. Invest., 64:495 (1979).
32. J.J. Grantham, J. Orloff, Effects of prostaglandin E_1 on the permeability response of the isolated collecting tubule to vasopressin, adenosine 3',5' monophosphate and theophylline, J. Clin. Invest., 47:1154 (1968).
33. S. Goldfarb, Effects of calcium on ADH action in the cortical collecting tubule perfused in vitro, Am.J. Physiol., 243:F481 (1982).
34. G. Frindt, E.E. Windhager, and A. Taylor, Hydroosmotic response of collecting tubules to ADH or cAMP at reduced peritubular sodium, Am. J. Physiol., 243:F503 (1982).
35. M. Lorenzen, G. Frindt, A. Taylor, and E.E. Windhager, Quinidine effect on hydroosmotic response of collecting tubules to vasopressin and cAMP, Am. J. Physiol., 252:F1103 (1987).
36. S.M. Jones, G. Frindt, and E.E. Windhager, Effect of peritubular [Ca] or ionomycin on hydroosmotic response of CCTs to ADH or cAMP, Am. J. Physiol., 245:F240 (1988).
37. H.R. Jacobson, and M.D. Breyer, Phorbol myristate acetate, dioctanoylglycerol, and phosphatidic acid inhibit the hydroosmotic effect of vasopressin on rabbit cortical collecting tubule, J. Clin. Invest., 8:590 (1987).
38. D.C.H. Harris, P.A. Gabow, S.L. Linas, D.E. Rosendale, S.P. Guggenheim, and R.W. Schrier, Prevention of hypercalcemia-induced renal concentrating defect and tissue calcium accumulation, Am. J. Physiol., 251:F642 (1986).
39. M.G. Brunette, J. Vary, and S. Carriere, Hyposthenuria in hypercalcemia. A possible role of intrarenal blood-flow (IRBF) redistribution, Pflugers Arch. 350:9 (1974).
40. N. Beck, H. Singh, and S.W. Reed, Pathogenic role of cyclic AMP in the impairment of urinary concentrating ability in acute hypercalcemia, J. Clin. Invest., 54:1049 (1974).
41. K. Takaichi, S. Uchida, and K. Kurokawa, High Ca^{++} inhibits AVP-dependent cAMP production in thick ascending limbs of Henle, Am. J. Physiol., 250:F770 (1986).
42. C.E. Dent, Some problems of hyperparathyroidism, Brit. Med. J., 2:1419 (1962).
43. H.M. Lloyd, Primary hyperparathyroidism. Analysis of the role of the parathyroid tumor. Medicine, 47:53 (1968).
44. C.E. Ganote, D.J. Philipsborn, E. Chen, and F.A. Carone, Acute calcium nephrotoxicity: an electron microscopical and semiquantitative light microscopical study, Arch. Pathol., 99:650 (1975).

HYPOKALEMIA

Neil A. Kurtzman

Department of Internal Medicine
Texas Tech University Health Sciences Center
Lubbock, Texas 79430

In healthy adults potassium intake averages about 60-100 mEq per day. Of this, 90% is excreted in the urine, the remaining 10% appears in the stool. Since potassium is the main intracellular cation, less than 2% of body potassium appears in extracellular fluid. Even though the great bulk of potassium is in intracellular fluid, there is a good relationship between the state of body potassium stores and the serum potassium. In general, the greater the potassium deficit, the greater the fall in serum potassium. This relationship is essentially linear. Virtually all the filtered potassium is reabsorbed by the kidney prior to the collecting tubule. Thus, all the potassium that appears in the urine is secreted in the terminal nephron.

METABOLIC CONSEQUENCES OF HYPOKALEMIA

One of the most important effects of potassium depletion is on glucose tolerance. The impaired glucose tolerance which is, at least in part, the consequence of decreased pancreatic insulin secretion may be responsible for some of the deleterious effects of prolonged diuretic therapy on the cardiovascular system.

Profound potassium depletion is associated with muscle weakness which may progress to frank rhabdomyolysis. The muscle weakness of hypokalemia may, if advanced, induce respiratory failure.

Potassium depletion has variable effects on vascular resistance depending upon its duration. When acute, there is increased vascular resistance, whereas chronic potassium depletion is associated with reduced vascular resistance.

The effects of potassium depletion on cardiac function are well known. When potassium depletion accompanies digitalis therapy, the effects may be lethal. The precise role of potassium depletion in the initiation of sudden death in patients taking diuretic therapy is suspected but not proven.

Potassium depletion has profound effects on renal function. In addition to inducing the characteristic morphologoc effects on the tubules, there is a whole array of functional abnormalities. These include reduced glomerular filtration rate, reduced renal blood flow, impaired urinary concentrating capacity, increased urinary prostaglandin excretion, sodium

Table 1. Clinical Causes of Hypokalemia

Edema	Hypertension	Neither
1. Congestive heart failure	1. Primary aldosteronism	1. Periodic Paralysis
2. Cirrhosis	2. Adrenogenital syndrome	2. Renal tubular acidosis
3. Nephrosis	3. Malignant hypertension	3. Vomiting
4. Diuretics	4. Primary reninism	4. Diarrhea
	5. Renal artery stenosis	5. Bartter's syndrome
	6. Licorice	6. Sweating
	7. Diuretics	7. Diuretics
	8. Liddle's syndrome	
	9. Carbenoxalone	

retention, altered response to parathyroid hormone, and altered PAH handling. In addition, potassium depletion increases renal renin release while decreasing aldosterone secretion from the zona glomerulosa of the adrenal.

ASSESSMENT OF THE HYPOKALEMIC PATIENT

Since most of the potassium is inside cells and since potassium can cross cell membranes at a very rapid rate, it is necessary to determine whether the hypokalemia seen in an individual patient is the result of redistribution or the result of potassium loss. The factors which control the transcellular movement of potassium include the adrenergic nervous system; beta stimulation moves potassium into cells while alpha stimulation has the reverse effect. Insulin moves potassium into cells, glucagon has the reverse effect. A fall in extracellular pH moves potassium out of cells, a rise has the opposite effect. The easiest way to determine if potassium depletion is the result of potassium loss or redistribution is to measure the urinary concentration of potassium. If it is low, then either potassium has been lost from an extrarenal site or has been redistributed. The history of the individual patient usually resolves this issue. If the urine is low in sodium, then urinary potassium loss may cease even if renal potassium wastage is the cause of the patient's hypokalemia. The tendency towards potassium wastage can be uncovered when adequate amounts of sodium are delivered to the distal nephron which will then secrete large amounts of potassium if stimulated to do so.

CLINICAL CAUSES OF HYPOKALEMIA (Table 1)

In general the easiest way to classify hypokalemic disorders is to determine whether hypokalemia occurs on the background of edema, hypertension, or is not associated with either. Edematous diseases associated with hypokalemia are congestive heart failure, nephrotic syndrome, and cirrhosis. In almost all patients with these disorders the hypokalemia arises when the patient is treated with diuretics. The hypokalemia results when adequate amounts of sodium are delivered to a collecting tubule which is exposed to large amounts of aldosterone. The aldosterone results from the contraction of effective arterial blood volume associated with these disorders. The increased delivery of sodium results from the treatment of these disorders with diuretics rather than as an intrinsic event.

Hypertensive patients commonly develop hypokalemia, most often as result of diuretic therapy. Hypokalemia, however, is the hallmark of primary aldosteronism. It is also seen in children with two forms of the adrenogenital syndrome, the 11- and 17-hydroxylase deficiency syndromes. Malignant hypertension is a profound form of secondary hyperaldosteronism

Table 2. Clinical Disorders of Potassium Depletion Associated with Acid-Base Abnormalities

Metabolic Alkalosis	Metabolic Acidosis
Diuretics	Diarrhea
Vomiting	Ketoacidosis
Penicillin or carbenicillin	Laxative abuse
Mineralocorticoid excess	Intestinal fistulas
	Renal tubular acidosis
	Salt-losing nephropathies

and is quite commonly associated with hypokalemia. Licorice administration can result in hypokalemia. This is the result of the glycyrrhizic acid which is contained in natural licorice. This substance has an action on the collecting tubule similar to that of aldosterone, though it is not a steroid. Carbenoxolone similarly exerts an effect on the distal nephron which resembles that of aldosterone. The rare disorder Liddle's syndrome is associated with hypokalemia. This syndrome results from stimulation to sodium absorption and potassium and hydrogen secretion in the collecting tubule which does not require the action of aldosterone. It is essentially an end organ disorder which resembles primary aldosteronism except that it is associated with almost zero levels of aldosterone. Patients with this disorder are sensitive to amiloride therapy but do not respond to spironolactone. The disorder is extremely rare.

Hypokalemia not associated with edema or hypertension may arise from a variety of disorders. Both the proximal and distal tubular acidosis may be associated with hypokalemia. The latter form of the disorder is the classical variant of distal renal tubular acidosis, the type commonly seen in children and families and which is associated with nephrolithiasis and nephrocalcinosis. The hypokalemic variety of periodic paralysis is well known and usually does not present a diagnostic dilemma. Both vomiting and diarrhea may be associated with hypokalemia. The rare disorder Bartter's syndrome is also associated with profound renal potassium wastage. And, of course, diuretic therapy is the leading cause of hypokalemia in this group of patients.

The hypokalemia associated with diuretics, vomiting, and occasionally seen in patients given large amounts of sodium penicillin is associated with metabolic alkalosis. Conversely, metabolic acidosis is seen in patients with diarrhea, ketoacidosis, laxative abuse, intestinal fistulas, renal tubular acidosis, and salt-losing nephropathy (Table 2). The metabolic acidosis associated with distal renal tubular acidosis and hypokalemia responds to bicarbonate therapy. This syndrome can be completely reversed by the administration of 60 to 100 mEq of bicarbonate a day, or even less. On the other hand, patients with proximal renal tubular acidosis may have their hypokalemia worsened when treated with bicarbonate. This is the result of increased distal delivery of sodium and bicarbonate which results from a proximal leak. The volume contraction these patients are afflicted with results in accelerated sodium-for-potassium exchange.

VOMITING

The hypokalemia of vomiting is the result primarily of renal potassium loss. The concentration of potassium in gastric fluid is quite low. When patients vomit and lose hydrochloric acid, serum bicarbonate rises. This is initially associated with an increased filtered load of bicarbonate. Much of this bicarbonate escapes reabsorption and appears in the urine.

The combination of sodium bicarbonate loss in the urine and hydrochloric acid loss in the gastric juice is the equivalent of salt, carbon dioxide, and water loss. This results in volume contraction; the ensuing volume contraction results in the release of excess amounts of aldosterone. The aldosterone in turn stimulates the distal exchange of sodium for potassium and results in renal potassium wastage. As the disorder progresses the ensuing hypokalemia suppresses adrenal aldosterone release. Thus, if studied late in the course of the syndrome patients with vomiting may have normal levels of aldosterone. It should be emphasized that normal levels of aldosterone in the face of severe hypokalemia are in effect increased.

BARTTER'S SYNDROME

Bartter's syndrome is a rare disorder characterized by hypokalemic metabolic alkalosis, normal or decreased blood pressure, resistance to the pressor effects of angiotensin II, and hyperplasia of the juxtaglomerular apparatus. The onset is usually in childhood, however, there is impaired urinary concentrating ability even with correction of hypokalemia. High renin and aldosterone levels are noted, potassium wastage occurs even in the absence of aldosterone, sodium restriction will eventually result in sodium conservation. Chloride wastage is virtually invariable, and prostaglandin excretion is high. Indomethacin therapy lowers renin and aldosterone and restores angiotensin sensitivity, but the hypokalemia persists. Finally, angiotensin II blockade lowers blood pressure.

A number of hypotheses have been offered to explain the pathogenesis of this syndrome. The two that have received the most attention are primary or potassium wastage, and chloride wastage. A theory which explains all the features of the disease is that the ascending limb of Henle's loop has defective chloride transport which results in salt wastage and volume contraction. Owing to the defect in chloride transport in the ascending limb potassium is also not reabsorbed and primary potassium wastage results which will persist even in the absence of aldosterone. The volume contraction, however, stimulates aldosterone release which only accentuates potassium wastage. If volume becomes contracted enough, the sodium delivered to the collecting tubule will be exchanged for potassium and hydrogen so that a sodium- but not chloride-free urine can be elaborated. Exactly what the mechanism for primary potassium wastage unrelated to a chloride defect would be and how it would cause all the manifestations of Bartter's syndrome has not yet been explained.

TREATMENT

The treatment of hypokalemia is obvious. Potassium should be replaced either orally or intravenously depending upon the clinical circumstances. If given intravenously the maximum rate of potassium administration in normal sized adults is 20 mEq per hour. Of course, a careful search should be made to determine the cause of the hypokalemia and specific treatment aimed at the cause should be instituted.

REFERENCES

Kurtzman N.A., and Gutierrez L.F.: Hypothesis: The Pathophysiology of Bartter's Syndrome. JAMA 234:758, 1975.

Batlle D.C., and Kurtzman N.A.: Syndromes of Aldosterone Excess and Deficiency. Med Clin N Amer 67:879, 1983.

Batlle D.C., and Kurtzman N.A.: Clinical Disorders of Aldosterone Metabolism. Disease-a-Month Vol 30, No 8, 1984.

Smith J.D., Bia M.J., and DeFronzo R.A.: Clinical disorders of potassium metabolism. In "Fluid, Electrolyte, and Acid-Base Disorders" Arieff A.I. and DeFronzo R.A., eds., Churchill Livingstone, New York 413, 1985.

Sabatini S., and Kurtzman N.A.: Metabolic Alkalosis. In "Clinical Disorders of Fluid and Electrolyte Metabolism," 4th ed., (Maxwell M.H., Kleeman C.R., and Narins R.G., eds) McGraw-Hill Book Company, New York 691, 1987.

Kurtzman N.A.: Renal tubular acidosis: a constellation of syndromes. Hosp Prac 22:173, 1987.

Alexander EA, Perrone RD: Regulation of extrarenal potassium metabolism. In "Clinical Disorders of Fluid and Electrolyte Metabolism", 4th ed., Maxwell M.H., Kleeman C.R., and Narins R.G., eds. McGraw-Hill Book Company, New York 105, 1987.

Field M.J., Berliner R.W., and Giebisch G.H.: Regulation of potassium metabolism. In "Clinical Disorders of Fluid and Electrolyte Metabolism", 4th ed., Maxwell M.H., Kleeman C.R., and Narins R.G., eds., McGraw-Hill Book Company, New York 119, 1987.

Raymond K.H., and Kunau R.T. Jr.: Hypokalemic states. In "Clinical Disorders of Fluid and Electrolyte Metabolism", 4th ed., Maxwell M.H., Kleeman C.R., and Narins R.G., eds., McGraw-Hill Book Company, New York 519, 1987.

INFECTION AND THE KIDNEY

THE RENAL RESPONSE TO INFECTION

Richard J. Glassock, Cynthia C. Nast, and Arthur H. Cohen

Department of Medicine and Pathology
Harbor-UCLA Medical Center
UCLA School of Medicine, Torrance, California

INTRODUCTION

Involvement of the kidneys, either primarily or secondarily, in the course of infectious diseases is a rather common event and has figured prominently in the history of nephrology. Indeed, in the pre-antimicrobial era, acute and chronic renal disease developing as a part of systemic infection was a frequent cause of mortality (1). With partial control of infectious diseases through antibiotic and chemotherapeutic agents, renal disease is now a less frequent cause of mortality in bacterial infections; however, it remains as an important cause of morbidity and mortality in viral, protozoal and helminthic infections particularly hepatitis B, malaria and schistosomiasis. The therapy of infection has also created iatrogenic renal diseases not recognized in the pre-antimicrobial era.

To discuss the renal response to infection in its broadest dimensions would require many hundreds of thousands of words, far more than is available in this Symposium. Therefore, we have chosen to analyze and will attempt to classify the mechanisms whereby a local or systemic infection and its consequences could result in renal injury using examples of bacterial, viral, fungal, protozoal or helminthic infections to illustrate important points. In addition, we will present a brief overview of the most recent kidney manifestation of infection now delineated as a new clinical pathologic entity; namely, the nephropathy associated with human immunodeficiency virus (HIV) infection.

MECHANISMS OF RENAL INJURY IN INFECTION

The processes which result in renal injury consequent to infection may be conveniently divided into <u>five</u> general classes. In four, the infection, along with a biologic response of the host are responsible for renal disease, and in one, the renal damage is a result of therapy rather than the infection itself. This latter process is included because of its great importance in determining overall renal morbidity and because it can frequently be confused with renal manifestations arising as a direct or indirect consequence of the infection being treated.

CLASS I: Direct microbial invasion (extra vascular or blood borne) of the renal parenchyma with resultant inflammation and structural damage due to a local host biological response. Bacterial infections of the urinary tract are common examples of this mode of injury (2). Microorganisms may gain access to the parenchyma directly from the circulation, as in hematogenous staphyloccocal pyelonephritis with microabscess formation or miliary tuberculosis. More commonly, organisms reach the kidney by the ascending route. Bladder infection by coliform bacteria may be transmitted to the kidney by retrograde flow of urine consequent to vesico-ureteric reflux (or alternatively via ureteric or renal lymphatic channels). Intrarenal reflux permits infected urine to flow into the papillae and thereby into the interstitium where the bacteria multiply, produce locally okasis endo- and exotoxins and evoke a polymorphonuclear leukocyte infiltrate. This inflammatory response, while tending to localize the infection, leads to the release of intracellular degradative enzymes and the production of toxic oxygen radicals which destroy tissue and induce scar formation. Residual non-viable bacterial antigens and/or the release of sequestered antigens (e.g. Tamm-Horsfall protein) may lead to delayed hypersensitivity reactions which perpetuate renal injury. Furthermore, it is possible, though not conclusively proven, that an auto-immune response (see below) to some normal or altered renal constituent participates in the prolongation of renal injury in the absence of continued viable bacteria.

CLASS II: Disseminated (blood-borne) infection with renal parenchymal injury resulting from a systemic host biological response.

Not involving antibody production: Systemic infections, by virtue of the release of biologically active substances from the organism itself, may initiate a series of complex events which can result in serious renal injury. The best known of these reactions is the syndrome of endotoxemia arising from gram negative bacteremia. Endotoxin (bacterial lipopolysaccharide) resides in the outer membrane of many gram negative organisms. Its lipid A component is responsible for many of its properties, including the activation of monocytes and the promotion of intra-vascular coagulation. Lipopolysaccharide causes macrophages to rapidly release cytokines, including tumor necrosis factor (TNF) interleukins 1 and 6, alpha interferon, platelet derived transforming growth factors, and colony stimulating factors. These soluble, cell-derived factors in turn dramatically influence the properties of other cells, including T and B lymphocytes, endothelial cells, polymorphonuclear leukocytes and fibroblasts. Activated monocytes and macrophages also begin to express procoagulant activity on their surface and thus participate in the promotion of intravascular coagulation. TNF may be central among these cell derived soluble factors in promoting diverse clinical features of the syndrome of endotoxemia since this cytokine directly or indirectly causes fever, release of acute phase proteins, shock and vascular tissue injury (3). Severe endotoxemia can result in ischemic acute tubular necrosis and when fibrinolysis is impaired the disseminated intravascular coagulation can lead to patchy or complete cortical necrosis. Lipopolysaccharide may also, through its action as a polyclonal B cell stimulator, lead to the production of a variety of auto antibodies (see below) (4).

Involving Antibody Production: When systemic infection involves a humoral antibody response and when soluble antigens of the infecting organisms are released into the body fluids, circulating immune complexes may be formed, some of which may possess properties favoring deposition in vascularized organs such as the kidneys, skin, joints and heart valves. Infectious endocarditis is such a disease and is uniformly associated with high levels of circulating immune complexes and is often accompanied by evidence of complement activation and an auto-antibody response to IgG containing immune complexes (rheumatoid factor). (5) The immune complexes, which deposit in glomerular capillaries and elsewhere, may contain the antigens of the infecting organisms. If renal disease is not severe, anti-microbial therapy, with elimination of the antigen, will result in cure of the renal disease. Similarly, certain chronic infections, most notably of Hepatitis B virus, may evoke a chronic immune complex disease with the antigen-antibody complexes comprising one or more of the protein antigens defined by the virion and the host antibody response. Malaria may be yet another example of such a chronic immune complex disease.

CLASS III: Localized extra renal infection with parenchymal renal injury resulting from a systemic host biological response.

Not Involving Antibody Production: Here the infection itself is well localized to a specific organ or tissue, and spread into the blood stream is not a necessary prerequisite. However, non-replicating products of the microorganisms which are released locally elicit a systemic response not involving antibody production. For example, localized gastrointestinal infection with a vero-toxin producing E. Coli results in a systemic response of intravascular coagulation leading to the consumption of procoagulant factors, thrombocytopenia bleeding, microangiopathic hemolytic anemia, and renal failure due to thrombosis within the small vessels of the kidney (Hemolytic-Uremia syndrome) (6). In an entirely different pathway, chronic bacterial suppurative infection (e.g. osteomyelitis, bronchiectasis, tuberculosis) leads to the production of interleukins by activated macrophages and the subsequent production of amyloid A protein by the liver. For poorly understood reasons, perhaps involving local amyloid P protein, amyloid fibrils resistant to proteolytic enzyme digestion form and/or deposit within the kidney and elsewhere and provoke disease (secondary amyloidosis) (7).

Involving Antibody Production and/or Cell Mediated Immunity: Here a localized infection leads to a systemic immune response to antigenic products of the infecting organism or by "molecular mimicry" to an auto antibody response to one or more normal tissue antigens. (8) The sharing of epitopes between microbial antigens and normal tissue antigens, which are usually short sequences of amino acids, is responsible for the "molecular mimicry". At times, non-viable antigens of infecting organism are liberated into the circulation and lodge at distant sites due to a biochemical affinity for tissue or extra-cellular matrix proteins. Post-streptococcal glomerulonephritis has been proposed as a possible example of this latter sequence of events, since some investigators have discovered an antigen, found exclusively in nephritogenic streptococci, called endostreptosin, can localize within glomeruli and bind with circulating antistreptosin antibody (9). Thus, the in-situ formation of immune complexes may be responsible for the disease. Alternatively or in addition, deposition of circulating immune complexes may be responsible for post-streptococcal glomerulonephritis, since immune complexes containing streptococcal antigens and activation of the alternative pathway of complement are commonly found in early stages of the disease.

CLASS IV: Localized extra renal infection resulting in direct immune or non-immune mediated damage to non-renal tissue with secondary delayed damage to renal structures. Here infection is playing a very remote and indirect role in the pathogenesis of renal disease. The renal injury results when irreversible structural alterations and a substantial loss of function of an organ or tissue leads to systemic metabolic pertubations which secondarily affect the kidney. A genetically preconditioned, possibly viral induced, auto-immune destruction of the Beta cells of the pancreatic islets leading to insulin-dependent diabetes mellitus and late onset diabetic nephropathy is the classical example of this mechanism (10). Virus induced hepatic necrosis which may result in cirrhosis with hepato-renal syndrome or secondary IgA Nephropathy (Hepatic glomerulosclerosis) is another.

CLASS V. Renal Disease Arising as a complication of the therapy of infectious disease. While not strictly a renal response to infection, renal disease developing secondary to an adverse effect of antimicrobial is a common accompanyment of infectious disease. It is quite often difficult to separate clinically from the more direct effect of infection, particularly those of a bacterial nature on the kidney. Two general subclasses of this mechanism are well recognized and will not be discussed further: first, a hypersensitivity reaction, antibody or cell mediated, to one or more epitopes of the antimicrobial agent, quite often Penicillin or a derivative (11). Acute interstitial nephritis, with infiltrates of eosinophilis and lymphocytes and plasma cells is the most frequent pathological finding. The immune response may be directed not only to the antimicrobial agent but also to normal or altered renal tissue. Acute renal failure is the most common clinical expression of this sub-class of mechanism. Second, direct nephrotoxic injury to one or more elements of the nephron leading to impaired renal excretory function may occur (12). Aminoglycoside antibiotics, pentamidine and acyclovir are most often incriminated. Acute tubular necrosis and non-oliguric acute renal failure are the most common pathologic and clinical manifestations respectively.

HUMAN IMMUNODEFICIENCY VIRUS (HIV) NEPHROPATHY: A Newly Discovered Prototype of Renal Response to Infection

In recent years, particularly from Nephrology Centers in Miami, New York City and Los Angeles, a new clinico-pathologic entity has been delineated in patients chronically infected with HIV, most but not all of whom have had full blown clinical evidence of Acquired Immuno Deficiency Disease (AIDS) (13). For unexplained reasons, this particular complication of HIV infection, called HIV-associated nephropathy, has not been observed in San Francisco, Bethesda, Pittsburgh, or Boston, Kansas City, to any great extent in other countries, despite the widespread occurrence of HIV infection (14, 15, (This Symposium). Since many patients acquire HIV infection through intravenous drug abuse, including heroin, the entity may be confused with heroin associated nephropathy, to be discussed later in this Symposium by Dr. Massry (16). However, we and others believe that the entity can occur in the absence of intravenous heroin abuse (at least as determined by a careful review of medical history) and this fact permits its separation from other causes of renal disease in patients with HIV infection who also abuse drugs intravenously. Furthermore, the lesion has been well documented in children with AIDS. HIV associated nephropathy is not the only renal lesion occurring in chronically HIV infected individuals. A wide spectrum of glomerular, tubular and vascular diseases occur in these patients, including acute endocapillary proliferative glomerulonephritis, membranous glomerulonephritis, amyloidosis, acute interstitial nephritis, acute tubular necrosis, and focal and segmental glomerulosclerosis related to chronic intravenous heroin abuse.

The major clinical features of HIV associated nephropathy are shown in Table I. Over the last four years 15 patients have been diagnosed as HIV associated nephropathy at our center in our own renal pathology laboratory (13).

The lesion has been observed in asymptomatic carriers of HIV, patients with AIDS related complex (ARC) and as a late manifestation of full blown AIDS. Not surprisingly, most individuals have been male (90% in our patients), and blacks predominate over white (60% of our patients are black). Whether this sex and racial prediliction is an epi-phenomenon of geography and case selection, or a manifestation of a true racial predisposition to disease is unknown. As stated above HIV associated nephropathy can arise in patients who have no known history of intravenous drug abuse (only 30% of our patients had any history of IV drug abuse) or opportunistic infections and also occurs in children. One of our patients was detected following nephrectomy for persistent hematuria resulting from accidental trauma. Children with HIV-associated nephropathy have been reported from Miami, Los Angeles and Montreal.

The presenting renal manifestations include heavy non-selective proteinuria, (ranging from 2.8 to over 20 grams per day in our patients), edema and severe hypo-albuminemia. Serum creatinine has been elevated at the time of diagnosis in the majority of cases (80% in our patients) and rapidly progresses to end stage renal failure in most but not all patients.

Other clinical features are generally related to an immunodeficiency state or to concomitant disease and include anemia, lymphocytopenia, and thrombocytopenia. Nephromegaly is uniformly observed. This feature is not usually seen among HIV sero-negative patients with nephrotic syndrome and chronic intravenous heroin abuse.

The pathologic findings in HIV nephropathy are quite distinctive in our experience and in three cases has lead to the diagnosis of asymptomatic HIV infection. Table II outlines the major pathologic findings (13).

By standard light microscopy the lesion consists of a combination of glomerular, tubular and interstitial abnormalities which taken together is quite unique. The glomerular lesion consists of typical focal, segmental and global glomerulosclerosis most commonly in early stages of evolution not greatly different from idiopathic or other secondary forms of focal sclerosis. Tubular abnormalties are prominent with active necrosis and regeneration accompanied by pronounced dilatation of many tubular segments. The lumina are filled with pale staining casts often with scalloped borders. Cellular protein reabsorption droplets are very prominent in the proximal tubules. The interstitium is edematous and contains a variable pleomorphic mononuclear infiltrate. By immuno-fluorescence, IgM, C3 and CIq are found in areas of segmental glomerulosclerosis. The giant tubular casts contain Ig, albumin and fibrin but are uniformly negative for Tamm-Horsfall protein, and are composed of precipitates of filtered plasma proteins. Ultra structurally, the major findings are in the visceral epithelial cells and vascular endothelial cells. The foot processes of the visceral epithelial cells are diffusely effaced and the enlarged cytoplasma contains many vacuoles, blebs or protein droplets. Endothelial cells of glomeruli and other vessels contain very large numbers of tubulo reticular inclusions. Electron dense deposits are uncommonly found. Abnormal nuclei with loose or aggregated chromatin are found infrequently; some are probably post-mortem artifacts. Except for focal and segmental glomerulosclerosis usually in advanced stages of formation, the other lesions are not found in heroin associated nephropathy in HIV sero-negative patients.

The pathogenesis of HIV associated nephropathy is unknown; while some believe that unrecognized intravenous drug abuse is primarily responsible for the renal lesion, other data suggest direct infection of renal epithelium by HIV in disease production. The latter pathogenesis is suggested by the following: a) The lesions are observed in male homosexuals and transfusion related HIV infection or others without a known history of intravenous drug abuse or opportunistic infection. b) The lesion may be the initial manifestation in asymptomatic HIV infected individuals, c) HIV nucleic acid virion can be detected in glomerular epithelial and tubular epithelial cells by in-situ cDNA hybridization and immunoperoxidase evaluation using anti-p24 antibodies (17) and d) HIV infection can be transmitted by a renal allograft.

Three possible mechanisms can be offered to explain the association of HIV infection with the lesion. These include: a) The lesion is a chance observation not casually related to HIV infection, b) The lesion is due to a systemic response (antibody or a non-immune response) to HIV infection. (Class II or III response with cross-reacting auto-immunity) or c) The lesion is due to direct HIV infection of the renal parenchyma with resultant structural damage (Class I response).

Insofar as autoimmunity is concerned, recent intriguing findings of Golding and co-workers are quite relevant (18). By comparing the amino acid sequences of a portion of the major envelope glycoprotein of HIV (gp 41) with the amino acid sequence of the ß 1 domain of Class II major histo-compatability complex determined antigens, they have found a septapeptide of nearly identical sequence. Antibodies to intact HIV in sera of patients with AIDS react with the septapeptide from Class II MHC antigens. Thus, "molecular mimicry" and auto immunity to autologous antigens conceivably play a role in the pathogenesis of renal disease.

The clinical course of HIV-associated nephropathy has usually been relentlessly and rapidly progressive in most cases. In patients with AIDS, death usually supervenes in a matter of months. Only one of the nine patients in our initial series followed for at least six months or to death retained native renal function.

Unfortunately, no treatment is available for this disorder. As no patient has been treated with anti-viral agents to our knowledge. The effect of a reduction in renal viral burden upon prognosis is unkown. A major question remains regarding the apparent wide discrepancy of the reported prevalence of HIV associated nephropathy. Some groups, including those from Amsterdam to be reported here, (this symposium) have not yet observed patients with this lesion. Some believe that it does not exist but rather is a consequence of unrecognized intravenous drug abuse, opportunistic infection or a chance occurrence. Heroin associated nephropathy which will be discussed later by Dr. Massry, appears to be a different entity. (This symposium) Table III compares and contrasts the clinical and pathologic findings in HIV associated nephropathy and heroin-associated nephropathy.

The occurrence of HIV associated nephropathy in non-intravenous drug abusers who are asymptomatic insofar as HIV infection is concerned, and (if confirmed by subsequent studies) the finding of the viral genome of HIV in the glomerular and tubular epithelial cells could be cited as an argument in favor of the existence of HIV associated nephropathy as a new clinical pathologic entity. Only time will tell whether this will be the true state of affairs.

TABLE I

Human Immunodeficiency Virus (HIV) Associated Nephropathy

Clinical Features

Observed in male homosexuals, intravenous drug abusers and recipients of blood contaminated with HIV. (? heterosexual partners of HIV infected persons).

May have clinical onset prior to, contemporaneously with or following clinical diagnosis of acquired immuno deficiency disease (AIDS).

Almost exclusively male sex; strong preponderance of blacks.

Present with poor-selective heavy proteinuria, edema, progressive renal failure and hypertension.

Anemia, absolute lymphopenia (and/or decrease $^{T}HI/^{T}Sc$ ratio), thrombopenia.

Bilaterally enlarged, echogenic kidneys.

Opportunistic infections (P. Cariini, Candida, M. avium intracellulare, herpes, toxoplasmosis)

Postive tests for antibody to HIV.

(T_{HI} = T-helper-inducer cells; T_{Sc} = T-suppressor-cytoxic cells).

TABLE II

Human Immunodeficiency Virus Associated Nephropathy Pathologic Features

---

Focal, segmental and global glomerulosclerosis

Diffuse foot process effacement with abnormal visceral epithelial cells (vacuoles)

Tubular cell necrosis and/or dysmorphism

Giant occlusive tubular casts (PAS negative or weakly positive, Tamm-Horsfall protein negative)

Tubulo-reticular structures in endothelial cells

Variable immunofluorescence findings (amorphous/granular IgM deposits)

Abnormal nuclei in glomerular and tubular cells (? artifact)

TABLE III

A Comparison of Human Immunodeficiency Virus (HIV) and Heroin Associated Nephropathies

	Heroin Associated	HIV Associated
Male Sex preference	+++	++++
Black/white ratio	++++	++
Nephrotic Syndrome	+++	+++
Rapid Progression to ESRD	+	+++
Nephromegaly	±	+++
Focal and Segmental glomerulo-sclerosis	+++	+++
Tubulo-Vesicular Structures	±	+++
Giant Tubular Casts	±	+++
Tubular Necrosis	±	+++
Interstitial Inflammation	+	+++
Visceral Epithelial Abnormalities	++	++
HIV detected in biopsies	?	+++

REFERENCES

1. Osler, William. The Principles and Practice of Medicine. 7th Edition. D. Appleton and Co. New York 1909.
2. Rubin, R. H., Tolkoff-Rubin, N.E. and Cotran, R.S. Urinary tract Infection, pyelonephritis and reflex nephropathy. in B. Brenner and F. Rector. (Editors). The Kidney. 3rd Edition. W. B. Saunders, Philadelphia. 1986. pg 1085-1141.
3. Old, L.J. Tumor necrosis factor. Science 230:630-632, 1985.
4. Morrison, D. and Ryan, J.L. Bacterial endotoxins and host immune responses. Adv. Immunol. 28:294-450, 1979.
5. Bayer, A.S. Theofilopoulos, A., Eisenberg, R., Dixon F.J. and Guze, L., Circulating immune complexes in infective endocarditis. N.Eng.J.Med. 295:1500-1505, 1976.
6. Karmali, M., Steele, B.T., Petrie, M. and Lim, C. Sporadic cases of hemolytic-uraemic syndrome associated with faecal cytotoxin and cytoxin producine escherichia coli in stools. Lancet 1:619-620, 1983.
7. Glenner, G. Amyloid deposits and amyloidosis. The ß-fibrilloses. N.Eng J. Med. 302:1283-1294, 1980.
8. Oldstone, M.B.A. Molecular mimcry and auto-immune disease. Cell 50:819-820, 1987.
9. Selegson, G., Lange, K., Majeed,H.A., Doel, H., Cronin, W., Bovie, R. Significance of endostreptosin antibody titers in post-streptococcal glomerulonephritis. Clin. Nephrol. 24: 69-75, 1985.
10. Kaldany, A., Busick, E.J. and Eisenbarth, G.S. Diabetes mellitus and the immune system. A. Marble, L. Krall, R. Bradley, A. R. Christlieb, J.S. Soeldner (Editors) Joslin's Diabetes Mellitus. 12th Edition. Lea & Febiger, Philadelphia 1985. pg 51-64.
11. Cotran, R.S., Rubin, R. and Tolkoff-Rubur, N.F. Tubulointerstitial diseases. in B. Brenner and F. Rector. The Kidney 3rd Edition. in W.B. Saunders, Philadelphia. 1986. Pg.1143-1174.
12. Humes, H.D. and Weinberg, J.M. Toxic nephropathies. in B. Brenner and F. Rector (Editors). The Kidney, 3rd Edition. W.B. Saunders, Philadelphia 1986. Pg. 1491-1532.
13. Cohen, A.H. and Nast, C. HIV-associated nephropathy. A unique combined glomerular tubular and interstitial lesion. Modern Pathology 1:87-97, 1988.
14. Balow, J.E., Macker, A.M., Rook, A.H. Paucity of glomerular disease in acquired immunodeficiency syndrome. Kidney Int. 29:178, 1986 (abstract).
15. Humphries, M.N., Schoenfeld, P.Y. Renal complications in patients with the acquired immune deficiency syndrome. Amer. J. Nephrol. 7:1-8, 1987.
16. Rao, T..K.S., Nicastri, A.D. and Friedman, E.A. Natural history of heroin-associated nephropathy. N. Engl. J. Med 290: 19-25, 1974.
17. Cohen, A.H., Sun, C.J., Shapshak, P. and Imagawan, D. Demonstration of human immunodeficiency virus in renal epithelium in HIV-associated nephropathy. Submitted for publication, 1988.
18. Golding, H.J., Robey, F.A., Gates, F.J., Linder, W., Beining, P.R. Hoffman, T., and Golding, B. Identification of homologous regions in human immunodeficiency virus I gp 41 and human MHC class IIß1 Dorman. I. Monoclonal antibodies against the gp 41-derived-peptide and patients sera react with native HLA Class II antigens, suggesting a role for autoimmunity in the pathogenesis of acquired immunodeficiency syndrome. J.Exp.Med 167: 914-923, 1988.

RENAL INVOLVEMENT IN HANTAVIRUS DISEASE

B.Čižman*, D.Ferluga**, S.Kaplan-Pavlovčič*, M.Koselj*, J.Drinovec*, and T.Avšič***

*Department of Nephrology, University Medical Center Ljubljana, Yugoslavia
**Institute of Pathology, and ***Institute of Microbiology Faculty of Medicine, Ljubljana, Yugoslavia

INTRODUCTION

Hantavirus disease (HVD) or hemorrhagic fever with renal syndrome is now regarded as an acute infectious disease with a variety of clinical manifestations (1,2). It is caused by viruses from the Bunyaviridae family (3). The prototype of this group is Hantaan virus which was first isolated in Korea in 1976 (4). Today we know more than 100 strains of this virus which are antigenically related. Seroepidemiological studies have revealed worldwide occurrence of the infection (5). The severe form of HVD is more often seen in the Far East (6). In Europe the mild form, known as nephropathia epidemica (NE),is found in Scandinavia (7) and Western Europe(8).

In Yugoslavia the first HVD case was reported in 1952 (9). Several epidemics occurred between 1958 and 1986 (10,11). The first written data concerning HVD in Slovenia,the north-western part of Yugoslavia, dates back to the year 1952. Since 1985 routine serological tests of the disease became possible at our institution.

In this paper we describe the clinical course of 10 serologically confirmed HVD patients. A comparision between clinical spectrum of the disease and histological findings in renal tissue was done in 6 cases.

MATERIAL AND METHODS

Patients

From 1983 10 patients with acute renal failure (ARF) in HVD were treated in the Department of Nephrology at University Medical Center Ljubljana. Their disease was suspected as leptospirosis, drug-induced interstitial nephritis, acute renal failure of unknown etiology and HVD. Clinical course of the disease was very different, 2 case reports are presented below.

Case report No. 1. An 18-year-old boy fell ill on 13 August 1985. 14 days before he had helped his parents working in a field and was presumably exposed to rodent excretions. He became acutely ill with signs of respiratory infection and was hospitalised at the general hospital for 2 days. After 4 days he was readmitted to the same hospital because of hematemesis, oliguria, hematuria and neurological disturbances. The next day hypotension, pulmonary edema and bradicardia developed and he was transferred to University Medical Center. The physical examination after the admission to intensive care revealed signs of shock, he was unconscious, dehydrated and because of respiratory failure, assisted ventilation was required. Laboratory data showed mild anemia, leukopenia, normal trombocytes, decreased protrombine time, high values of urea and serum creatinine (1900 µmol/l), normal liver enzymes and mildly elevated LDH. Urine analysis showed 3-plus proteinuria and microhematuria. Hemodialysis were performed,and in 3 days the patient improved his condition. Ultrasound revealed enlarged kidneys with distended parenhyma. On the 16th day of the disease percutaneous renal biopsy was performed. The polyuric phase of ARF lasted almost 2 weeks and the patient was released with mild renal insufficiency (serum creatinine 180 µmol/l). Serological tests for antibodies to Hantaan virus (76/118 strain) showed a four fold increase between the 1st and 2nd sera.

Case report No.2. A 35-year-old carpenter became sick on 26 Oct. 1986 with high fever (39,6°C), headache, mialgia and blurred vision. On the 4th day he was hospitalised at the general hospital and, next day because of anuria and hematuria transferred to our Department. On admission he was well, but lumbar regions were sensitive to palpations. Laboratory data showed trombocytopenia, decreased prothrombine time and elevated serum creatinine 790 µmol/l. Liver enzymes were slightly abnormal. Urinalysis revealed a protein excretion of 1.7 gr per day and microeritrocyturia. Ultrasound of the kidneys was normal. After parenteral hidration and furosemid diuresis began to increase. The clinical course became rapidly favourable. On the 8th day after admission serum creatinine returned to normal. In serological examinations higher titers to Puumala virus were observed.

Serological technique

Human sera were screened by indirect immunofluorescent antibody test (IFA) using different hantaviruses: prototype Hantaan 76/118, CG 18/20, Prospect Hill - Ph 1, Fojnica and Vranica. All sera were also tested for the presence of antibodies against leptospirosis by using the agglutination lysis test.

Histological methods

For light microscopic studies percutaneous renal biopsy specimens were fixed in Duboscq-Brazil and embedded in Paraplast. 3-4 um thick sections were stained with hematoxylin-eosin, Masson's trichrome, periodic acid/ Schiff, periodic acid/silver methamine, and according to iron Perl's and elastica Gieson-Weigert's technique. A semiquantitative assessment was made for the severity of each pathological feature.

Direct immunofluorescence was performed on cryostat frozen sections using commercially available FITC-labeled reagents(Dakopatts, Denmark) specific for human immunoglobulin-IgG, -IgA, -IgM and complement fraction C3, C1q, C4 and fibrin/fibrinogen.

Samples for electron microscopy were fixed in buffered 2 % osmium tetroxide and embedded in Epon. Ultrathin sections stained with uranium acetate and lead citrate were examined in electron microscope Phillips 201 C.

RESULTS

There were 8 men and 2 women whose ages ranged from 18-36 with a mean age of 26. Most of the patients became ill during summer, one in October and two in late spring. In the first phase of HVD, which lasted from

4 to 6 days different signs and symptoms were observed - table 1. Most of the patients were treated in this phase with antipiretics, analgetics,and some of them with antibiotics. In the 2nd part of this febrile phase hemorrhagic manifestations occurred in 5 patients. These included conjunctival injection (4 patients),skin and soft palate petechias (2 patients), epistaxis (2 patients), hematemesis in one patient and melena in another one. All patients had microhematuria.

Acute renal failure developed in the period from 4th to the 8th day of the disease and usually coincided with hospital admission or transfer to our department. Characteristics of ARF are shown in table 2.

On admission 2 patients were hypertensive predominantely due to hypervolemia,2 were hypotensive and others had normal blood pressure. One patient developed cyanosis and flushing of the face with progressive dyspnea and this necessitated intubation and assisted ventilation. Three patients had bradycardia (42-48/min) and two developed tachycardia. In laboratory data trombocytopenia ($34x10^9/l$ - $103x10^9/l$) was found in 5 patients and decreased protrombine time (0.48-0.57) in three cases. Leucocytosis was observed in 3 and leucopenia in one case. ESR was accelerated between 17-50 mm/h in 8 patients. Mild liver disfunction (SGOT 47-95 U/l and SGPT 66-228 U/l) was documented in 6 patients. Elevated LDH was found in all 5 patients, who were tested. Complement level and its various fractions were normal in all but 1 patient. Renal size was increased on ultrasound in nearly all patients.

Table 1. Signs and symptoms in the febrile phase of HVD (n=10)

Signs and symptoms	No of pts
fever	10
headache	8
pain in the throat	5
myalgia and arthralgia	4
abdominal and loin pain	8
nausea and vomiting	7
blurred vision	2
diarrhea	2
neurologic disturbances	2

Table 2. Acute renal failure in patients with HVD (n=10)

Patient	Oliguria day	Oliguria ml/24^h	Proteinuria (g/day)	Creatinine (μmol/l)	Polyuria (day)
F.Š.			5.4	270	7
M.V.	6	100	0.3	1130	11
V.T.	7	250	21.3	1130	17
B.H.	7	300	0.7	460	10
J.H.	6	100	+++	1900	16
A.B.	5	100	1.7	745	9
M.K.	4	175	1.3	1320	16
A.Š.	6	150	1.5	800	11
M.P.	6	200	4.8	790	16
A.P.	5	200	+++	1030	8

The treatment of acute renal failure is shown in table 3. Hemodialysis was required in 5 patients, in one predominantely due to hypervolemia. Two patients needed prolonged treatment. Secondary complications were observed in 4 patients which included pancreatitis and pneumonia in one case, pancreatitis, bacteriemia and uroinfection in another 3 cases. One patient was treated with corticosteroids because of the suspicion of drug induced interstitial nephritis found in renal biopsy. There was no effect on renal function and after 14 days the treatment was discontinued. Recovery of renal function was complete in all but one patient who had diminished urine concentration ability, mild renal insufficiency - serum creatinine 180 µmol/l and mild hypertension.

Ultrasound guided percutaneous renal biopsy was performed in 6 patients between 9th and 16th day from the onset of the disease. It was performed at the end of oliguric phase or at the beginning of the polyuric phase of ARF. Complications after renal biopsy occurred in 2 cases - mild lumbar pain and macrohematuria in one case and microhematuria in another one.

Histological observations

Renal cortex as well as medulla were available for light microscopic studies in 4 cases and cortical tissue only in 2 cases. The results are summarized in table 4.

Table 3. Treatment of acute renal failure in patients with HVD (n=10)

Patient	Acute renal failure inf.+furosemid	dopamin	HD	Infection	Recovery
F.Š.	-	-	-	-	N
M.V.	+	+	3	-	N
V.T.	+	+	7	+	N
B.H.	-	-	-	-	N
J.H.	-	+	5	+	RI
A.B.	+	-	-	-	N
M.K.	+	+	7	+	N
A.Š.	+	+	-	-	N
M.P.	+	+	2	+	N
A.P.	+	-	-	-	N

N = normal, RI = mild renal insufficiency, HD = hemodialysis

Table 4. Tubulo-interstitial lesions in renal tissue in HVD patients (n=4)

Biopsy (day)	Renal tissue	Tubuli deg.	necrosis	reg.	Interstitium congestion	hemorrhagia
10	cortex	+	0	+	+-	0
	medulla	+	+	+	++	++
16	cortex	+	+	+	+-	0
	medulla	++	+++	++	++	++
9	cortex	+	0	+	+-	0
	medulla	+	+-	+	+++	++
10	cortex	++	+-	+-	0	0
	medulla	+	++	+	++	+++

0 = none, +- = minimal, + = slight, ++ = moderate, +++ = severe

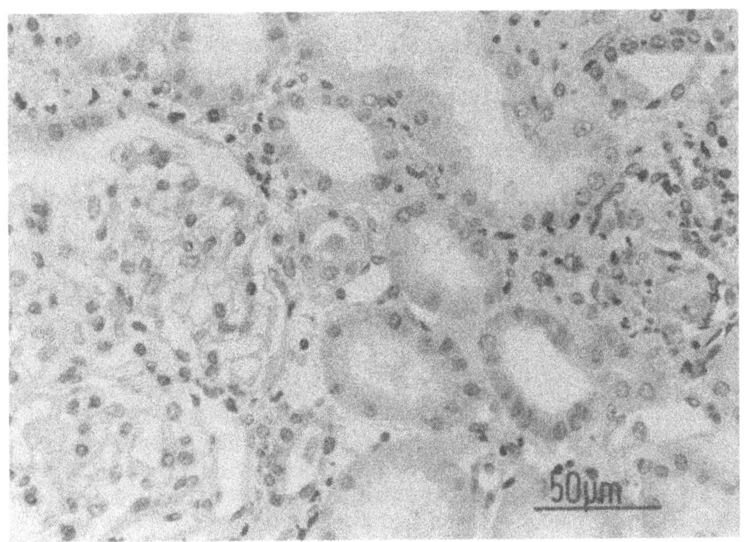

Fig. 1. Focally accentuated tubulo-interstitial inflammatory lesions and only insignificant glomerular changes. Hematoxylin-eosin, x105

In the renal cortex focal to diffuse, minimal to moderate degenerative and regenerative tubular epithelial changes accompanied by interstitial edema and inflammatory mixed cell infiltrates of varying intensity were observed. (Fig. 1.) Significantly more pronounced tubular necrosis and marked congestion of the intertubular capillaries and focal or widespread interstitial hemorrhagies were found in the medulla. (Fig. 2.)

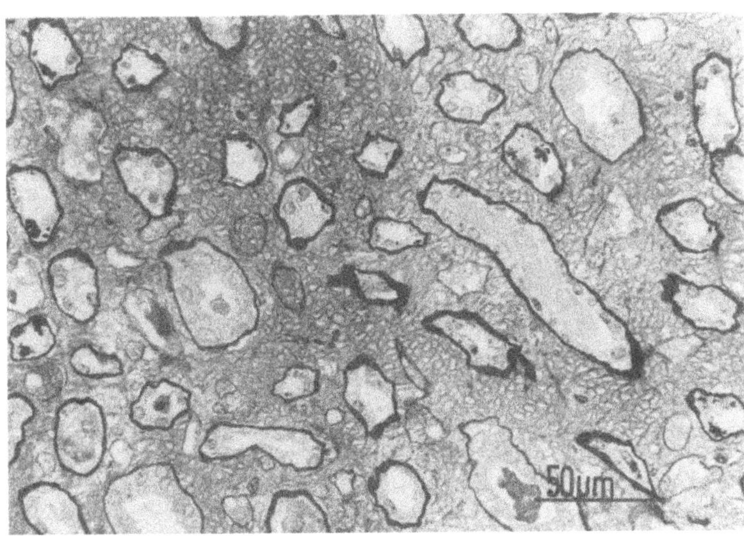

Fig. 2. Congestion of intertubular capillaries and widespread interstitial hemorrhagia of the renal medulla. Periodic acid/silver methamine x105

Immunofluorescence studies showed patchy to diffuse, slight to moderate granular deposits of IgM, IgG, and C3 along the peripheral glomerular basement membrane in only one case, in all other cases the findings were completely negative or insignificant.

The preliminary electron microscopic examinations revealed degenerative changes of the endothelial cells pronounced especially in the intertubular capillaries of the renal medulla.

DISCUSSION

A clinical picture of our patients with HVD showed marked variations ranged from mild to severe forms of the illness. The symptoms which were common to practically the whole group were abrupt onset of fever and headache in the first phase and onset of loin and abdominal pain in the second phase. Half of the patients had hemorrhagic phenomena. The mild form of HVD occurred in 2 patients and moderate in 3 patients and were practically the same as perceived in patients with NE in Scandinavia and Western Europe (7,8). The severe form of the disease was similar to those observations in the Far East and in the observation of Greek patients (6, 12,13). In this severe form more hemorrhagic manifestations occurred, neurological involvement was more frequent and more severe acute renal failure developed. Two patients were in shock, which represent a higher percentage as observed with other groups (6,12). ARF was presented in all patients, it was oliguric in all but one case. In some patients it was suspected at the beginning that ARF was result of drug induced interstitial nephritis because of administration of antipiretics and antibiotics in the first phase of HVD. This dilemma was also observed with another groups (14,15). Secondary complications were practically the same as observed (12) or in acute renal failure (16). Pancreatitis in our 2 patients could be the result of virus propagation or alcohol consumption in already known heavy drunkard before onset of the disease. There were no fatalites presumably because no hemorrhagic complications arose and efficient supportive treatment was provided. Treatment of the patients was symptomatic, antibiotics and corticosteroids had no influence on renal function. Hemodialysis treatment was safe and efficient.

Positive serological tests for anti-hantavirus antibodies confirmed the clinical diagnosis of HVD. Two different reactivity patterns were observed: sera with higher titers for Hantan virus and sera with higher titers for Puumala virus. All of the patients were serological negative for leptospirosis.

Our microscopic studies showed besides generally mild and unspecific tubulo-interstitial inflammatory changes in the renal cortex much more pronounced and significant lesions of the medulla showing hemorrhagic necrotizing interstitial nephritis. This observation was almost the same as observed in other studies (14,15,7). Electron microscopic degenerative changes were additionally observed suggesting capillary toxicosis.These findings could be the pathophysiologic disturbance of Hantan virus. The results of our immunofluorescence studies are not in accordance with the suggestion that immune complexes may play an important role in the pathogenesis of HVD (17).

Comparision between the pathological changes in renal tissue and clinical course in 4 patients with HVD is shown in table 5.

Table 5. Comparision between clinical course of HVD, severity of ARF and histological changes in renal tissue in HVD patients (n=4)

Patient	Severity of ARF	Clinical course of HVD	Histologic changes	Renal function at follow-up
B.H.	+	+	+	N
J.H.	+++	+++	+++	RI
A.Š.	++	+	+	N
M.K.	+++	+++	++	N

N = normal renal function, RI = renal insufficiency
+ = mild, ++ = moderate, +++ = severe

CONCLUSIONS

The clinical course in our patients was different and showed variations in severity of HVD. Although our group of patients was small we could conclude that existed good correlation between the severity of ARF and histological changes under light microscopy predominantely in renal medulla. Immunofluorescent changes were found only in one specimen. Symptomatic treatment was efficient, no one died. Recovery of renal function was complete in all but one patient. Further studies are needed to find the long-term influence of Hantaan virus on renal tissue and to compare this with clinical observation.

REFERENCES

1. Desmyter J., van Ypersele de Strihou C., van der Groen G., Hantavirus disease. Lancet 2: 158, 1984.
2. PHLS Report: Haemorrhagic fever with renal syndrome: Hantaan virus infection, Brit Med J 290: 1410, 1985.
3. C.S. Schmaljohn , J.M. Dalrymple, Analysis of Hantaan virus RNA: Evidence for a new genus of Bunyaviridae. Virology 131: 482-491, 1983.
4. H.W. Lee, P.W. Lee, K.M. Johnson, Isolation of the etiologic agent of Korean hemorrhagic fever. J Infect Dis 137: 298-308, 1978.
5. H.W. Lee, Hemorrhagic fever with renal syndrome. History, Hantaan virus and Epidemiological features. Scand J Infect Dis (Suppl) 36: 82-85,1982.
6. H.W. Lee, Korean hemorrhagic fever. Prog med Virol 28: 96-113, 1982.
7. J. Lähdevirta, Nephropathia Epidemica in Finland. A clinical,histological and epidemiological study. Ann Clin Res 3 (Suppl 8): 1-154,1971.
8. C. van Ypersele de Strihou, G. van der Groen, J. Desmyter: Hantavirus Nephropathy in Western Europe: Ubiquity of Hemorrhagic Fevers With Renal Syndrome, in: Advances in Nephrology 15, 143-171, 1986.
9. Z. Radošević, I. Mohaček, The problem of nephropathia epidemica Myhrman-Zetterholm in relation to acute interstitial Nephritis. Acta Med Scand 149, 221-228, 1954.
10. J. Gaon, M. Karlovac, M. Gresikova at al, Epidemiological features of hemorrhagic fever, Folia Med Facult Med Univ Saraviensis, 3, 23-42, 1968.
11. B. Antonijević, A. Gligić, Hemoragične groznice s bubrežnim sindromom. Vojnosanit Pregl 39: 205, 1982.
12. J. Lähdevirta, Clinical features of HFRS in Scandinavia as compared with East-Asia. Scand J Infect Dis (Suppl) 36: 93-95, 1982.
13. A. Antoniadis, J.W. Le Duc, S. Daniel-Alexiou, Clinical and epidemiological aspects of hemorrhagic fever with renal syndrome in Greece, Eur J Epidemiol 3, 295-301, 1987.
14. C. van Ypersele de Strihou, Acute oliguric interstitial nephritis. Kidney Int 16: 751-765, 1979.

15. M. Zeier, K. Andrassy, R. Waldherr und E. Ritz, Akutes Nierenversagen durch Hantavirus, Dtsch med Wschr 111, 207-210, 1986.
16. W.F. Finn, Recovery from acute renal failure in: Acute renal failure, B.M. Brenner and J.M. Lazarus eds., Churchill Livingstone, New York 1988.
17. E.J. Jokinen, J. Lähdevirta, Y. Collan, Nephropathia epidemica: immunohistochemical study of pathogenesis. Clin. Nephrol. 9, 1-5, 1978.

Acknowledgement

The authors wish to express their sincere thanks to Irena Cotman for her excellent technical preparation of this manuscript.

Request for reprints of this paper should be sent to:

Borut Čižman, M.D.
Department of Nephrology
University Medical Center
Zaloška 7
61000 Ljubljana, Yugoslavia

GLOMERULAR LESIONS AND OPPORTUNISTIC INFECTIONS OF THE KIDNEY IN AIDS: AN AUTOPSY STUDY OF 47 CASES

H.J. van der Reijden[1], M.E.I. Schipper[2],
S.A. Danner[3] and L. Arisz[1]

1. Renal Unit, Department of Internal Medicine
2. Department of Pathology
3. AIDS Unit, Department of Internal Medicine

Academic Medical Center, University of Amsterdam
Meibergdreef 9, 1105 AZ Amsterdam, The Netherlands

SUMMARY

AIDS-associated nephropathy (AAN) causing acute renal failure has been described in patients with AIDS. It is characterized by massive proteinuria and focal segmental glomerulosclerosis.

From 1982 until 1987, 177 patients with AIDS were seen in our center. Most of them were homosexual or bisexual men. One patient was also an intravenous drug addict. One patient was a black female. None suffered from a nephrotic syndrome or needed hemodialysis during their illness.

In 47 of the 110 patients who died an autopsy was performed.

On microscopical examination of kidney tissue obtained at autopsy, no abnormalities were seen in 12 patients and slight abnormalities were found in 35 patients. Glomerular changes, mostly fibrous caps in Bowman's space, were present in 22 patients. Mesangial and intracapillary lesions were seen in only 5 patients. Tubular atrophy was found in 14 patients and sparse interstitial inflammation in 15 patients.

A renal localisation of disseminated opportunistic infections was found in 11 patients: CMV (n=4), tuberculosis (n=2), Mycobacterium avium intracellulare (n=1) and Cryptococcal infection (n=4). In one patient a renal localisation of a Kaposi sarcoma and in another patient a renal localisation of a disseminated non-Hodgkin lymphoma was found.

In conclusion the clinical picture of AAN with acute renal failure was not found in our center. As is the case with héroin associated nephropathy, AAN seems to be confined to certain areas in the USA, suggesting that racial or local co-factors, are important for the pathogenesis of AAN in AIDS.

General autopsy findings

Forty-two patients died of opportunistic infections like disseminated Cytomegalovirus infection or Mycobacterium avium intracellulare infection, pneumocystis carinii pneumonia or generalized cryptococcosis (table 2).

Five patients died of disseminated Kaposi's sarcoma. A total of 11 patients showed at autopsy beside opportunistic infections also Kaposi sarcoma lesions, usually localized in the gastrointestinal tract, the skin, the respiratory system and the lymph nodes. In two patients also a disseminated non-Hodgkin lymphoma, probably Burkitt-type or non-classifiable was found. Two patients died of a generalized TBC infection.

Brain pathology, without opportunistic infections in the other parenchymatous organs, was present in four patients (3 cases of cerebral toxoplasmosis and 1 case of progressive multifocal leucoencephalopathy).

Table 1. Clinical data in 47 patients with AIDS

Male	46
Female	1
Age*	41,2 yr (24-63)
Race	all caucasian (except the female)
IV drugs	1 (also homosexual)
Serum creatinine*	
- at presentation	82 micromol/l (42-186)
- terminal	106 micromol/l (32-513)
Serum albumin*	
- at presentation	38 gr/l (19-51)

* mean (range)

Table 2. Autopsy findings in 47 AIDS patients

Main cause of death	no.	kidney localisation
Pneumocystis carinii pneumonia	21	-
Cytomegalovirus infection	18	4
Mycobacterium avium intracellulare	11	1
Cryptococcal infection	6	4
Kaposi sarcoma	5	1
non-Hodgkin lymphoma	2	1
Tuberculosis	2	2
Other	6	-

INTRODUCTION

In patients with AIDS recently a new entity has been described consisting of a nephrotic syndrome with progression to uraemia in weeks to months, with enlarged kidneys and focal and segmental glomerulosclerosis on biopsy. This entity, indicated as AIDS-associated nephropathy (AAN)[1-4] seems to be confined to certain areas in the United States and has a greater incidence in black patients with AIDS and HIV positive intravenous drugaddicts[5,6]. Since HIV positive patients with either a nephrotic syndrome or chronic renal failure were not seen in our AIDS unit we performed an autopsy study in 47 AIDS patients to analyse the incidence of specific HIV-associated renal lesions. All these patients died of opportunistic infections and/or disseminated Kaposi's sarcoma.

PATIENTS AND METHODS

From 1982 until 1987, 177 patients with AIDS (according to the present CDC criteria)[7] were seen in our center. All patients but one were male and 96% were homosexual or bisexual men. One patient was also an i.v. drug abuser. All but one (the female) were caucasian.

None of these patients suffered from severe renal failure or nephrotic range proteinuria at presentation. The serum creatinine concentrations were less than 200 micromol/liter.

Eventually 110 patients died and in 47 of them an autopsy was performed.

At autopsy pieces of both kidneys were fixed in formalin, in Tel's and Karnofski's fixative and frozen in liquid nitrogen. Light microscopical examination was performed on hematoxylin-eosin, elastica van Giesson and methenamine silver stained sections of both kidneys.

All slides were examined by one pathologist (MS).

RESULTS

Kidney function

The serum creatinine concentrations at presentation in the 47 AIDS patients ranged from 42 to 186 micromol/l. Only two patients presented with concentrations above 110 micromol/l, caused by dehydration due to diarrhoea (table 1).

In the period prior to their death, serum creatinine levels ranged from 32-422 micromol/liter. None of the patients developed a nephrotic syndrome or needed renal replacement therapy.

Proteinuria was analysed by paper dip-stick method (Albustix®). All urine samples tested except one were negative, trace or one plus positive (1 gr/l). One patient presented with four plus proteinuria but had a normal serum albumin concentration, as was the case in those 9 patients whose urine was not tested. In the urinary sediment no abnormalities were found in any of the patients.

Table 3. Clinical and histological data on 35 AIDS patients with abnormal histology of the kidneys.

Pat. no.	Age years	Diagnosis [1] presentation	Diagnosis [1] autopsy	Serum creatinin[2] presentation	Serum creatinin[2] terminal	Albu stix	PA findings[3] in kidneys
1.	24	KS,MAI	CRC,KS	88	65	neg	INT
2.	41	PCP	PML	65	43	+	FC
3.	36	CrS	CrS,MAI	42	32	tr.	INT
4.	38	KS	KS	58	105	neg	FC,TA,INT
5.	36	KS	KS	52	49	+	ISCH,TA,INT
6.	42	CRC	CRC,NHL	78	103	neg	ISCH,TA,INT
7.	46	TOXO	TOXO,PML	90	80	neg	FC
8.	41	CMV	CMV	78	122	neg	FC
9.	46	TOXO	TOXO	85	51	neg	FC,TA
10.	33	PCP	CMV,CRC	186	85	neg	FC,INT
11.	31	PCP	PCP,KS	72	138	tr.	CRC,FC,TA
12.	33	PCP	CMV	74	513	+	FC
13.	42	PCP	PCP,CMV	77	59	tr.	MES,INT
14.	39	PCP	PCP,PML	78	70	neg	FC
15.	37	KS	KS,TBC	79	55	tr.	FC
16.	36	KS	KS	65	57	neg	TBC,FC
17.	30	CRC	CRC,CMV	nt.	nt.	+	MES
18.	48	PCP	CMV,TOXO	79	122	nt.	CRC,INT
19.	42	PCP	KS,CMV	109	124	nt.	FC,TA
20.	40	EBV	CMV,MAI	76	68	tr.	CMV,TA
21.	54	TOXO	TOXO,CMV	80	49	tr.	CMV,TA,FC,INT
22.	43	KS	KS	73	69	tr.	CMV
23.	26	PCP	TOXO	69	64	nt.	KS,FC
24.	62	PCP	PCP,CMV	97	65	neg	TA
25.	37	KS,PCP	KS,PCP	79	93	neg	FC,MES,TA,INT
26.	30	PCP	MAI,TOXO,TBC	79	110	nt.	FC,MES,TA
27.	42	PCP	MAI,PCP	77	79	++++	FC,TA,INT
28.	48	KS	KS	77	49	nt.	MAI,FC
29.	44	KS	KS,PCP	65	65	tr.	FC
30.	31	PCP	PCP	91	95	nt.	ISCH,TA
31.	50	CrS	CMV	107	90	nt.	MES
32.	60	Candida	CRC	77	87	neg	CMV,FC
33.	63	TBC	TBC	117	102	neg	CRC,FC,INT
34.	43	PCP	CRC	67	57	tr.	TBC,ISCH,FC,INT
35.	47	KS	NHL	83	115	nt.	CRC,INT

Legends:

1 KS Kaposi sarcoma, CRC cryptococcal infection, PCP pneumocystis carinii pneumonia, MAI mycobacterium avium intracellulare infection, CrS cryptosporidiosis, NHL non-Hodgkin Lymphoma, TOXO cerebral toxoplasmosis, PML progressive multifocal leucoencephalopathy, CMV cytomegalo virus infection, EBV Epstein Barr Virus infection, nt. not tested, tr. trace.

2 micromoles per liter.

3 INT interstitial infiltrate, FC fibrous caps, TA tubular atrophy, MES mesangial or intracapillary proliferation, ISCH ischaemic changes.

Histological findings in the kidneys

The renal lesions in 35 patients consisted of slight abnormalities, only evident in the methenamine silver staining, except the opportunistic infections which were already found in the hematoxylin-eosin stained slides (table 3).

Ischaemic changes like hyalinization of glomeruli, were present in four patients. These patients had serum creatinine concentrations lower than 103 micromol/l just before death.

The kidneys of 22 patients showed fibrous caps in the Bowman's space.

Mesangial and intracapillary lesions were found in five patients.

Slight tubular changes like atrophy and a sparse inflammatory infiltrate in the interstitium was present in respectively 14 and 15 patients, mostly the same group.

In 11 patients a renal manifestation of a disseminated opportunistic infection was found. Cryptococcal infection was present in the kidney of 4 patients (Fig. 1.), CMV in 4 patients (Fig. 2.), tuberculosis in 2 patients and MAI in one patient.

A renal manifestation of Kaposi's sarcoma was found in one patient (Fig. 3.) and another patient showed a non-Hodgkin lymphoma in the kidney. In 12 patients no abnormalities were found.

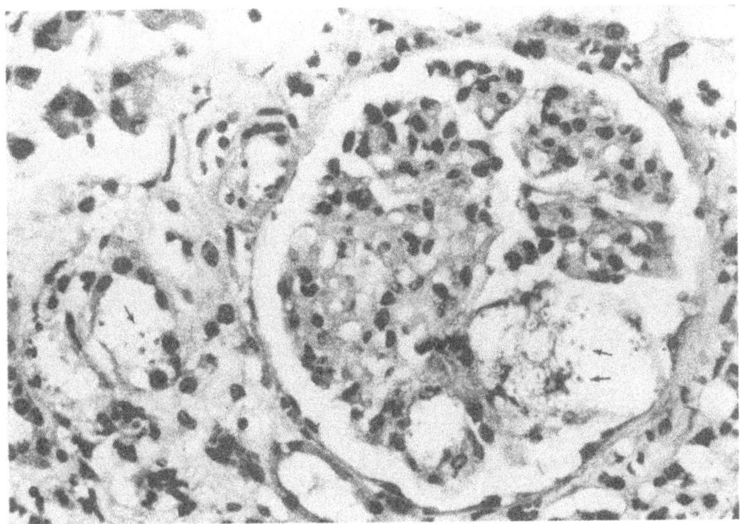

Fig. 1. Cryptococcal infection of the glomerulus (arrows).

DISCUSSION

In our attempt to detect a specific HIV-associated renal lesion, such as AIDS-Associated Nephropathy (AAN), we found neither clinical evidence (like a nephrotic syndrome), nor microscopical evidence for this disease in the Amsterdam series of AIDS patients.

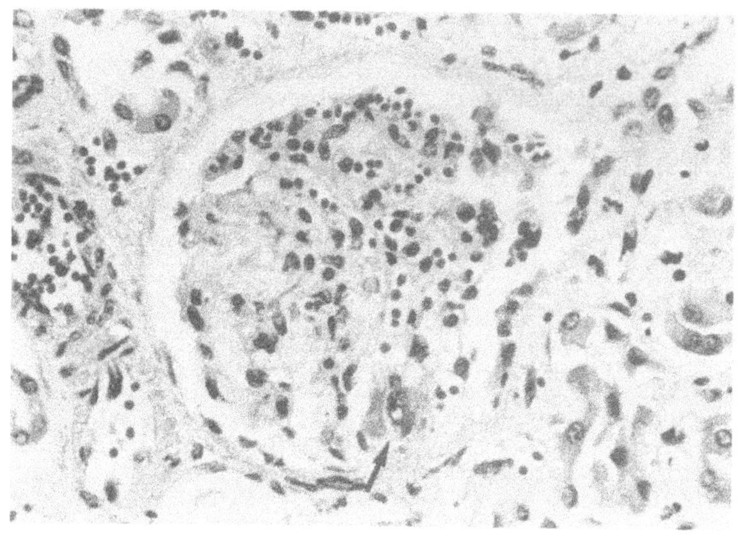

Fig. 2. Glomerulus with CMV inclusion body (arrow).

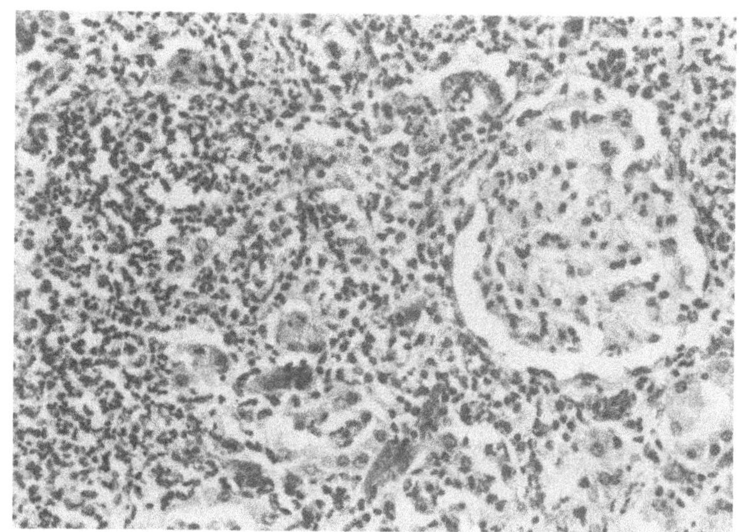

Fig. 3. Kidney with infiltration of Kaposi sarcoma.

Focal and segmental glomerulosclerosis (FGS) has been defined as the pathological lesion characteristic for AAN[1,3] the same as in heroin associated nephropathy (HAN)[8,9]. In a recent study comparing AAN and HAN, FGS was found in both groups[9].

The same tubular and glomerular abnormalities found in our patients, were seen by Bauer et al.[2] in the AAN group (i.e. dilatation of Bowman's space, tubular degenerative changes and sparse interstitial infiltrates) but not in HAN. At the ultrastructural level nuclear bodies (type III to V) are described more frequently in AAN. They may suggest a viral etiology but they are also not specific for AAN[10].

However AAN was not found in San Francisco[11] and in other USA centres and equally it could not be demonstrated in our series. This remains to be elucidated as is the case with the differences in the prevalence of HAN, which was found in the same centers as AAN is reported nowadays[8,12,13].

Possibly racial factors e.g. the black and hispanic race and i.v. drug abuse play a major role in the development of FGS and thus in AAN. Since both these factors are almost absent in our series this might be the explanation of not finding AAN, despite a large number of microscopical abnormalities.

In the kidneys of our patients there was evidence of a (disseminated) opportunistic infection in 10/47 patients (21%), according the incidence mentioned in literature (0-42%)[4,9].

It was not possible to correlate the renal lesions with the prevalence of different opportunistic infections during the disease (table 4).

Those microscopical abnormalities found might all be remnants of septic periods and interstitial nephritis due to opportunistic infections of the kidney and the frequent use of nephrotoxic medication in AIDS.

Table 4. Histological findings correlated with opportunistic infections of the kidneys

Histological findings	no.	Opportunistic infections
Ischaemic	5	1
Fibrous caps	22	7
Mesangial	5	-
Interstitial	15	5
Tubular	14	3
None	13	1

REFERENCES

1. V. Pardo, R. Menesses, L. Ossa, D.J. Jaffe, J. Strauss, D. Roth, J.J. Bourgoignie, AIDS-related glomerulopathy: occurrence in specific risk groups, Kidney Int 31(5):1167-73 (1987).
2. F. Bauer, R.E. Cutler, AIDS and renal disease: clinical and pathological features, Dial and Transpl 17(1):37-8 (1988).
3. T.K.S. Rao, L.R. Mallis, E.A. Friedman, Nephropathy as the initial manifestation of human immunodeficiency virus (HIV) disease, abstract, Kidney Int 1:205 (1988),
4. E. Rousseau, P. Russo, N. Lapointe, S. O'Regan, Renal complications of acquired immunodeficiency syndrome in children, Am J Kidney Dis 11(1):48-50 (1988).
5. T.K.S. Rao, E.A. Friedman, A.D. Nicasti, The types of renal disease in the acquired immunodeficiency syndrome, N Engl J of Med 316:1062-8 (1987).
6. K. Welch, W. Finkebeimer, Ch.E. Alpers, W. Blumenfeld, R,L, Davis, E.A. Smuckler, J.H. Beckstead, Autopsy findings in the Acquired Immunedeficiency syndrome, JAMA 252(9):1152-9 (1984).

7. Revision of the CDC surveillance case definitions for the aquired immunodefiency syndrome. MMWR 36 (suppl. no.15) (1987).
8. T.K.S. Rao, A.D. Nicastri, E.A. Friedman, Natural history of héroin-associated nephropathy, N Engl J Med 290:19-23 (1974).
9. P. Chandler, A. Soni, A. Suri, R. Bhagwat, J. Yoo, G. Treser. Renal ultrastructural markers in AIDS-associated nephropathy, Am J Pathol 126(3):513-26 (1987).
10. P. Chandler, G. Treser, Ultrastructural markers of AIDS nephropathy, Kidney 31:335 (1987).
11. S. Mazbar, M.H. Humphries, AIDS-associated nephropathy is not seen at San Francisco General Hospital, abstract, Kidney Int 1:202 (1988).
12. E.E. Cunningham, M.A. Zielezny R.C. Venuto, Heroin-associated nephropathy; A nationwide problem, JAMA 250:2935-6 (1983).
13. G.D. Lundberg, Why does uremia in herion abusers occur predominatly among blacks, JAMA 250:2965-7 (1983).

DRUGS-INDUCED NEPHROPATHIES

SELECTED ASPECTS OF DRUG USE IN RENAL FAILURE

William M. Bennett, and
Lawrence W. Elzinga

Division of Nephrology and Hypertension
Oregon Health Sciences University
Portland, Oregon U.S.A.

INTRODUCTION

The kidney is the major organ involved in the elimination of drugs and their pharmacologically active metabolites. Thus, the frequency and severity of adverse drug reactions are increased in patients with renal insufficiency. Updated recommendations for the use of relevant drugs in patients with varying degrees of renal dysfunction are available (1-3). This paper will review selected aspects of this large subject, emphasizing topics of recent interest and for which new information is available.

Narcotic Analgesics in Chronic Renal Failure

It has been widely recognized by nephrologists that patients with renal failure are often "sensitive" to morphine and other narcotics despite their predominant elimination from the body by hepatic metabolism. Small doses frequently produce profound respiratory depression and a decreased level of consciousness. Using modern analytical methods, parent morphine does not accumulate in renal failure; however, there is retention of pharmacologically active metabolites such as morphine 6-glucuronide which may be of clinical significance (4,5). In experimental animals morphine 6-glucuronide is four times as active as morphine with a prolonged duration of action (5). The half-lives of absorption as well as elimination of parent morphine are actually shortened in renal failure (6,7). It is now becoming clear that at least part of the "increased sensitivity" to morphine in renal dysfunction may be due to the kidneys' role in drug metabolism. In the isolated perfused rat kidney, significant morphine metabolism has been documented (8). In cadaver renal transplant patients with initial allograft dysfunction, plasma morphine concentrations are higher than living related donor recipients with initial function and non-anesthetized controls (9). Whatever the mechanism, clinicians should administer small doses of morphine to postoperative renal failure patients with the need for narcotic analgesia.

Meperidine has a prolonged elimination half-life in renal failure due to a lower plasma clearance and an increased volume of distribution. An active metabolite, normeperidine also has decreased excretion. Accumulation of normeperidine may lead to seizures in patients with renal insufficiency (10). Prolonged effects of codeine have also been reported in renal failure (9). Newer narcotic analogues have not had detailed studies in renal failure patients. The accumulation of pharmacologically active metabolites is the probable explanation for the adverse effects of all opiod analgesics in renal insufficiency (9).

Pharmacologic Management of Urinary Tract Infections in Patients with Compromised Renal Function

Successful treatment of infection of the urinary tract in patients with reduced renal function depends on adequate delivery of appropriate antibiotics to the site of infection in the renal parenchyma or urine. Renal dysfunction does not usually become a limiting factor until glomerular filtration rate drops to less than 15-20 ml/min. In general, antibiotics which are almost exclusively filtered at the glomerulus, such as the aminoglycosides, achieve low concentrations in urine when glomerular filtration rate is less than 10-15 ml/min (11). However, because of renal aminoglycoside uptake by tubular cells, persistent bacteriocidal concentrations may be obtained in parenchyma for long periods in experimental animals (11). However, it is currently unclear whether this is true in the scarred and chronically diseased renal interstitium of patients with chronic renal disease. Antibiotics which are secreted into the urine by tubular cells usually achieve sufficient concentrations to achieve clinical cures of urosepsis even in patients with end-stage renal disease (12). Examples of such drugs include beta lactam antibiotics and trimethoprim-sulfamethoxazole. There are few studies with newer fluoroquinolone antibiotics in this setting, but on theoretical grounds they should be effective.

For treatment of renal infections, care should be taken not to adjust dosage too far downwards for the reduced renal function because antibacterial efficacy may be lost despite "usual therapeutic" blood levels. Moderate drug accumulation of beta lactam antibiotics such as penicillins, cephalosporins and carbapenems is usually well tolerated even in end-stage renal disease although the patient should be monitored carefully for complications such as seizures. With moderate renal dysfunction, trimethoprim may raise serum creatinine by competition for tubular secretory pathways. This does not reflect reduced renal function since glomerular filtration rate is unaffected by trimethoprim. Nitrofurantoin should be avoided in renal failure patients because retention of metabolites can result in severe peripheral neuritis (1,3). Care must be taken to replace body stores of drugs removed by hemodialysis in patients with severe urosepsis and renal failure.

Fungal infection of the renal parenchyma is a particularly difficult problem. Although amphotericin B is effective *in vitro* against the infecting organism, the total dose necessary to achieve cure leads to nephrotoxicity which in turn limits tissue penetration of the drug (13). Very limited data exists regarding ketocomazole and flucytosine for renal fungal infections. With broad spectrum antibiotic use in immunocompromised hosts and diabetic patients, fungal colonization of the lower urinary tract is common. Clinical recognition of the potential risk of ascending infection should be emphasized since timely local measures such as bladder installation of amphotericin B can prevent ascending involvement of the renal parenchyma or obstruction of the ureter by fungus balls.

Treatment of Infection in Patients with Autosomal Dominant Polycystic Kidney Disease (APKD)

Patients with APKD make up approximately 10 percent of all patients with end-stage renal disease. In addition to the above considerations which are applicable because of renal dysfunction *per se*, serious morbidity and even mortality may occur when the renal cysts themselves become infected because of poor antibiotic delivery. In APKD, cyst epithelium retains characteristics of the nephron site of origin (14). The majority of cysts have leaky epithelium typical of the proximal nephron segments although documentation of the site of origin can only be demonstrated in some of these cysts. Furthermore, not all of these "nongradient" cysts have attachments to nephron segments (15). This limits drug delivery by filtration requiring that an effective drug gain entry to cysts by diffusion and active transport if ion pumps are still functional. Aminoglycosides and beta lactam drugs achieve unreliable concentrations under these circumstances probably because they are water soluble and diffuse poorly across lipid membranes (16). Elzinga et al. recently demonstrated that trimethoprim-sulfamethoxazole achieves concentrations in cyst fluid adequate to kill test organisms in an *in vitro* assay. Efficacy was achieved rapidly independent of renal function (17). Other effective antibiotics are chloramphenicol and on theoretical grounds other lipid soluble agents (18,19).

A small percentage of cysts in APKD arise from a distal nephron site of origin. The tight epithelium is able to maintain steep electrochemical gradients for hydrogen ion, sodium and creatinine. To deliver antibiotics to these cysts, drugs with high pKa may be required (20). Again, trimethoprim-sulfamethoxazole and chloramphenicol are effective. Because of the wide variety of potential urinary pathogens not sensitive to available drugs with the proper pharmacologic properties to achieve penetration into all types of nephron cysts, the newly developed fluoroquinolones are particularly exciting. Elzinga and Bennett have obtained cyst fluid, blood and urine at surgery in patients with APKD treated with ciprofloxacin. Fluid was tested for bacterial killing against representative test organisms before the drug was begun and after therapeutic doses adjusted for renal function (21). Results are depicted below:

Concentration and Efficacy
Ciprofloxacin in Cyst Fluid
from Patients with Polycystic Disease

Cyst Type	N	Ciprofloxacin ([illegible]/ml)	Pre-drug Fluid vs *E. coli*	Post-drug Fluid vs *E. coli*
Nongradient	18	4.5±0.8	< 1:2	1:128
Gradient	19	25.1±7.9	< 1:2	1:256
Indeterminant	20	8.3±2.1	< 1:2	1:128

Other fluoroquinolones have not been vigorously evaluated in this regard. Norfloxacin seems to be less effective than ciprofloxacin when studied in this manner (21). It should be emphasized that these studies with uninfected patients do not insure clinical cures in patients with cyst infections although early anecdotal experience is encouraging.

Prompt clinical diagnosis is crucial for preservation of kidney function and reduction of morbidity. A patient with APKD who has unexplained fever, abdominal pain or constitutional symptoms may have renal infection even when urine cultures are sterile (22). CAT scan is sometimes useful to detect cyst infection in APKD. Cyst wall thickening and an increased density of cyst contents are findings suggestive of infected cysts. Organisms involved in cyst infection are usually gram-negative aerobic bacteria but gram-positive cocci, and anaerobes are possible pathogens. Further studies concerning infecting organisms and effective antibiotics are needed. With refractory infection, surgical drainage may be necessary to avoid systemic sepsis and major morbidity (23).

Patients with acquired renal cysts developing in the course of chronic renal failure occasionally develop parenchymal and cyst infection from ascending and hematogenous routes. Limited information suggests that therapeutic considerations relevant to APKD apply to this form of cystic disease as well.

Aminoglycoside Dosing in Renal Failure

Despite expert pharmacokinetic monitoring aminoglycoside-induced renal dysfunction occurs in approximately 15 percent of therapeutic courses of these widely used antibiotics (24). It has been presumed that maintenance of aminoglycoside blood levels within the narrow "therapeutic range" would both maximize antibacterial efficacy and minimize nephro- and oto-toxicity. Recent information, however, suggests that dosing strategies designed to achieve high peak serum levels and long "sub-therapeutic periods" may be equally efficacious and, in addition, may reduce further renal and eighth nerve damage.

Multiple experimental studies have shown that the height of the serum peak level can be dissociated from renal damage. If a given daily dose is given once per day as opposed to a multiple dosing regimen, renal damage is minimized with the former strategy (25). This is presumably related to quantitatively less transport of drug from the tubular lumen into the renal tubular cells due to less anionic phospholipid receptor occupancy (25). Recently, however, Bennett et al. have been able to dissociate renal aminoglycoside concentrations from nephrotoxicity by use of a polymer of aspartic acid residues (26). Thus, although the explanation for the dissociation of peak serum levels from nephrotoxicity is unclear, the phenomenon could be exploited as a useful strategy to reduce clinical nephrotoxicity (27). Similar considerations apply to oto-toxicity although the experimental data are limited.

Even if a change in dosing regimen to larger, less frequent doses reduced the adverse renal and otologic effects of aminoglycosides, it would not be clinically advantageous if antibacterial efficacy were lost. It has been assumed that it is necessary to maintain serum aminoglycoside concentrations above the minimum inhibitory concentration of the infecting pathogen for the entire 8-12 hour dosage interval. Although logical, this has never been proven. Even with concentration-dependent bacterial killing and high peak levels achieved after a single large dose of aminoglycoside, it has been assumed that efficacy would be lost if serum aminoglycoside concentrations fell below the MIC for a prolonged period.

In 1981, Bundtzgen et al. reported persistent suppression of bacterial growth following *in vitro* exposure of aerobic gram-negative bacilli to aminoglycosides (28). This phenomenon was termed the "post-antibiotic effect" (PAE). In contradistinction to the effect of aminoglycosides, the beta-lactam antibiotics produced very short or no *in vitro* PAE with gram-negative bacilli. Blaser et al. employed a two-compartment, *in vitro* kinetic model system to demonstrate superiority of intermittent dosing as opposed to continuous aminoglycoside administration even though the latter maintained a constant "therapeutic level" (29). Two groups have addressed the issue of an *in vivo* PAE. Kapusnik and Sande evaluated the influence of aminoglycoside dosing regimens on experimental Pseudomonas pneumonia in sedated guinea pigs (30). With a constant total dosage, one daily tobramycin proved as efficacious as every four hour tobramycin. Based on in vivo regrowth of bacteria in the lung and measurements of the total time serum drug levels were below the MIC for the Pseudomonas strain used, a PAE exceeding 16 hours was reported. Possible concomitant drug-induced toxicity was not assessed. Pechere et al. reported similar studies in mice, but the measured endpoints differed (31). Pechere failed to demonstrate an in vivo PAE, but this result may reflect the use of survival, rather than lung bacterial colony counts, as an endpoint. Based on the presence of a PAE in vitro and probably in vivo, and encouraged by the earlier studies which demonstrated less toxicity with large single dose, the possibility has emerged that changing the aminoglycoside dosage regimen may allow for both equal or better efficacy and less nephrotoxicity.

We substantiated these data experimentally using a rat model of subcutaneous abscess. As before, experimental aminoglycoside toxicity could be attenuated by administering the selected total daily dose with a single large dose as opposed to multiple smaller drug administrations. There was no ototoxicity despite the high peak serum levels. The presence of infected, as compared to sterile subcutaneous abscesses, did not influence the magnitude of renal injury. Importantly, there was no evidence of loss of antibacterial activity with the reduced frequency of administration of drug which implies the presence of an in vivo post-antibiotic effect. These results suggest that it may be possible to administer aminoglycosides to patients less often and enjoy the triple benefits of less risk of toxicity, no loss of antibacterial activity, and reduced expense. Careful controlled clinical trials testing these strategies are needed. In adjusting drug dosage for pre-existing renal insufficiency, less frequent rather than reduced dosage methods are probably superior.

ACKNOWLEDGEMENTS

The author's studies cited here were supported by a grant from the Polycystic Kidney Research Foundation, Kansas City, Missouri. The secretarial assistance of John Davis is appreciated.

REFERENCES

1. W.M. Bennett, G.R. Aronoff, T.A. Golper, G. Morrison, I. Singer, and D.C. Brater, "Drug Prescribing in Renal Failure: Dosing Guidelines for Adults," American College of Physicians, Philadelphia (1987).
2. W.E. Reed and S. Sabatini, The use of drugs in renal failure, Seminars in Nephrology 6:259-295 (1986).
3. D.C. Brater, "Drug Use in Clinical Medicine," B.C. Decker, Toronto (1987).
4. R.J. Osborne, S.P. Joel, and M.L. Slevin, Morphine intoxication in renal failure: role of morphine-6-glucuronide, Br Med J 292:1548-1549 (1986).
5. J. Sawe, and I. Odar-Cederlof, Kinetics of morphine in patients with renal failure, Eur J Clin Pharmacol 32:377-382 (1987).
6. G.R. Park, M.P. Shelly, A.R. Manara, and K. Quinn, Sedation in intensive care: morphine and renal failure, Intensive Care Med 13:365-366 (1987).
7. D.F. Woolner, D. Winter, T.J. Frendin, E.J. Begg, K.L. Lynn, and G.J. Wright, Renal failure does not impair the metabolism of morphine, Br J Clin Pharmacol 22:55-59 (1986).

8. P.J. Ratcliffe, J.W. Sear, C.W. Hand, and R.A. Moore, Morphine transport in the isolated perfused rat kidney, Proc EDTA-ERA 22:1109-1114 (1985).
9. G.L. Chan and G. Matzke, Effects of renal insufficiency on the pharmacokinetics and pharmacodynamics of opiod analgesics, Drug Intell Clin Pharm 21:773-783 (1987).
10. K Chan, J Tse, F Jennings, and M. Orme, Pharmacokinetics of low dose intravenous pethidine in patients with renal dysfunction, J Clin Pharmacol 27:516-522 (1987).
11. W.M. Bennett, M.N. Hartnett, R. Craven, D.N. Gilbert, and G.A. Porter, Gentamicin concentrations in blood, urine and renal tissue of patients with end-stage renal disease, J Lab Clin Med 30:389-394 (1977).
12. W.M. Bennett and R. Craven, Ampicillin and trimethoprim-sulfamethoxazole treatment of urinary tract infections in patients with severe renal disease, JAMA 236:946-950 (1976).
13. C. Langston, D.A. Roberts, G.A. Porter, and W.M. Bennett, Renal phycomycosis, J Urol 109:941-944 (1973).
14. R. Huseman, A. Grady, D. Welling, and J. Grantham, Macropuncture study of polycystic disease in adult human kidneys, Kidney Int 18:375-385 (1980).
15. J.J. Grantham, J.L. Geiser, and A.E. Evan, Cyst formation and growth in autosomal dominant polycystic kidney disease, Kidney Int 31:1145-1152 (1987).
16. R.S. Muther and W.M. Bennett, Cyst fluid antibiotic concentrations in polycystic kidney disease: differences between proximal and distal cysts, Kidney Int 20:519-522 (1981).
17. L. Elzinga, T. Golper, A.L. Rashad, M.E. Carr, and W.M. Bennett, Trimethoprim-sulfamethoxazole in cyst fluid from autosomal dominant polycystic kidneys, Kidney Int 32:884-888 (1987).
18. S.J. Schwab, Efficacy of chloramphenicol in refractory cyst infections in autosomal dominant polycystic kidney disease, Am J Kidney Dis 5:258-261 (1985).
19. W.M. Bennett, L. Elzinga, J.P. Pulliam, A.L. Rashad, and J.M. Barry, Cyst fluid antibiotic concentrations in autosomal dominant polycystic kidney disease, Am J Kidney Dis 6:400-404 (1985).
20. S. Schwab, D. Hinthorn, and J.J. Grantham, pH-dependent accumulation of clinamycin in polycystic kidneys, Am J Kidney Dis 3:63-66 (1983).
21. W.M. Bennett, T.A. Golper, and L.W. Elzinga, Fluoroquinolones in patients with polycystic kidney disease, Aust NZ J Med (in press).
22. S.J. Schwab, S.J. Bander, and S. Klahr, Renal infection in autosomal dominant polycystic kidney disease, Am J Med 82:714-718 (1987).
23. R. Sweet and W. Keane, Perinephric abscess in patients with polycystic kidney disease undergoing chronic hemodialysis, Nephron 23:237-240 (1979).
24. G.R. Matzke, R.L. Lucarotti, and H.S. Shapiro, Controlled comparison of gentamicin and tobramycin nephrotoxicity, Am J Nephrol 3:11-17 (1983).
25. W.M. Bennett, G.W. Wood, D.C. Houghton, and D.N. Gilbert, Modification of experimental aminoglycoside nephrotoxicity, Am J Kidney Dis 3:292-296 (1986).
26. W.M. Bennett, C.A. Wood, S.J. Kohlhepp, P.W. Kohnen, D.C. Houghton, and D.N. Gilbert, Experimental gentamicin nephrotoxicity can be prevented by polyaspartic acid, Kidney Int 33:353 (1988).
27. C.A. Wood, D.R. Norton, S.J. Kohlhepp, P.W. Kohnen, W.M. Bennett, G.A. Porter, D.C. Houghton, R.E. Brummett, and D.N. Gilbert, The influence of tobramycin dosage regimen on nephrotoxicity, oto-toxicity and antibacterial efficacy in a rat model of subcutaneous abscess, J Infect Dis (in press).

28. R.W. Bundtzgen, A.U. Gerber, D.L. Cohen, and W.A. Craig, Postantibiotic suppression of bacterial growth, Rev Infect Dis 3:28-37 (1981).
29. J. Blaser, B.B. Stone, and S.H. Zinner, Efficacy of intermittent versus continuous administration of netilmicin in a two-compartment in vitro model, Antimicrob Agents Chemother 27:343-349 (1985).
30. J. Kapusnik, C. Hackbarth, H. Chambers, K. Scott, T. Carpenter, and M. Sande, Efficacy of once daily versus intermittent dosing of tobramycin in neutropenic and normal, sedated guinea pigs with experimental Pseudomonas pneumonia [Abstract 548], in: Program and Abstracts of the 25th Interscience Conference on Antimicrobial Agents and Chemotherapy, Washington, D.C., American Society for Microbiology (1985).
31. M. Pechere, R. Letarte, and J-C Pechere, Efficacy of different dosing schedules of tobramycin for treating a murine Klebsiella pneumoniae bronchopneumonia, J Antimicrob Chemother 19:487-491 (1987).

THE ANALGESIC AGENTS AND RENAL DISEASE

Sandra Sabatini

Departments of Internal Medicine and Physiology

Texas Tech University Health Sciences Center

Lubbock, Texas 79430

INTRODUCTION

In 1827 the active ingredient in willow bark, an extract useful to the ancients for analgesia, was found to contain a precursor of salicylic acid (salicin)(1) . In 1899 Dreser synthesized aspirin (acetylsalicylic acid), and since that time numerous congeners have been introduced into clinical medicine (1,2). These include phenacetin, acetanilid, and acetaminophen. In the 1960's, a new series of compounds was introduced, the nonsteroidal anti-inflammatory agents. Some of these are chemically related to acetanilid (i.e., phenylbutazone and indomethacin), while others are not (i.e., meclofenamate, ibuprofen, and piroxicam). Many compounds have been screened in the laboratory, and virtually all have anti-inflammatory, antipyretic, and analgesic effects similar to those of the salicylates. The compounds inhibit the biosynthesis of prostaglandins in many tissues, including the kidney, and it is thought that this inhibition is the mechanism whereby they exert their analgesic effects (3).

In 1950, Zollinger and Spühler (4) described a series of patients having renal dysfunction, including papillary necrosis, and in every case, ingestion of the non-narcotic pain reliever, Saradon®, was recorded. Saradon® is composed of antipyrine (150 mg), phenacetin (250 mg), and caffeine (250 mg). Since that original description, several studies have confirmed an increased incidence of renal dysfunction in humans following excess use of the non-narcotic analgesics (5-11).

DEFINITION AND CLINICAL COURSE

Although the hallmark of renal lesion induced by the non-narcotic analgesics is papillary necrosis, it is not the only lesion caused by some or all of these agents (Table 1). The lesions described in Table 1 are acute effects usually seen after short term ingestion of the drug (12,13). They are generally, although not always, reversible. The chronic ingestion of non-narcotic analgesics results in papillary necrosis (14-18). Papillary necrosis is a clinical syndrome described as an ischemic infarction of the inner medulla and papilla of the kidney. In general, the illness begins as a febrile one associated with dysuria and flank pain. In very severe cases, if all the papillae are infarcted, anuria may occur. In most cases sepsis ensues. Examination of the urine reveals hematuria, pyuria, and bacteruria; sometimes fragments of the renal papilla may be found. Renal function may deteriorate rapidly and despite vigorous hemodialysis many patients will die from infection. If only some of the papillae are infarcted, the characteristic "ring sign" will be seen on intravenous pyelography. Renal function may stabilize if the offending agent is removed.

Clinically, papillary necrosis is seen not only following abuse of the non-narcotic analgesics, but also in patients with obstructive uropathy, diabetes mellitus, and sickle cell disease (19-22). The lesion has been described in neonates with respiratory distress syndrome (23). The general characteristics of the adult patients at risk for developing papillary necrosis, the localization of the renal lesion, and other associated findings are summarized in Table 2. Unlike the patient with

Table 1. Acute Renal Effects of the Non-Narcotic Analgesics

	ASA	Acetaminophen	NSAID*
Acute Tubular Necrosis	+	+	+
Acute Cortical Necrosis	−	−	?
Acute Interstitial Nephritis	+	−	+
Nephrotic Syndrome	−	−	+
Acute Glomerulonephritis	?	?	?
Renal Prostaglandin Inhibition	+	−	+

ASA = Acetylsalicylic acid
*NSAID = Nonsteroidal Anti-inflammatory Drugs
(Summarized from Refs 12, 13)

Table 2. Diseases Associated with Renal Papillary Necrosis in Humans.

Characteristics	Analgesic Abuse	Obstructive Uropathy	Sickle Cell Disease/Trait	Diabetes Mellitus
Sex Distribution (%)				
Male	≅ 15	≅90	50	25
Female	85	≅10	50	75
Age (%)				
20-30 (y)			20	
30-50 (y)	most >30 y		60	
>50 (y)		≅90-95	≅20	75
Duration	2-3 kg index over 3 yrs	variable	variable	≅10 yr
Infection (%)	15-30	≅90	±	82
Obstruction (%)	±	100	±	18
Location of Lesion				
Unilateral	--		most	35%
Bilateral	most	variable	--	65%
Other	- Headache 85% - GI Symptoms 40% - Anemia 65% - Personality Disorder 75% - Bladder Cancer 10% - Urochrome Pigmentation to skin and viscera - ESRD 2≅30% worldwide		- Not seen in Hgb AC - Ages 2 yr to 80 yr	- Autopsy prevalence cause of death 4-5%

(Summarized from Refs 19-21, 27)

obstructive uropathy (an older male) or sickle cell disease or trait (any age and either sex), the typical patient with analgesic nephropathy is a female of greater than 30 years with pain, anemia, a personality disorder, and gastrointestinal complaints. The pain is usually headache or dyspepsia. The anemia is usually secondary to gastrointestinal bleeding. A yellow pigmentation of the skin may be present and is thought due to deposition of a phenacetin metabolite in the skin (24). Transitional cell carcinoma of the bladder is probably also the result of a metabolite(s) of phenacetin (25,26). In virtually all of the patients with analgesic nephropathy the drugs are taken surreptitiously; the amount of drug ingested and the duration are often denied.

From retrospective data, Murray and Goldberg (5) suggest that nephropathy occurs after the cumulative ingestion of 2-3 kg of index drug. Controversy exists as to which agent is the toxic one in humans. Probably all are, although most of the published literature relates specifically to phenacetin (for review see Ref 17).

NATURE OF THE PROBLEM

The use of non-narcotic analgesics both in the United States and worldwide is extrordinarily widespread. In the United States alone it is estimated that the per capita consumption of non-narcotic analgesics is 10 gm/year. Unlike the 1960's and before when virtually all nonprescription preparations were combinations containing phenacetin, the compounds most frequently ingested now are acetylsalicylic acid, acetaminophen, and the newer "nonsteroidal anti-inflammatory" agents (e.g., phenylbutazone, ibuprophen, indomethacin). While all compounds are thought to share a common mechanism of action, they have quite diverse chemical structures and quite different physico-chemical properties (1). They are thought to produce analgesia by inhibiting

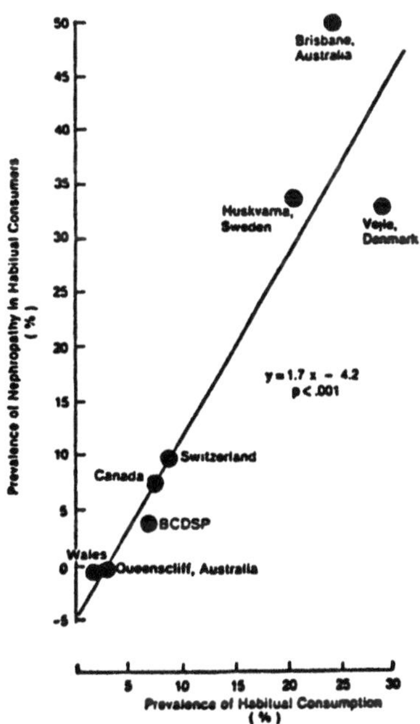

Figure 1. Prevalence of nephropathy in patients versus the prevalence of daily non-narcotic analgesic consumption. Nephropathy is minimally defined as an increase in serum creatinine; BCDSP is the Boston Cooperative Drug Surveillance Program (Adapted from Ref 17).

Table 3. Prevalence of Analgesic Nephropathy and Renal Papillary Necrosis

Locale	Analgesic Nephropathy in Renal Failure (%)	Renal Papillary Necrosis on Autopsy (%)
Queensland, Australia	30	21
New Zealand	13	> 4
Southeastern United States	10	1.7
Scotland	4.6	0.6
Northeastern United States	2.2	0.2

(Summarized from Ref 17)

prostaglandin synthesis in a wide variety of tissues (1,2,27-29); thus, unlike morphine and opium, which produce analgesia by altering the perception of pain and central nervous system (30), these compounds produce analgesia by decreasing local inflammation.

Figure 1 shows the prevalence of analgesic nephropathy as a function of analgesic consumption, and it is clear that a highly significant correlation exists (17). In this graph the prevalence of nephropathy is defined by one of several criteria: elevated serum creatinine, abnormal concentrating ability, or papillary necrosis. The Brisbane data (i.e., the highest point) was autopsy proven papillary necrosis; the control population in Brisbane had a prevalence of only 1.8%, a highly significant difference. Little published information is available for the United States. In 1976, Murray and Goldberg (5,31) surveyed 30 large centers. They identified 328 new cases of analgesic nephropathy and ≅20% of patients with interstitial disease were thought secondary to analgesic abuse. In the southeastern part of the United States the highest prevalence was noted, approximately 35% (32,33). In the northeastern part of the country the prevalence is much lower. The reason(s) for this difference is not clear. Some believe there is under-reporting in the northeast, while others feel this truly represents differences in the pattern of drug use.

The prevalence of analgesic nephropathy and documented papillary necrosis is shown in Table 3. As recently reanalyzed by Buckalew and Schey (17) in nineteen studies the association is clear. When these same investigators reviewed the world wide literature from 1967 to 1981 regarding the prevalence of patients with analgesic nephropathy in End Stage Renal Disease, the geographic variation is readily apparent (Table 4). These patients presumably all have papillary necrosis and, in Australia, are thought to comprise ≅30% of dialysis and transplant patients. In the northeastern United States and Canada they comprise far less (17,31,34).

There is a population of patients who regularly consume large amounts of aspirin and nonsteroidal anti-inflammatory agents under medical supervision. These are patients with rheumatoid arthritis. Two large studies have examined the prevalence of papillary necrosis (autopsy diagnosis or clinical diagnosis) as compared to a control population (35,36). In general, these data show that the greatest risk is for those patients taking phenacetin-containing compounds. For example, 30% of patients taking phenacetin had an autopsy diagnosis of papillary necrosis versus 8.3% for the patients on phenacetin-free compounds ($P<0.05$)(36). A clinical diagnosis of papillary necrosis was made in 13% consuming phenacetin-containing compounds versus 0.97% in those

Table 4. Prevalence of Analgesic Nephropathy in Dialysis and Transplant Patients

Locale	Years	Prevalence %
Australia	1967-1974	29.5
Belgium	1980	18
Switzerland	1979	17.5
New Zealand (Wellington)	1969-1971	12.5
Winston-Salem, USA	1974-1976	10
Germany	1979	5
Scotland	1968-1969	4.5
New Zealand (Auckland)	1966-1969	3.7
Washington, DC, USA	1979	2.8
Canada	1976	2.5
Philadelphia, USA	1981	1.7

(Summarized from Ref 17 and includes results obtained from 12 published studies; See Ref 17, Table 3, for original citations).

taking aspirin alone ($P<0.05$)(35). Ten year follow-up of rheumatology clinic patients on aspirin alone shows that they appear to be at low risk although an autopsy diagnosis of non-obstructive interstitial nephritis was significantly higher in patients consuming aspirin as compared to nonusers (22% vs 9%, respectively)(37).

Restriction of phenacetin has led to a decrease in incidence of papillary necrosis in some countries and not in others (16,38-44). In Finland, for example, the autopsy diagnosis of papillary necrosis decreased from ≅9% to 3.8% after 1965. In that same year the drug was only available by prescription. In Australia, on the other hand, this does not appear to be the case even though the two common nonprescription combinations (Bex and Vincent's) have removed phenacetin from the formula and replaced them with acetominophen and salicylamide, respectively (both contain aspirin and caffeine) (42-44).

PATHOPHYSIOLOGY OF DRUG INDUCED PAPILLARY NECROSIS

Function of the Papillary Collecting Duct and the Juxtamedullary Nephrons

The papillary collecting duct, while small in surface area, plays a major role in the final regulation of the urine. This segment has been studied using micropuncture, microcatheterization, and microperfusion techniques. The collecting duct reabsorbs sodium, secretes potassium, and is the nephron site thought responsible for adaptation to a high potassium diet (45-48). Several studies suggest that the papillary collecting duct may be the final regulator of calcium, magnesium, and phosphate transport (49-52). Water reabsorption and maximal urinary concentration occur in the papillary collecting duct. In the absence of vasopressin both the papillary collecting duct and the medullary thick ascending limb contribute to maximal urinary dilution. All segments of the collecting duct (cortical, medullary, and papillary) contribute to urinary acidification, however, the papillary collecting duct appears to contribute least (46,53-56).

The medulla and papilla contain at least three types of interstitial cells. Cytoplasmic lipid inclusions are characteristic of the Type

I cells. Biochemically these have been found to contain mainly triglycerides with small amounts of cholesterol esters and phospholipids (57,58). The triglycerides are unusually rich in the long chain fatty acids, homo-γ-linolenic and arachidonic acids. This has led to the theory that the Type I cells are specifically involved in the production and storage of the renal prostaglandins. Although the interstitial cells are capable of prostaglandin synthesis, they are by no means unique. At least 50% of prostaglandin synthetic activity comes from the collecting duct cells *per se* (59,60). The Type I cells have also been said to function as mechanical support, to synthesize extracellular matrix, and to aid in urinary concentration and blood pressure control (61-64). The Type II cells, lesser in number, are probably phagocytic cells (65), and the Type III cells, pericytes, have no known function (66).

The juxtamedullary nephrons in humans comprise ≅20-30% of the one million nephrons found in each kidney. The nephrons are located deep within the cortex at the zone separating cortex from medulla. The juxtamedullary nephrons have long loops of Henle, unlike their counterparts in the superficial cortex. The juxtamedullary nephrons are larger in size, have a higher single nephron GFR, and different transport characteristics. These nephrons transport bicarbonate at higher rates, are less reliant upon carbonic anhydrase, and are thought to be the nephrons responsible for potassium adaptation (67-70). It is apparent that a lesion which selectively destroys the juxtamedullary nephrons, as occurs in papillary necrosis, should be associated with predictable alterations in renal function.

Models of Papillary Necrosis

The pathogenesis of papillary necrosis in humans has remained problematic. There seems no question that all of the non-narcotic analgesics are capable of causing the lesion in humans. The usual animal models (dog, rat, and rabbit) are surprisingly resistant to large quantities of salicylates, phenacetin, and the nonsteroidal anti-inflammatory agents. These compounds must be given in large quantities over long periods of time (18,71-73). For example, Nanra and Kincaid-Smith (71) demonstrated that papillary necrosis occurred in only one-half of the rats given acetylsalicylic acid after 10-60 weeks; the concentration of drug necessary to produce this was 500 mg/kg/day. In 1978 Molland (72) found that phenacetin and its primary metabolite, acetaminophen, resulted in an incomplete form of papillary necrosis after a one year administration; however, when combined with salicylates complete papillary necrosis occurred in 80% of the rabbits. Other investigators, however, have failed to confirm these findings in experimental animals, thus hampering our insight into the pathophysiology (18,74-76). At best, the animal models are highly variable and require long-term administration of very large quantities of the non-narcotic analgesics. Surgical papillectomy has been studied by a few investigators (77-79). While important observations have emerged, the technique is difficult, and small changes in the level at which papillectomy is performed may produce widely varying effects on renal function.

Certain alkylating agents chemically induce papillary necrosis (80-85). The best studied is 2-bromoethylamine hydrobromide (BEA), a small halogenated hydrocarbon with the following chemical structure:

$$BrCH_2CH_2NH_2 \cdot HBr \rightarrow CH_2\text{—}CH_2 \text{ (bridged by } NH\text{)} + 2HBr$$

The compound is derived from ethylamine and is readily soluble in water.

It is thought to rapidly undergo ring closure, as shown, to a more stable compound. The compound has the advantage that a single intravenous injection produces papillary necrosis in virtually 100% of animals (86-92). The lesion also occurs in animals after intraperitoneal injection although the incidence is somewhat less (unpublished observations).

Morphology of Papillary Necrosis

Radiologically, the diagnostic sign of papillary necrosis in humans is the "ring sign". This represents the calcified papilla as seen on intravenous pyelography. When these kidneys are examined morphologically there is absence of the papilla, usually at the inner stripe of the outer medulla, tubular atrophy and cortical scarring. It is thought by most authorities that the cortical scarring often seen is secondary to degeneration seen after the long looped nephrons are lost.

In the 1970's Heptinstall and coworkers (87,88) temporally examined renal disease in rats given BEA. At 24 hrs the terminal portions of the collecting duct showed areas of necrosis and denudation of their epithelial lining. There was engorgement of the vasa recta. The thin limbs, particularly near the papillary tip, had lost their nuclei; however, the interstitial cells appeared normal. By the fourth day the entire papilla showed necrosis of all its constituent parts. There was a zone of demarcation between the papilla and the inner stripe of the outer medullary zone. The necrotic papilla had no epithelial lining and tubules were recognizable only as empty shells. By 21 days, complete calcification at the inner stripe of outer medulla was present and the papillary tip was often found lying free in the pelvis. The superficial glomeruli and the superficial cortex appeared normal initially; focal abnormalities were seen late, probably reflecting atrophy and scarring of the glomeruli containing long loops of Henle. We have confirmed these findings and have made additional observations using scanning electron microscopy (91). At 24 hrs, we found normal appearing surface morphology of the papillary tip, the juxtamedullary and superficial glomeruli. After 4 weeks, however, scanning electron microscopy revealed distinctly abnormal juxtamedullary glomeruli. These glomeruli were scarred and sclerotic; the superficial glomeruli, however, appeared completely normal (91).

Functional Changes in Papillary Necrosis

In humans with papillary necrosis renal insufficiency, salt wastage, hyperkalemia, and metabolic acidosis are often described. Table 5 summarizes pathophysiologic changes that occur during the development of the lesion in experimental animals given BEA. In intact animals, GFR at 1 day and 1 month is normal in nonhydropenic rats having moderate amounts of salt in their diet (89-92). This is in contrast to hydropenic animals which consistently show a decrease in GFR (89,92). If followed long enough all animals will die in renal failure. At 24 hrs SNGFR from the superficial glomeruli is normal (90). At 1 month, however, SNGFR in the superficial cortex is increased while that of the juxtamedullary nephrons is markedly depressed (90). This, we believe, sets the stage for the inexorable decline in renal function and ultimate progression to chronic renal failure.

Medullary and papillary plasma flow has been measured following BEA administration (93-95). Both were found to be normal at 24 hr and slightly increased at 6 hr. A microangiographic study, however, showed decreased flow to the vasa recta early in the course of the BEA-induced lesion (2 to 18 hr) which returned to normal after the first day (96).

Table 5. Summary of the Effects of Papillary Necrosis on Renal Function

Hemodynamics/Glomerular Function		
	Increased:	Medullary Plasma Flow (early)
		Superficial SNGFR (late)
	Decreased:	GFR (late)
		Juxtamedullary SNGFR (late)
	No Change:	Medullary Plasma Flow (late)
		GFR (early)
		Superficial SNGFR (early)
Electrolyte Excretion		
	Increased:	NaCl
		Calcium
		Phosphate
	Decreased:	Potassium (during high K adaptation)
	No Change:	Potassium (normal diet)
		Magnesium
Acid Excretion		
	No Change:	HCO_3 Reabsorption
		Titratable Acid Excretion
		NH_4 Excretion
		Minimum Urine pH
Water Homeostasis		
	Increased:	Urine Volume
	Decreased:	Response to AVP
		Urine Osm
		$T^{c}_{H_2O}$
	No Change:	C_{H2O}

(Summarized from Refs 89-95,97).

Salt wastage occurs early in the course of papillary necrosis (92). If dietary salt is withdrawn 3-4 days after the lesion is produced, animals do not adapt normally. They continue to excrete urine containing substantial amounts of sodium and chloride; under these conditions, volume contraction becomes apparent and many animals develop frank renal failure. These findings are similar to that reported by Shimamura in 1976 (97) using the same model, and by Wilson in 1972 (77) using the surgical papillectomy model.

Potassium homeostasis is abnormal in papillary necrosis. One previous study in animals having surgical papillectomy and renal failure shows that they are unable to excrete an acute potassium load normally (78). In BEA induced papillary necrosis, potassium excretion is similar to that seen with controls if animals are on a normal diet; following sulfate infusion, potassium excretion rises normally (89). If the animals are stressed, however, quite different results are seen. Following potassium deprivation, animals with BEA-induced papillary necrosis are unable to conserve potassium normally and develop hypokalemia (89). Following chronic potassium adaptation, induced by additional dietary intake, the superimposition of papillary necrosis leads to hyperkalemia and a marked decrease in potassium excretion (89). Mortality in potassium-adapted animals subsequently given papillary necrosis is significantly higher than in potassium adapted animals alone. The cellular basis for this effect appears to be due to the loss of Na-K ATPase activity (98), although segmental analysis of nephron ATPase activity has not yet been performed in animals during the early stages of papillary necrosis. In normal rats Na-K ATPase activity of microdissected juxtamedullary proximal tubule is the same as that of the superficial proximal tubule (99).

Whether the abnormalities in potassium homeostasis represent only a loss of collecting duct function is not yet clear. While the inability to adapt to chronic potassium loading could be the consequence of deranged collecting duct function (46), loss of juxtamedullary nephrons could also explain these findings. Jamison and coworkers (100) have found that the thin limbs of the deep nephrons secrete considerable potassium, and this is enhanced by chronic potassium loading. Selective loss of the juxtamedullary nephrons theoretically could alter potassium balance enough to explain the observations discussed above.

There are no documented abnormalities of calcium, phosphate, and magnesium excretion in humans with analgesic-induced papillary necrosis, however, both the juxtamedullary nephron and the collecting duct have been postulated to be important in the regulation of these divalent ions (50,51,101,102). The juxtamedullary nephrons have been demonstrated to have a greater absorptive capacity for calcium as compared to the superficial nephrons (101). Calcium wastage occurs in the BEA model of papillary necrosis (90) as well as in animals with papillectomy (49). In all likelihood the effect on calcium excretion is due to alteration in juxtamedullary nephron function. Papillary necrosis also results in phosphaturia (90). The phosphaturia is totally abolished by parathyroidectomy indicating that the presence of parathyroid hormone is, in some manner, required for this phenomenon. Parathyroidectomized animals with papillary necrosis are able to adapt normally to phosphate deprivation, a finding in marked contrast to results obtained with low sodium diet in which salt wastage consistently occurs.

Recent micropuncture studies have shown that during magnesium deprivation, fractional magnesium excretion in the final urine is lower than that in the late distal tubule (52). These results suggest that the collecting duct (or the juxtamedullary nephron) is important in the final regulation of urinary magnesium excretion. We examined magnesium handling in animals with established papillary necrosis, and found excretion to be the same as control; furthermore, if animals were placed on a zero magnesium diet they did not develop magnesuria despite the presence of papillary necrosis. These data show that the absence of the papillary structures and juxtamedullary nephrons is not associated with altered magnesium handling or phosphate homeostasis (in the TPTX animal). Apparently, normal homeostasis of these divalent ions can easily be maintained by the superficial proximal tubule, cortical thick ascending limb, and cortical collecting tubule.

Many patients with analgesic nephropathy or other clinical conditions associated with papillary necrosis develop hyperchloremic metabolic acidosis. They also have a decrease in glomerular filtration rate and, the acidosis is often described as being out of proportion to the decline in renal function. The metabolic acidosis could solely be the result of renal failure (103), or it could be due to a selective defect in acid excretion as a result of damage to the collecting duct or the juxtamedullary nephrons.

Micropuncture and microcatheterization studies have shown that the collecting duct is capable of significant acidification of the urine (104,46). In the papillectomized rat (with renal failure) total acid excretion and ammonium excretion is lower than that of control animals or animals with partial nephrectomy (78). We examined acidification in rats with papillary necrosis in two separate studies: one group was studied at 24 hr, the second group was studied 1 month after established papillary necrosis (89,91). Proximal tubule acidification was completely normal as assessed by bicarbonate and phosphate reabsorption. Distal tubule function was also normal. Animals were able to lower the urine pH normally in response to ammonium chloride; also, they were able to respond normally to sodium sulfate and to raise the urine pCO_2. Ammonium excretion, titratable acid excretion, and net acid excretion in animals with papillary necrosis was the same as control animals. These studies were carried out under acute clearance experiments as well as carefully controlled balance conditions. The only finding that we were able to discern was that baseline bicarbonate excretion was slightly higher in animals with chronic papillary necrosis when studied under balance conditions (91). This is likely due to the higher baseline urinary flow rates observed in animals with papillary necrosis.

These findings further document the lack of effect of the deeper segments as major regulatory sites for acid-base homeostasis. Recent evidence suggests that the cortical collecting tubule and perhaps the medullary collecting tubule are the major sites for urinary acidification (53,54). The papillary collecting tubule does not respond to acidemia with increased proton ATPase activity (56); it contains variable amounts of enzyme activity depending on the site dissected. Segments dissected after entry into the ducts of Bellini contain very little enzyme activity (55). Segments dissected higher contain ≅3-fold more (56). In summary, the presence of hyperchloremic metabolic acidosis in a patient with analgesic nephropathy and mild renal insufficiency should provoke the physician to search for another underlying cause to explain the acidosis. The other causes may include, for example, hyporeninemic hypoaldosteronism or urinary tract obstruction (105).

Patients with analgesic nephropathy often complain of polyuria and have a urinary concentrating defect unresponsive to vasopressin. Perhaps the most striking finding noted in animals with BEA-induced papillary necrosis is that of polyuria. Urine volume in rats increases from 10 to 40 ml in the first 24 hr period after the induction of papillary necrosis and remains high throughout the course of the lesion (89-92). Urine osmolality averages 600 mOsm/kg H_2O as compared to normal rats which have a urine osmolality of 1800 mOsm/kg H_2O. Overnight water deprivation with or without the exogenous administration of vasopressin does not correct the defect in concentrating ability induced by BEA (89). Free water reabsorption is decreased in animals with papillary necrosis, but free water clearance is normal (89).

ROLE OF URINARY CONCENTRATING ABILITY IN THE GENERATION OF PAPILLARY NECROSIS

There are reports in the literature showing that analgesic-induced papillary necrosis occurs with increasing frequency during the hot summer months and is more severe following volume contraction (73,106, 107). These observations suggest that the ability to concentrate the urine may be important in the generation of the lesion.

In a series of experiments we studied the role of urinary concentrating ability on the generation of BEA-induced papillary necrosis (92). A variety of animals models were selected in which urinary concentrating ability, urinary flow rate, and papillary solute concentration were distinctly abnormal (Table 6). Morphology and adaptation to a zero sodium diet were studied for 7-10 days following the administration of BEA. The control animals used in this study were hetero-

Table 6. Summary of the Effect of Urinary Concentrating Ability on the Generation of Papillary Necrosis (PN)

Condition	UV	PSC	NaCl Wastage after BEA	Histologic PN after BEA
Sprague-Dawley Rat	NL	↑	+	+
Heterozygous BB Rat	NL	↑	+	+
Homozygous BB Rat	↑	↓	No	No
Chronic AVP Replacement to Homozygous BB Rat	NL	↑	+	+
Furosemide-treated Sprague-Dawley Rat	NL	↓	+	+
Abrupt Withdrawal of AVP to Homozygous BB Rat	↑	NL	+	+
Sprague-Dawley Rat drinking 5% glucose	↑	↓	No	No

UV = urine volume; PSC = papillary solute concentration; BB = Brattleboro Rat (central diabetes insipidus); NL = Normal (absolute values are not given); (Summarized from Refs 89-92)

zygous Brattleboro rats, animals which have endogenous vasopressin and have the ability to concentrate their urine normally following water deprivation. These animals, when given BEA, develop the typical morphologic lesion of papillary necrosis; the functional lesion associated with this is the inability to conserve sodium when it is withdrawn from the diet.

When their homozygous Brattleboro litter mates were given BEA and then placed on a zero sodium diet neither the morphologic nor functional lesion of papillary necrosis developed. These animals adapted normally to sodium deprivation, excreting a sodium free urine. Homozygous Brattleboro rats have no endogenous vasopressin and their urine osmolality is ≅250 mOsm/kg H_2O. Since the absence of vasopressin *per se* may in some manner have prevented papillary necrosis we replaced the homozygous Brattleboro rat with vasopressin for 14 days. During this time urine flow rate fell to values identical to normal animals and urinary osmolality rose. When BEA was given, all the animals developed the characteristic morphologic and functional lesions of papillary necrosis. Sprague-Dawley rats undergoing a water diuresis (5% glucose drinking water), when given BEA, did not develop salt wastage or papillary necrosis.

Animals with central diabetes insipidus (i.e., homozygous Brattleboro rats) and those undergoing a water diuresis (5% glucose to Sprague-Dawley rats) have a functional alteration which consists of two parts:

1) elaboration of dilute urine for extended periods of time which is associated with a decrease in papillary solute gradient, and
2) a very high urine flow rate.

The protective effect observed in the BEA-treated homozygous Brattleboro rats could be the consequence of either the high urine flow rate, the decrease in papillary solute concentration, or both. To separate these possibilities we performed two additional sets of experiments. Furosemide was given to Sprague-Dawley rats on a chronic basis; this resulted in an isotonic urine and a decreased papillary osmolality (92). After 14 days the furosemide was withdrawn and BEA was administered. In other words, the compound was given to animals with a decreased papillary

Table 7. Possible Mechanisms of Papillary Necrosis

1. Direct cellular injury
2. Reduction or redistribution of renal blood flow
3. Prostaglandin inhibition
4. Free radical formation
5. Hypersensitivity/Immunologic

osmotic gradient but a normal rate of urine flow. These animals developed all the features of papillary necrosis. Cumulative sodium excretion was markedly increased in comparison to their sham-treated litter mates (92).

To examine the other variable, i.e., an increase in urine flow rate in the absence of a prolonged decrease in papillary tonicity, we studied the effect of abrupt withdrawal of vasopressin to vasopressin-replaced homozygous Brattleboro rats. Animals were treated with vasopressin for 7-14 days. The vasopressin was stopped and when urine flow increased (≅18 hr later), the animals were then studied. This maneuver resulted in an increase in urine volume on the background of a previously normal papillary solute osmotic gradient. When these animals were given BEA, the characteristic lesion of papillary necrosis resulted (92).

Thus, it appears that to prevent the nephrotoxic effect of BEA both a prolonged increase in urine flow and a decrease in papillary solute gradient must be present. The lesion of papillary necrosis will result if only one of the two maneuvers is attempted. The exact interrelationship between these two variables in the causation or prevention of papillary necrosis remains to be elucidated. While these maneuvers have not been tested in humans, their applicability is of obvious interest.

POSSIBLE MECHANISMS ON THE DEVELOPMENT OF PAPILLARY NECROSIS

Table 7 summarizes some of the possible mechanisms leading to papillary necrosis. There is abundant evidence in the literature suggesting that the non-narcotic analgesics cause direct cellular injury. The salicylates have been shown to inhibit the hexose monophosphate shunt in the medulla, however, acetaminophen has no such effect (108,109). In dog medullary slices only the combination of salicylic acid and acetaminophen alters metabolism (109,110). The salicylates decrease protein synthesis probably due to inhibition of amino acyl-tRNA synthetase. Salicylates also deplete the cell of adenosine triphosphate (115). A cortico-medullary gradient has been shown to occur following both salicylates and acetaminophen under certain experimental conditions (111-113). This means that the concentration of drug at the papillary tip is several fold higher than that seen in the cortex. If volume contraction is present this concentration gradient is even higher.

Molland (114) has postulated that a decrease in papillary blood flow could lead to ischemia of the deeper parts of the kidney and subsequently result in cellular necrosis. This mechanism is certainly applicable to patients with sickle cell disease in which there is sludging and sickling of the papillary vasa recta, and in diabetics in whom there is extensive nephrosclerosis. Renal blood flow has been examined in experimental papillary necrosis in only a few studies and the results are conflicting. In one study blood flow was decreased, but other studies show blood flow to be unchanged as compared to control

(93-96). Anoxia and ischemia could easily still occur in the face of normal measurements if the affinity of hemoglobin for oxygen is decreased. Salicylates decrease erythrocyte 2,3-diphosphoglyceride in dose-dependent manner. Such a decrease would be the same as an absolute fall in papillary blood flow and could, thus, easily lead to ischemia and infarction. Phenacetin and acetaminophen may cause methemoglobinemia and sulfhemoglobin formation (1). With therapeutic doses of the drug, 1-3% of hemoglobin is converted to methemoglobin, and this usually is of no clinical consequence. With chronic abuse, however, methemoglobinemia may be prominent and could contribute to renal ischemia. BEA _per se_ alters the hemoglobin molecule _in vitro_ (116); whether this occurs with the non-narcotic analgesics is not yet known.

The kidney synthesizes all known prostaglandins and thromboxanes. The major role of these products appears to be in the control of renal blood flow and glomerular filtration rate, the stimulation of renin secretion, and the modulation of sodium and water excretion (1,3,27,29, 70,117). Salicylates and the nonsteroidal anti-inflammatory agents inhibit renal cylco-oxygenase and prevent prostaglandin synthesis. In conventional doses these agents reduce renal synthesis of prostaglandins by 75% within 1 hr of parenteral administration (117). Acetaminophen, however, does not inhibit the renal prostaglandins. Thus, while the theory of prostaglandin inhibition is intriguing and could be a common unifying thread for all these agents, clearly this explanation is not complete. It may be that these compounds, particularly acetaminophen, also alter leukotriene synthesis in the kidney. While the role of these compounds in the kidney is not understood, it appears that leukotriene C_4 has profound effects on renal hemodynamics (118).

The metabolites of acetaminophen bind to proteins of renal tissue and deplete the cell of glutathione (119,120). Free radical formation also results from acetaminophen and its more stable metabolite, 3,5,-dimethyl acetaminophen (121). The free radical then reacts with oxygen to form superoxide, resulting in alterations of membrane lipids. Free radicals stimulate endogenous phospholipase activity in isolated brain capillaries (122). Phospholipase activation results in phospholipid degradation with accumulation of free fatty acids and lysophospholipids (123). This results in membrane dysfunction. Inhibition of glucose-6-phosphate activity and altered membrane permeability have been demonstrated (124-126). Free fatty acids have been shown to cause calcium efflux from liver and kidney mitochondria (127). Whether all these effects are solely the result of changes in calcium is not yet clear, as free radicals _per se_ can alter membrane permeability independent of calcium (128). As many of these observations were made in the renal superficial proximal tubule and other tissues, the relationship to papillary necrosis is not yet known.

There is no good evidence suggesting that the non-narcotic analgesics cause papillary necrosis either by a hypersensitivity reaction or by immunologic mechanisms. Of interest, however, are the several reports of serum-induced papillary necrosis (129,130). We have tried to examine this model but have been unable to consistently reproduce the renal lesion.

Therapy and Prognosis

The therapy of papillary necrosis is primarily supportive (131). If the offending agent can be identified it should be discontinued. This often is not possible owing to the nature of those abusing the drug. Adequate urinary drainage should be maintained and patients should be treated aggressively for sepsis. Coverage for both gram positive and gram negative organisms is probably prudent. While dialysis can maintain patients in the face of complete anuria, many will die of infection. If they survive, renal function may stabilize for a time; many will eventually require maintenance hemodialysis. Psychologic counseling may be of some value as a number of these patients have a psychiatric history. In the "at risk" patient who must use the non-narcotic analgesics regularly a prolonged water diuresis may minimize the risk for subsequent development of papillary necrosis.

ACKNOWLEDGEMENTS

This work was supported in part by a grant from the National Institutes of Health, #R01-DK36119. Dr. Sabatini is the recipient of a Research Career Development Award, #K04-DK-05127. The author would like to thank Ms Sondra Rogers for her excellent typographical assistance.

REFERENCES

1. RJ Flower, S Moncada, and JR Vane, in: The Pharmacological Basis of Therapeutics (ed 7), AG Gilman, LSGoodman, TW Rall, et al, eds, MacMillan, New York, 1985
2. Symposium on Analgesics, Georgetown University, Ann Intern Med 141:271, 1981
3. Symposium Proceedings, MJ Dunn and C Patrono (eds), Am J Med 81(2B):1, 1986
4. HU Zollinger and O Spühler, Schweiz Z Allg Pathol 13:806, 1950
5. T Murray and M Goldberg, Ann Rev Med 26:537, 1976
6. O Nordenfelt and N Ringerts, Acta Med Scand 170:385, 1961
7. K Larsen and CE Moller, Acta Med Scand 164:53, 1959
8. FJ Gloor, Kidney Int 13:27, 1978
9. RS Nanra, J Stuart-Taylor, and AH de Leon, et al, Kidney Int 13:79, 1978
10. G Eknoyan, WY Qunibi, and RT Grisson, et al, Medicine 61:55, 1982
11. Symposium Proceedings, M Zimmermann and DM Long (eds), Am J Med 75:1, 1983
12. DM Clive and JS Stoff, N Engl J Med 9:563, 1984
13. MH Gault, TC Rudwal, and WD Engles, et al, Ann Intern Med 68:906, 1968
14. T Murray and M Goldberg, Ann Intern Med 82:453, 1975
15. RM Murray, Kidney Int 13:50, 1978
16. UD Dubach, B Rosner, and PS Levy, et al, Kidney Int 13:41, 1978
17. VM Buckalew Jr, and HM Schey, Medicine 65:291, 1986
18. G Eknoyan, Sem in Nephrol 4:65, 1984
19. PS Ellis and HM Pollack, Sem in Nephrol 4:77, 1984
20. SK Mujais, Sem in Nephrol 4:40, 1984
21. CA Vaamonde, Sem in Nephrol 4:48, 1984
22. IW McCall, N Maule, and P Desal, et al, Radiology 126:99, 1978
23. MD Lelong-Tissier, M Benazet, and JD Ropert, et al, Arch Fr Pediatr 36:287, 1979
24. DM Kriber, Br J Med 2:615, 1967
25. U Bengtsson, S Johansson, and L Angervall, Kidney Int 13:107, 1978
26. TA Gonwa, WT Corbett, and HM Schey, et al, Ann Int Med 93:249, 1980
27. M Hamberg, Biochem Biophys Res Commun 49:720, 1972
28. B Samuelsson, E Granström, and M Hamberg, et al, Annu Rev Biochem 47:997, 1978
29. MJ Dunn, Annu Rev Med 35:411, 1984
30. JH Jaffe and WR Martin, in: The Pharmacological Basis of Therapeutics (ed 7), AG Gilman, LS Goodman, and TW Rall, et al, eds, MacMillan, New York, 1985

31. TG Murray and M Goldberg, Kidney Int 13:64, 1978
32. TA Gonwa, RW Hamilton, and VM Buckalew Jr, Arch Intern Med 141:462, 1981
33. TG Murray, PD Stolley, JC Anthony, et al, Arch Intern Med 143:1687, 1983
34. DR Wilson amd MD Gault, Can Med Assoc J 127:500, 1982
35. I Ferguson, F Johnson, and B Reay, et al, Med J Aust 1:950, 1973
36. AAH Lawson and N Maclean, Ann Rheum Dis 25:441, 1966
37. RD Emkey and JA Mills, JAMA 247:55, 1982
38. A Kasanen, Ann Clin Res 5:369, 1973
39. M Sillanpää, A Kasanen, and A Elonen, Acta Med Scand 212:3123, 1982
40. RM Murray, Br Med J 4:131, 1972
41. CE Maybeck and B Wichmann, Acta Med Scand 205:599, 1979
42. JH Stewart, Kidney Int 13:72 1978
43. JH Stewart, SW McCarthy, and BG Storey, Br Med J 1:440, 1975
44. RS Nanra, J Stuart-Taylor, and AH de Leon, Kidney Int 13: , 1978
45. K Ullrich, Circulation 21:869, 1960
46. K Hierholzer, Am J Physiol 201:318, 1961
47. J Diezi, P Michand, and J Aceues, et al, Am J Physiol 224:623, 1973
48. W Rau and E Frömter, Pflügers Arch 351:99, 1977
49. FW Finkelstein and AS Kliger, Am J Physiol 233:F97, 1977
50. JH Stein and JH Reineck, Kidney Int 6:1, 1974
51. ZS Agus, PJS Chiu, and M Goldberg, Am J Physiol 232:F545, 1977
52. SL Carney, NLM Wong, and GA Quamme, et al, J Clin Invest 65:180, 1980
53. TD McKinney and MB Burg, Am J Physiol 234:F141, 1978
54. ME Laski and NA Kurtzman, J Clin Invest 72:2050, 1983
55. S Sabatini and NA Kurtzman, Clin Res 35:637A, 1987
56. S Sabatini and NA Kurtzman, Clin Res 36:46A, 1988
57. E Anggard, S-O Bohman, and JE Griffin, et al, Acta Physiologica Scandinavia 84:231, 1972
58. IN Bojensen, in: The Renal Medulla and Hypertension. AK Mandal and S-O Bohman eds, Plenum Medical Book Co, New York, 1980
59. RM Zusman, in: The Renal Medulla and Hypertension. AK Mandal and S-O Bohman, eds, Plenum Medical Book Co, New York, 1980
60. S-O Bohman, Prostaglandins 14:729, 1977
61. TR Beck, A Hassid, and MJ Dunn, J Phar Exp Ther 215:15, 1980
62. WS Sternberg, E Farber, and CE Dunlap, J Histochemistry and Cytochemistry 4:266, 1956
63. S-O Bohman, J Ultrastructure Reas 47:329, 1974
64. EE Muirhead, Hypertension 2:444, 1980
65. RE Bulger and BF Trump, Am J Anatomy 118:685, 1966
66. RR Bruns and GE Palade, J Cell Bio 37:244, 1968
67. JP Frommer, ME Laski, and DE Wesson, et al, J Clin Invest 73:1034, 1984
68. JH Reineck, R Parma, and JL Barnes, et al, Am J Physiol 239:F187, 1980
69. JP Frommer, DE Wesson, and M Laski, et al, Am J Physiol 249:F107, 1985.
70. BM Brenner, LD Dworkin, and I Ichikawa, in: The Kidney (3rd ed), BM Brenner and FC Rector, eds, Saunders, Philadelphia, 1986
71. RS Nanra and P Kincaid-Smith, Br Med J 3:559, 1970
72. EA Molland, Kidney Int 13:5, 1978
73. E Abraham, A Rubenstein, and N Levin, Nature 200:695, 1963
74. JR Leonards, V Inter Cong Nephrol, H Villareal, S Karger (eds), Basel, p 50
75. MA McIver and JB Hobb, Med J Aust 1:197, 1975
76. BM Phillips, RW Hartnagel, and JL Leeliny, et al, Aust-NZ J Med Suppl 6:48, 1976
77. DR Wilson, Can J Physiol Pharmacol 50:662, 1972
78. FW Finkelstein and JP Hayslett, Kidney Int 6:419, 1974

79. TL Hardy, Br J Exp Pathol 51:591 1970
80. C Levaditi, Arch Int Pharmacodyn 8:45, 1901
81. EE Mandel and H Popper, AMA Arch Pathol 52:1, 1970
82. M Fuwa and D Waugh, Fed Proc 26:517, 1967
83. DJ Davies, Arch Pathol 86:377, 1968
84. M Fuwa and D Waugh, Arch Pathol 85:404, 1974
85. FE Cuppage and A Tate, Lab Invest 31:593, 1974
86. A Oka, Virchows Arch [Pathol Anat] 214:149, 1913
87. G Murray, RG Wyllie, and GS Hill, et al, Am J Pathol 67:285, 1972
88. GS Hill, RG Wyllie, and M Miller, et al, Am J Pathol 68:213, 1972
89. JAL Arruda, S Sabatini, and PK Mehta, et al, Kidney Int 15:264, 1979
90. S Sabatini, PK Mehta, and S Hayes, et al, Am J Physiol 241:F14, 1981
91. S Sabatini, V Alla, and A Wilson, et al, Pflugers Arch 393:262, 1982
92. S Sabatini, S Koppera, and J Manaligod, et al, Kidney Int 23:705, 1983
93. K Solez, M Miller, and PA Quarles, et al, Am J Pathol 76:521, 1974
94. R Vanholder, N Lameire, and W Eeckhaut, et al, Arch Int Physiol Biochem 89:63, 1981
95. RL Clark, Invest Radiol 10:438, 1975
96. JT Cuttino, FU Goss, and RL Clark, et al, Invest Radiol 16:107, 1981
97. T Shimamura, Exp Mol Pathol 25:1, 1976
98. S Sabatini, J Pharmacol Exptl Therapeutics 232:214, 1985
99. S Sabatini and NA Kurtzman, Clin Res 35:663A, 1987
100. RL Jamison, FB Lacy, and JP Pennell, et al, Kidney Int 9:323, 1976
101. RL Jamison, NR Frey, and FB Lacy, Am J Physiol 227:745, 1974
102. FG Knox, H Osswald, and GR Marchand, et al, Am J Physiol 233:F261, 1977
103. S Sabatini, Med Clin North Am 67:845, 1983
104. J Buerkert and D Martin, Kidney Int 19:235A, 1981
105. DC Batlle, JAL Arruda, and NA Kurtzman, N Engl J Med 3045:373, 1981
106. B Sakar and P Kincaid-Smith, Br Med J 1:161, 1969
107. RS Nanra, JD Hicks, and JH McNamary, et al, Med J Aust 1:293, 1970
108. MH Gault and NT Shadhidi, Clin Pharm Ther 15:521, 1974
109. W Davidson, L Daffest, and W Shippey, Clin Res 21:227, 1973
110. WM Kluwe and JB Hook, Kidney Int 18:648, 1980
111. LW Bluemle and M Goldberg, J Clin Invest 47:2507, 1968
112. KH Beyer and RT Gelanden, Arch Int Pharmacodyn 231:180, 1978
113. MH Gault, in: Proceedings, IV Amer Soc Nephrol, Washington DC, (abst)
114. EA Molland, Kidney Int 13:5, 1978
115. AG Dawson, Biochem Pharmacol 24:1407, 1975
116. WT Morrisen, AD Pressley, and JG Adams, et al, Hemoglobin 5:403, 1981
117. M Dunn and EJ Zambroski, Kidney Int 18:609, 1980
118. KF Badr, C Baylis, and JM Pfeffer, et al, Clin Res 31:698, 1983
119. JF Newton, DA Pasino, and JB Hook, Toxicol Appl Pharmacol 78:39, 1985
120. CR Fernando, IC Calder, and KN Ham, J Med Chem 23:1153, 1980
121. RP Mason and V Fischer, Fed Proc 45:2493, 1986
122. AM Au, PH Chan, and RA Fishman, J Cell Biochem 27:449, 1985
123. KR Chien, A Han, and A Sen, et al, Circ Res 54:313, 1984
124. E Matthys, Y Patel, and J Kreisberg, et al, Kidney Int 26:153, 1984
125. DR Chien, J Abrams, and A Serroni, et al, J Biol Chem 253:4809, 1978
126. MS Paller, JR Hoidal, and TF Ferris, J Clin Invest 74:1156, 1984
127. I Roman, P Gmaj, and C Nowicka, et al, Eur J Biochem 102:615, 1979
128. WB Weglicki, BF Dickens, and IT Mak, Biochem Biophys Res Commun 124:229, 1984
129. A Ljungvist and J Richarson, Lab Invest 15:1395, 1966
130. JC Lee, SW French, and JP Wizgird, et al, J Lab Invest 17:458, 1967
131. S Sabatini, Sem in Nephrol 8:41, 1988.

LITHIUM INDUCED POLYURIA AND POLYDIPSIA

Giuseppe Passavanti, Erasmo Buongiorno, Giuseppina De Fino, Giulio Rutigliano*, Michele Giannattasio, and Pasquale Coratelli
Institute of Nephrology and Institute of Psychiatry*
University of Bari, Bari (Italy)

Introduction

It is well known that lithium carbonate, which is frequently used in the treatment of psychiatric disorders, can induce a syndrome characterized by polyuria and polydipsia (1). According to the various investigators, these clinical findings appear in a range between 20% and 70% of the patients treated (2,3,4,5,6,7). Lithium-induced polyuria and polydipsia may be due to primary polydipsia with secondary polyuria or to primary polyuria with secondary polydipsia. In support of the above-mentioned alternatives, it has been reported that lithium may stimulate thirst or may interfere with the ADH-dependent mechanisms. Experimental studies on rats have demonstrated that lithium can stimulate thirst (8,9,10,11). Other experimental studies on rats have demonstrated that lithium can deplete the posterior pituitary gland and the supra-optic nuclei of their neuro-endocrine material (12,13), showing that lithium may interfere with the synthesis, deposit and/or release of the ADH hormone, causing central diabetes insipidus. On the other hand, another cause which has been suggested is an interference by the lithium with the tubular renal action of the ADH, causing nephrogenic diabetes insipidus (14,15,16,17). In contrast, however, some authors were unable, under somewhat different experimental conditions, to detect a lithium-induced inhibition of the ADH -stimulated water flow in toads' urinary bladders (18).

In the present report the mechanisms which cause the above-mentioned syndrome are investigated, bearing in mind the controversies in literature regarding its pathogenesis.

Patients and Studies

Patients

46 patients on long-term lithium carbonate treatment entered the study, divided into two homogeneous groups according to age, sex and duration of treatment. The first group was composed of 17 non polyuric patients, 8 males and 9 females,aged 39.4 $\pm$ 11.2 years, on lithium treatment for 50 $\pm$ 40 months, with serum creatinine of 1.04 $\pm$ 0.12 mg/dl and creatinine clearance of 98.91 $\pm$ 14.79 ml/min/1.73 m^2. The second group was composed of 29 polyuric patients, 13 males and 16 females,aged 41.5 $\pm$ 11.6 years, on lithium treatment for 71 $\pm$ 44 months,with serum creatinine of 0.99 $\pm$ 0.19 mg/dl and with creatinine clearance of 92.25 $\pm$ 8.94 ml/min/1.73 m^2.

None of the patients included in the study had a history of urinary tract infections or of other renal disease, and proteinuria, haematuria, glycosuria or hypertension were not found in any of them.

Patients with episodes of acute lithium intoxication, and patients on other drugs in addition to lithium, were excluded.

1st Study

The renal concentrating ability was assessed in the 46 patients by means of a 15-hour dehydration test in the following manner: all the patients fasted from 6 p.m. until 9 a.m. the following day; at 6 a.m., 12 hours after the last fluid and food had been ingested,the patients emptied their bladder and the urinary osmolality and creatinine were then measured on the urine samples collected from 6 a.m. until 9 a.m.; at 9 a.m., blood samples were taken to determine plasma sodium, osmolality and creatinine.

The choice of a 15-hour dehydration test was based on the observation, in our laboratory, that urinary osmolality had reached maximal levels within this period of time in 18 normal subjects.

A longer period of water deprivation (WD), in fact, did not modify the osmolality values reached in the urine samples collected from 6 a.m. until 9 a.m. (Tab. 1).

Urinary and plasma osmolality were determined by freezing-point depression on a Fiske OS™ Osmometer; serum lithium levels (expressed as a mean of the determinations performed monthly during the period of therapy on blood samples drawn in the morning, 12 hours after the last dose) were measured by an Elvi 665 flame photometer.

Table 1. Urinary osmolality (Uosm mOsm/Kg) during WD in 18 normal subjects (* compared with the values of the 1st sample)

SUBJECT	Sex	1st sample	2nd sample	3rd sample	4th sample
1. C.A.	F	1195	1190	1087	928
2. C.A.	F	1015	1059	1029	1127
3. P.G.	M	956	948	948	997
4. C.C.	F	986	1000	1047	960
5. L.A.	M	1037	1027	969	937
6. C.A.	M	1139	914	1072	1185
7. T.G.	M	1116	1115	1129	1154
8. S.A.	M	989	946	958	1009
9. L.G.	M	999	1126	1180	1140
10. T.G.	M	985	952	955	853
11. D.L.C.	F	1310	1282	1061	1016
12. S.C.	F	1077	977	1063	1040
13. G.C.C.	M	1034	1083	1092	1094
14. C.F.	M	932	982	1065	1134
15. C.P.	M	1037	1032	1020	1111
16. D.F.G.	F	945	996	1012	829
17. F.C.	F	1111	1288	1164	1137
18. G.L.	M	888	844	891	894
Mean		1041.72	1042.27	1041.22	1030.27
± SD		103.07	120.81	77.23	111.10
± SEM		24.29	28.47	18.20	26.18
			N.S.*	N.S.*	N.S.*

1st sample: Uosm on the samples collected from 6 a.m. to 9 a.m. (12th - 15th h of WD)
2nd sample: " " " " 9 a.m. " 12 a.m. (15th - 18th " ")
3rd sample: " " " " 12 a.m. " 3 p.m. (18th - 21th " ")
4th sample: " " " " 3 p.m. " 6 p.m. (21th - 24th " ")

2nd Study

28 of the 46 lithium-treated patients (12 non-polyuric and 16 polyuric) all non-smokers and/or non-drinkers, were given the same dietary intake of calories (36-40 Kcal/Kg b.wt.), of protein (1-1.2 g/Kg b.wt.), of NaCl (9-11 g/day), and therefore the same calculated osmolar intake, about 900 mOsm/day.

In both groups of patients, the urine volume, urinary osmolality and osmolal excretion/day, urinary sodium and sodium excretion/day, fractional excretion of sodium, water intake, plasma sodium and osmolality before fluid intake and breakfast in the morning, and urinary ADH excretion were evaluated.

We chose the urine ADH dosage for evaluation as it offers a number of advantages with regard to the plasma ADH dosage: ADH is more stable in the urine than in plasma and furthermore, since ADH is secreted episodically, its plasmatic levels may vary very rapidly in response to test stimuli, while the assay of ADH in the urine provides an integrated estimate of the hormone secretion.

The measurement of ADH excretion was performed with a commercially available RIA Kit (Bühlmann laboratories AG, Basel Switzerland), after the ADH had been extracted from the urine according to the method described by Tausch et al (19), using disposable SEP-PAK columns packed with octadecasilyl--silica (C_{18} SEP-PAKS, Waters Associates, Inc., Milford, Ma).

Final recovery by extraction was evaluated for each sample by adding labeled ADH, and the concentration of ADH found in each sample was corrected for its recovery. The overall recovery was 85.25 ± 6 %. The intra-assay and inter-assay coefficient of variation was 6.6% and 8.4% respectively.

3rd Study

As the results of the 2nd study supported the existence of lithium-induced nephrogenic diabetes insipidus, a 3rd study was subsequently carried out to define the mechanism by which lithium may induce this condition. This study was performed in order to evaluate the possibility that the lithium-induced ADH-resistant tubulopathy may be due to an enhancement by lithium of the renal prostaglandin action.

12 of the 16 polyuric patients submitted to urine ADH measurement were divided into two groups.

6 patients (1st group) were studied on WD before and on the sixth day of indomethacin (3 mg/Kg b.wt.), prostaglandin synthesis inhibitor, administered in three daily doses for 6 days.

The other six patients (2nd group) with an identical mean maximal urinary osmolality to that of the 1st group received 40 mcg of DDAVP intranasally at the 15th h of WD, before and on the sixth day of indomethacin.

Three urine samples were collected to evaluate the urinary osmolality: from 12th to 15th h (1st sample), from 15th to 18th h (2nd sample) and from 18th to 21st h (3rd sample) of WD.

Statistics

All results are expressed as the mean $\pm$ the standard deviation. The significance was evaluated with the Student t-test. Linear regression analysis by the least-squares fit method was used to determine the correlation between the two variables. The reliability was determined by the correlation coefficient (r).

Results

1st Study

The response to the dehydration test in the 46 lithium-treated patients revealed the existence of a renal concentrating defect in the 29 polyuric patients (Table 2).

Table 2 . Response to dehydration test in 29 lithium-treated polyuric patients

PATIENTS	URINE OSMOLALITY (mOsm/Kg)	PLASMA OSMOLALITY (mOsm/Kg)	PLASMA SODIUM (mEq/l)	URINE VOLUME (ml/min)	CREATININE CLEARANCE (ml/min/1.73m2)
1. C.A.	515	296	144	1.05	77
2. F.G.	393	297	145	1.94	82
3. L.D.A.	558	299	143	0.99	76
4. S.A.	460	303	146	1.05	78
5. M.G.	355	298	148	1.71	70
6. D.C.G.	478	310	147	1.60	96
7. L.F.A.	627	305	146	1.19	75
8. P.S.	444	295	146	1.50	70
9. P.N.	594	301	147	0.98	114
10. Q.V.	420	303	146	0.91	78
11. T.O.	491	296	147	0.69	129
12. S.M.	299	301	148	1.48	91
13. T.O.	479	296	146	0.89	90
14. L.D.A.	523	295	145	0.96	75
15. R.C.F.	639	294	144	1.16	104
16. V.O.	452	297	146	1.14	99
17. L.F.	661	295	145	0.83	108
18. M.G.	355	299	149	1.71	70
19. T.O	440	297	146	1.50	70
20. D.L.	593	300	148	0.98	76.5
21. S.A.M.	318	302	149	1.27	88
22. C.M.	399	296	145	1.61	92
23. P.R.	440	296	145	1.05	101
24. D.G.N.	254	305	149	3.61	127
25. A.I.	626	299	150	0.82	80
26. P.A.	514	301	147	1.10	122
27. D.M.	305	296	146	2.04	102
28. A.C.	353	296	145	1.47	85
29. F.L.	414	296	145	1.55	77
MEAN	462.03	298.75	146.31	1.33	89.74
± S.D.	± 110.78	± 3.79	± 1.69	± 0.56	± 17.56

The maximal urinary osmolality was 462.03 ± 110.78 mOsm/Kg, in comparison with values of 919.70 ± 101.39 ($p < 0.0001$) in the 17 non-polyuric patients (Table 3).

The urine volume was 1.33 ± 0.56 ml/min and 0.57 ± 0.19 ml/min respectively ($p < 0.001$).

Plasma osmolality and plasma sodium were 298.75 ± 3.79 mOsm/Kg and 146.31 ± 1.69 mEq/l in the polyuric patients, 291.23 ± 1.30 mOsm/Kg and 141.88 ± 0.69 mEq/l in the non-polyuric patients, with statistically different values in each data group ($p < 0.0001$).

Creatinine clearance corrected for body surface was normal and there was no difference in either patient group (89.74 ± 17.56 in the polyuric patients and 97.52 ± 12.91 ml/min/1.73 m^2 in the non-polyuric patients).

Table 3. Response to dehydration test in 17 lithium-treated non-polyuric patients

PATIENTS	URINE OSMOLALITY (mOsm/Kg)	PLASMA OSMOLALITY (mOsm/Kg)	PLASMA SODIUM (mEq/l)	URINE VOLUME (ml/min)	CREATININE CLEARANCE (ml/min/1.73 m^2)
1. P.N.	964	290	141	0.58	91
2. T.M.	1105	291	142	0.63	95
3. L.L.	996	291	141	0.51	90
4. B.F.	828	293	142	0.30	98
5. D.M.M.	865	291	141	0.47	97
6. D.G.N.	875	290	142	0.66	94
7. S.C.	882	290	142	1.02	100
8. M.A.	804	293	143	0.44	106
9. R.A.	887	290	142	0.61	92
10. G.N.	859	292	142	0.72	89
11. T.G.B.	1088	292	142	0.55	86
12. M.C.	871	294	143	0.77	85
13. R.A.	932	292	142	0.55	81
14. M.A.	800	290	141	0.71	119
15. M.S.	1087	290	142	0.33	90
16. D.E.R.	983	290	141	0.22	127
17. R.P.	809	292	143	0.68	118
MEAN	919.70	291.23	141.88	0.57	97.52
± S.D.	± 101.39	± 1.30	± 0.69	± 0.19	± 12.91

None of the polyuric patients was unable to complete the dehydration test because of severe thirst or loss of more than 3% of body weight.

The evaluation of the lithium carbonate dose and the lithaemia revealed that the patients who presented the renal concentrating defect were the ones with a significantly higher daily dose and higher lithaemia (Tab. 4).

Table 4. Lithium dosage and average serum lithium level in two groups of patients

	AVERAGE DOSE Li_2CO_3 (mg/day)	AVERAGE DOSE Li_2CO_3 (mg/Kg b.wt.)	AVERAGE SERUM LITHIUM (mEq/l)
NON POLYURIC PATIENTS n = 17	1058.82 ± 282.97	14.83 ± 3.16	0.61 ± 0.15
	$p < 0.005$	$p < 0.0001$	$p < 0.0001$
POLYURIC PATIENTS n = 29	1313.79 ± 258.73	20.75 ± 3.87	1.12 ± 0.22

These data suggest the existence of a dose-effect relationship, individuating in the higher lithaemia levels a "trigger" factor in the pathogenesis of the polyuric-polydipsic syndrome. In fact, by correlating the daily dose of lithium carbonate taken by each patient with the maximal urinary osmolality, an inverse relationship was observed (Fig.1), and this was still more evident when the dose was expressed in mg/kg b.wt. (Fig. 2).

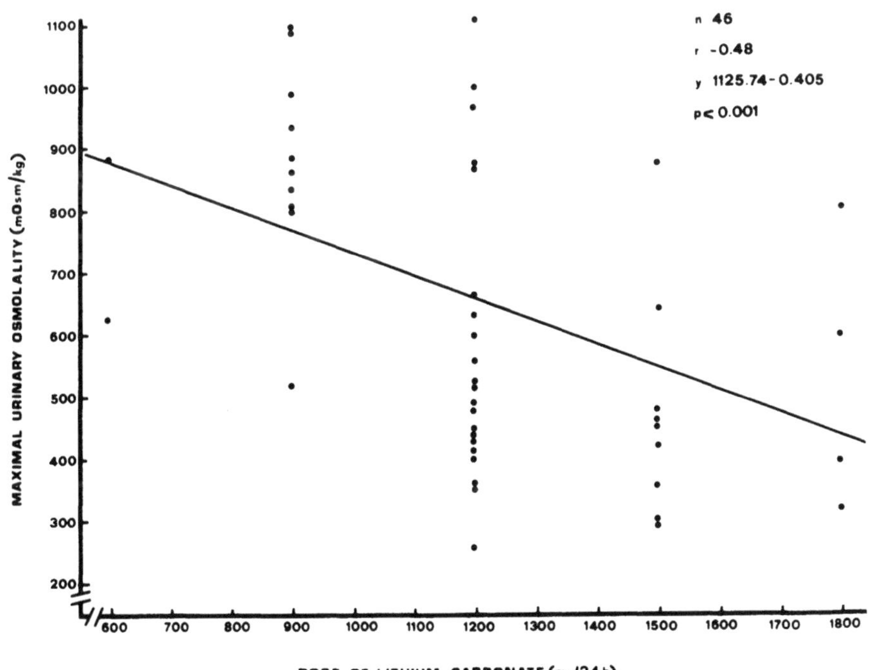

Fig.1. Relationship between dose of lithium carbonate (mg/24 h) and maximal urinary osmolality in 46 patients on long-term lithium treatment

On the same lines, an inverse correlation was observed between lithaemia and maximal urinary osmolality (Fig. 3).

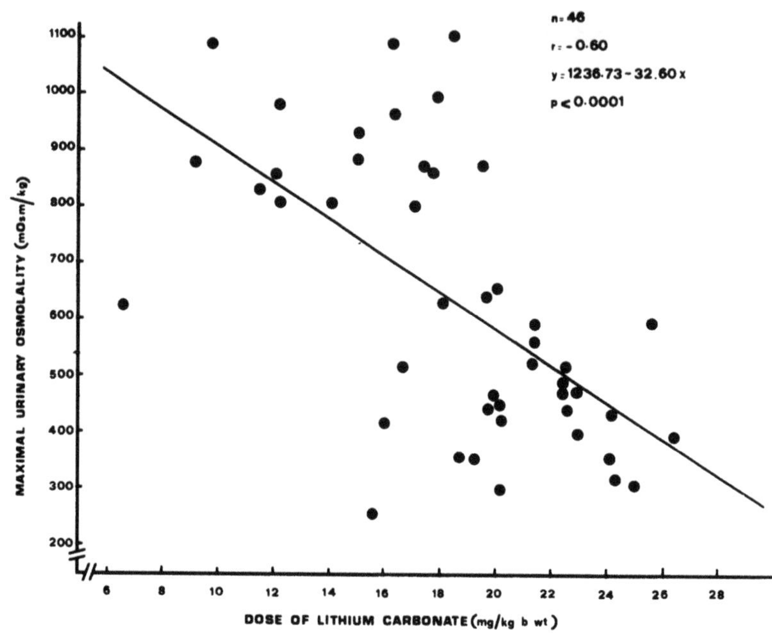

Fig.2. Relationship between dose of lithium carbonate (mg/Kg b.wt.) and maximal urinary osmolality in 46 patients on long-term lithium treatment

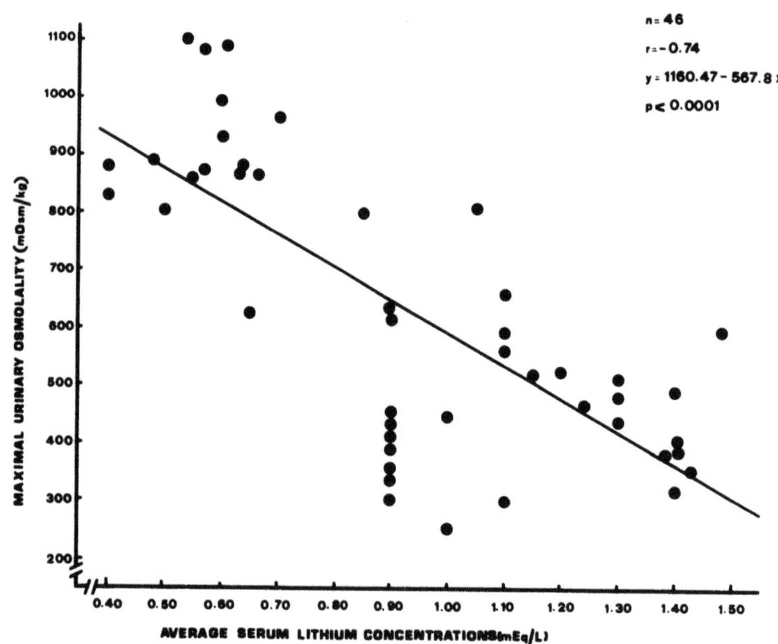

Fig.3. Relationship between average serum lithium concentrations and maximal urinary osmolality in 46 patients on long-term lithium treatment

2nd Study

In the patients submitted to urine ADH measurement we observed that the polyuric patients presented, contrarily to the non polyuric, significantly higher values of plasma osmolality (295.2 ± 2.4 mOsm/Kg vs 288.7 ± 1.6; p ∠ 0.001) and urinary ADH excretion levels (253 ± 88 ng/day vs 81 ± 29; p ∠ 0.0001) (Table 5).

Table 5. Dietetic details and water-solute balance in 28 selected lithium treated patients

	NON POLYURIC PATIENTS n 12		POLYURIC PATIENTS n 16
CALORIE INTAKE	36 - 40 Kcal/kg		
PROTEIN INTAKE	1 - 1.2 g/kg		
NaCl INTAKE	9 - 11 g/day		
CALCULATED OSMOLAR INTAKE	≃ 900 mOsm/day		
URINE VOLUME	1 510 ± 136	p<0.001	3 237 ± 1 208 ml/day
URINARY OSMOLALITY	638 ± 53	p<0.001	322 ± 102 mOsm/kg
URINARY OSMOLAL EXCRETION	953 ± 83	N.S.	946 ± 137 mOsm/day
URINARY SODIUM	123.5 ± 15.4	p<0.0001	69.5 ± 16 8 mEq/l
URINARY SODIUM EXCRETION	186 ± 20	N.S.	180 ± 30 mEq/day
SODIUM FRACTIONAL EXCRETION	0.94 ± 0.11	N.S.	0.90 ± 0 18
WATER DRINKING	729 ± 128	p<0.001	2 417 ± 1 232 ml/day
PLASMA SODIUM	140 ± 1.6	p<0.001	144.4 ± 2 mEq/l
PLASMA OSMOLALITY	288.7 ± 1.6	p<0.001	295.2 ± 2.4 mOsm/kg
URINARY ADH EXCRETION	81 ± 29	p<0 0001	253 ± 88 ng/day

values are mean ± SD

These results suggested a nephrogenic pathogenesis of the renal urinary concentrating impairment.

The existence of an ADH-resistant tubulopathy in polyuric patients was also supported by the discovery of an inverse correlation between urinary osmolality and ADH excretion levels, contrarily to the non-polyuric patients (Fig.4).

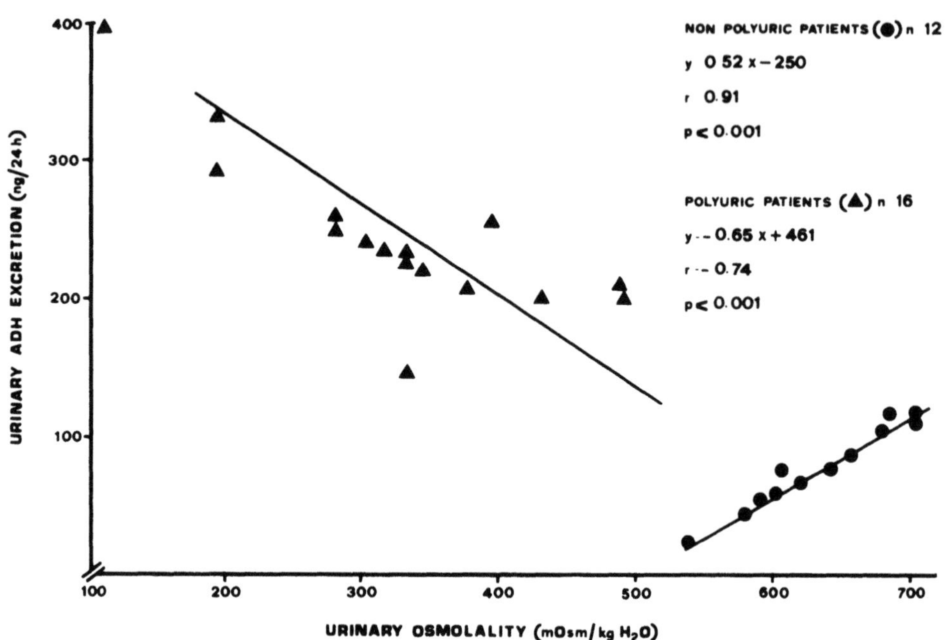

Fig.4 . Relationship between urinary osmolality and urinary ADH excretion

3rd Study

In the patients of the 1st group the Uosm was 472.50 ± 91.06 in the 1st, 494.66 ± 114.36 in the 2nd and 493.66 ± 99.62 mOsm/Kg in the 3rd sample, showing a urinary concentrating defect, which did not modify with the continuation of WD.

When the same patients were treated with indomethacin, however, the Uosm increased from 469.16 ± 118.86 mOsm/Kg in the first to 548.83 ± 114.09 in the 2nd ($p < 0.01$) and to 635.5 ± 109.3 in the 3rd sample ($p < 0.001$)(Fig. 5).

In the patients of the second group, who had received DDAVP at the 15th h of WD, the Uosm again did not modify with the continuation of WD (490.67 ± 47.86 in the 1st; 509.33 ± 44.21 in the 2nd; 535.16 ± 93.39 in the 3rd sample).

But when these patients were treated with indomethacin, the urinary osmolality increased very significantly, from 491.50 ± 125.25 in the 1st to 734.83 ± 148 in the 2nd ($p < 0.001$) and to 832.50 ± 118.86 in the 3rd sample ($p < 0.0001$). The latter values approach those found in the non-polyuric patients, which were 915.33 ± 9.64 in the 1st, 920.16 ± 115.30 in the 2nd, 944 ± 92.69 in the 3rd sample (fig.5).

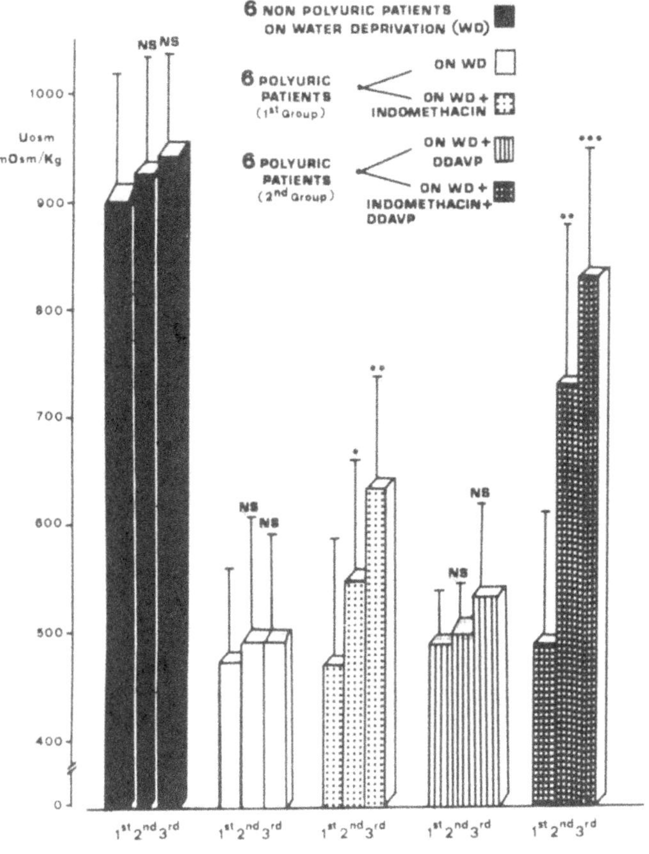

1st = Uosm ON THE SAMPLES COLLECTED FROM 12th TO 15th HOUR OF WD
2nd = Uosm ON THE SAMPLES COLLECTED FROM 15th TO 18th HOUR OF WD
3rd = Uosm ON THE SAMPLES COLLECTED FROM 18th TO 21th HOUR OF WD

Fig.5. Effect of indomethacin on the urinary osmolality (Uosm) in 12 patients with lithium-induced nephrogenic diabetes insipidus • $p < 0.01$ •• $p < 0.001$ ••• $p < 0.0001$

Discussion

Lithium may cause primary polydipsia (8,9,10,11), but lithium-induced primary polydipsia does not appear to have an important role in the genesis of polyuria in humans (2,7,20,22,34,67).

The possibility of central diabetes insipidus has also been suggested in some cases (2,7,14), but in most patients lithium seems to inhibit the renal action of the antidiuretic hormone (2,7,14,21,22,23). The latter pathogenesis was confirmed in our polyuric patients, in comparison with the non-polyuric patients, by significantly higher values of plasma osmolality and ADH urinary excretion, with a higher water intake. In addition, the lithium interference with the free water reabsorption results to be related to the use of higher doses and to maintenance serum levels in the higher therapeutic range, in accordance with Hullin's data (23) and in contrast with Donker's (24).

ADH is believed to induce its effect on the distal tubules and collecting ducts through the following mechanisms (25,26,27): 1) ADH binds to a membrane receptor, activating the adenylate cyclase enzyme; 2) the activated adenylate cyclase induces the production of cAMP; 3) through the cAMP-activation of a protein kinase, the membrane permeability to water is increased.

However, the means by which lithium reduces the ADH response has still not been defined. In other words, it is not clear whether lithium acts proximally or distally to the cAMP production, in interfering with the hydro-osmotic effect of ADH.

Studies on toads' urinary bladders have demonstrated that lithium antagonizes the hydro-osmotic effect of ADH, but not of dibutyryl cAMP, thus the lithium site of action is most likely to be proximal to cAMP generation (14). In dog, rabbit and rat renal medullary homogenates, lithium was found to impair the ADH- induced generation of cAMP (28,29,30) and in human renal medullary tissue it has been shown that lithium inhibits ADH-stimulated adenylate cyclase (31).

However, other Authors (32) were unable to detect any lithium effect on urinary or renal medullary cAMP levels in dehydrated rats (when the endogenous levels of ADH should have been high), and in other experimental studies the infusions of dibutyryl cyclic AMP were ineffective in concentrating the urine in lithium- treated rats, suggesting that at least one lithium action involves interference with the cellular mediation of vasopressin at a step beyond the formation of cAMP (2).

On the other hand, it has also been suggested that lithium may impair the water flow response to ADH or cAMP by stimulating cAMP phosphodiesterase to decrease the intracellular cAMP pool, but some Authors have found no lithium effect on the phosphodiesterase activity in human renal medullary homogenates (31).

Furthermore, other sites of action cannot be excluded.

Since it has been shown that lithium increases urinary prostaglandin E_2 excretion in dogs (33) and rats (11), and it has been established that there is antagonism between prostaglandin E and ADH (34,35,36,37), we postulated that the lithium-induced renal defect of the urinary concentrating mechanism might also be mediated by an enhanced prostaglandin effect on the renal medulla , which could depress the normal formation of cAMP.

If a renal prostaglandin imbalance is at the origin of ADH-resistant tubulopathy induced by lithium, the prostaglandin inhibition by means of indomethacin should cause an improvement in the ability to respond to ADH when polyuric patients are submitted to the dehydration test.

With the indomethacin we found a consistent increase in the urinary osmolality, and significantly higher values than those obtained with WD alone.

These results suggest that the lithium effect may be mediated via the augmentation of the prostaglandin action and, since indomethacin causes an increase in intracellular cAMP (38), it is conceivable that the prostaglandin blockade induces an increase in the urinary osmolality by reducing the lithium action in blocking cAMP generation, suggesting a lithium prostaglandin-mediated interference proximally to cAMP generation.

The most widely accepted view, in fact, is that prostaglandin E antagonizes the renal ADH-response through an inhibitory effect at the level of the AVP receptor-guanine nucleotide complex which may impair the cAMP production (35,39,40,41,42,43).

Our results seem to support a pathogenetic role of lithium-induced prostaglandin disorder, at the origin of the urinary concentrating defect, even if we consider the other possibility, according to which the lithium may interfere at the distal step to cAMP production.

In fact there are studies suggesting that prostaglandin E may exert its effects through specific receptors located in both the luminal and basolateral membranes (44).

However, an increase in urinary osmolality during treatment with indomethacin can be observed in normal subjects (45) and, furthermore, in hypophysectomized animals the combined administration of ADH and indomethacin induces greater increases in urinary osmolality than those obtained by the administration of ADH alone (46,47,48).

Nevertheless, we feel that considerations on the data in literature are outside the context of our experimental study, in which the administration of indomethacin freed the ADH tubular block.

The results of our study have allowed us to draw the following conclusions: 1) a high proportion of patients taking oral lithium carbonate develops a urinary concentrating impairment which, according to our data, is referred to the higher serum lithium levels; 2) the study excludes both primary polydipsia and central diabetes insipidus as possible pathogenetic factors in the polyuric-polydipsic syndrome in patients on long-term lithium treatment; 3) on the other hand, the study supports the notion that lithium treatment primarily affects the distal tubules and collecting ducts by producing a vasopressin-resistant impairment of the renal concentrating ability; 4) although the mechanism of the lithium action has not been entirely clarified, in our study the ADH resistance was significantly reversed by indomethacin, which suggests a lithium-induced prostaglandin imbalance as a pathogenetic factor in the urinary concentrating defect in patients undergoing long-term lithium therapy.

Acknowledgments

This research was supported by Ministero Pubblica Istruzione Grant 87/2300. The Authors wish to thank Ms.M.C.V. Pragnell B.A. for her help in revising the English.

References

1. M. Schou, Lithium in psychiatric therapy, Psychopharmacologia.1: 65 (1959).
2. J.N. JR Forrest, A.D. Cohen, J. Torretti, J.M. Himmelhoch, F.H. Epstein, On the mechanism of lithium-induced diabetes insipidus in man and the rat, J. Clin. Invest. 53: 1115 (1974).
3. M. Schou, P.C. Baastrup, P. Grof, P. Weis, J.Angst, Pharmacological and clinical problems of lithium prophylaxis, Br. J. Psychiatry 116: 615 (1970).
4. J.L. Marini, M.H. Sheard, Sustained-release lithium carbonate in a double-blind study: serum lithium levels, side effects, and placebo response, J. Clin. Pharmacol. 16: 276 (1976)
5. W.O. Williams, A.Z. Györy,Aspects of the use of lithium for the non-psychiatrist, Aust. NZ J. Med. 6: 233 (1976).
6. P.L. Padfield, S.J. Park, J.J. Morton, A.E. Braidwood, Plasma levels of antidiuretic hormone in patients receiving prolonged lithium therapy, Br. J. Psychiatry 130: 144 (1977).
7. P.H. Baylis, D.A. Heath, Water disturbances in patients treated with oral lithium carbonate, Ann. Intern. Med. 88: 607 (1978).
8. J.N. Galla, J.N. Forrest, B. Hecht, M. Kashgarian, J.P. Hayslett, Effect of lithium on water and electrolyte metabolism, Yale J. Biol. Med. 48: 305 (1975).
9. D.F. Smith, S. Balagura, M. Lubran, Antidotal thirst: a response to intoxication, Science 167: 297 (1970)
10. D.F. Smith, S. Balagura, Sodium appetite in rats given lithium, Life Sci. 11: 1021 (1972).
11. M.H. Miskind, R.E. Greenspan, W.H. Bay, T.F. Ferris, Studies on lithium-induced polyuria, Clin.Res. 25: 596 A (1977).
12. G.L. Ellman, G.L. Gan, Lithium ion and water balance in rats, Toxicol. Appl. Pharmacol.25: 617 (1973).
13. S. Hochman, Y. Gutman, Lithium: ADH antagonism and ADH independent action in rats with diabetes insipidus, Eur. J. Pharmacol. 28: 100 (1974).
14. I.Singer, D. Rotenberg, J.B. Puschett, Lithium-induced nephrogenic diabetes insipidus: in vivo and in vitro studies, J.Clin.Invest. 51: 1081 (1972).
15. I. Singer, E.A. Franko, Lithium-induced ADH resistance in toad urinary bladders, Kidney Int. 3: 151 (1973).
16. C.A. Harris, F.A. Jenner, Some aspects of the inhibition

of the action of antidiuretic hormone by lithium ions in the rat kidney and bladder of the toad Bufo marinus, Br. J. Pharmacol. 44: 223 (1972).
17. C. Torp-Pederson, N.A. Thorn, Acute effects of lithium on the action and release of ADH in rats, Acta Endocrinol. (Kbh) 73: 665 (1973)
18. P.J. Bentley, A. Wasserman, The effects of lithium on the permeability of an epithelial membrane, the toad urinary bladder, Biochim. Biophys. Acta 266: 285 (1972).
19. A. Tausch, H. Stegner, R.D. Leake, H.G. Artman, and D.A. Fisher, Radioimmunoassay of arginine vasopressin in urine: development and application, J. Clin. Endo. & Metab. 57: 777 (1983)
20. P.D. Miller, S.L. Dubovsky, K.M. McDonald, F.H. Katz, G.L. Robertson, R.W. Schrier, Central, renal and adrenal effects of lithium in man, Am. J. Med. 66: 797 (1979).
21. P.L. Padfield, J.J. Morton, G.B.M. Lindop and G.C. Timbury, Lithium-induced nephrogenic diabetes insipidus; changes in plasma vasopressin and angiotensin II, Clin. Nephrol. 3: 220 (1975).
22. P.L. Padfield, S.J. Park, J.J. Morton and A.E. Braidwood, Plasma levels of antidiuretic hormone in patients receiving prolonged lithium therapy, Brit. J. Psychiatry 130: 144 (1977).
23. R.P. Hullin, V.P. Coley, N.J. Birch, T.H. Thomas, D.B. Morgan, Renal function after long-term treatment with lithium, Br.Med.J. 1: 1457 (1979).
24. A.J.M. Donker, E. Prins, S. Meijer, W.J. Sluiter, J.W.B.M. Van Berkestijn and L.C.W. Dols, A renal function study in 30 patients on long-term lithium therapy, Clin.Nephrol. 12: 254 (1979).
25. M.Cox, I. Singer, Lithium and water metabolism, Am.J.Med. 59: 153 (1975).
26. D.Schlondorf, J.A. Satriano, Interactions of vasopressin, cAMP, and prostaglandins in toad urinary bladder, Am.J.Physiol. 248: F454 (1985).
27. K.H. Raymond, M.D. Lifschitz, Effect of prostaglandin on renal salt and water excretion, Am.J.Med. 80 (1A): 22 (1986).
28. T.P. Dousa, O. Hechter, The effect of NaCl and LiCl on vasopressin-sensitive adenyl cyclase, Life Sci 9: 765 (1970).
29. N.P.Beck, S.W. Reed, B.B. Davis, Effects of lithium on renal concentration of cyclic AMP, Clin. Res. 19: 684 (1971).
30. A.Geisier, O.Wraae, O.V. Olesen, Adenyl cyclase activity in kidneys of rats with lithium-induced polyuria, Acta Pharmacol. Toxicol. (Kbh) 31: 203 (1972).
31. T.B. Dousa, Lithium: interaction with ADH dependent cyclic AMP system of human renal medulla, Clin.Res. 21: 282 (1973).
32. G.Eknoyan, G.R. Corey, J. Loomis, W.N. Suki, M.Martinez-

Maldonado, Lithium-induced diabetes insipidus: effect on urinary cyclic AMP excretion and renal tissue adenylate cyclase activity, Clin.Res. 22: 524 (1974).

33. G.W. Rutecki, J.V. Nally, W.H. Bay, T.F. Ferris, The acute effects of lithium (Li) on renal function (abstract), Xth Annual Meeting American Society of Nephrology, Washington, D.C., November 20-22 (1977).
34. J.Orloff, J.S. Handler, S. Bergstrom, Effect of prostaglandin PGE_1 on the permeability response of toad bladder to vasopressin, theophylline, and adenosine 3' - 5'- monophosphate, Nature 205: 397 (1965).
35. J.J. Grantham, J.Orloff, Effect of prostaglandin E_1 on the permeability response of the isolated collecting tubule to vasopressin, adenosine 3' - 5'- monophosphate, and theophylline, J.Clin. Invest. 47: 1154 (1968).
36. F. Marumo, J.S. Eelman, Effects of Ca++ and prostaglandin E_1 on vasopressin activation of renal adenyl cyclase, J.Clin.Invest. 50: 1613 (1971).
37. A. Kalisker, D.C. Dyler, Inhibition of the vasopressin-activated adenyl cyclase from renal medulla by prostaglanins, Eur. J. Pharmacol. 20: 143 (1972).
38. G.M. Lum, G.A. Aisenbrey, M.J. Dunn, T. Berl, R.W. Schrier, K.M. McDonald, In vivo effect of indomethacin to potentiate the renal medullary cyclic AMP response to vasopressin, J.Clin.Invest. 59:8 (1977).
39. R. Locher, W. Vetter, L.H. Block, Interactions between 8-L-arginine vasopressin and prostaglandin E_2 in human mononuclear phagocytes, J.Clin.Invest 71: 884 (1983).
40. R.B.Clark, R.W. Butcher, Desensitization of adenylate cyclase in cultured fibroblasts with prostaglandin E_1 and epinephrine, J.Biol.Chem. 254: 9373 (1979).
41. S. Kassis, P.H. Fishman, Different mechanism of desensitization of adenylate cyclase by isoproterenol and prostaglandin E_1 in human fibroblasts, J.Biol.Chem. 257: 5312 (1982).
42. R.M. Burch, P.V. Malushka, 45Ca fluxes in isolated toad bladder epithelial cells: effects of agents which alter water or sodium transport, J.Pharmacol. Exp. Ther. 224: 108 (1983).
43. S.P. Nadler, S.C. Hebert, B.M. Brenner, Cholera toxin, forskolin, and PGE_2 interactions in isolated perfused rabbit cortical collecting tubules (abstr.) Am.Soc.Nephrol. 17: 233 (A) (1984).
44. D. Schlondorff, C.P. Carvounis, Jacoby M., J.A. Satriano, and S.D. Levine, Multiple sites for interactions of prostaglandin and vasopressin in toad urinary bladder, Am. J. Physiol. 241: F625 (1981)
45. L.Somova, S. Zaharieva, M.Ivanova, Humoral factors involved in the regulation of sodium-fluid balance in normal man. Acta Physiol. Pharmacol. Bulg. 10: 29 (1984).
46. J.R. Anderson, T. Berl, K.M. McDonald, and R.W. Schrier, Evidence for an in vivo antagonism between vasopressin

and prostaglandin in the mammalian kidney, J.Clin. Invest. 56: 420 (1975).

47. T.Berl, A.Raz, H. Wald, J. Horowitz, and W. Czaczkes, Prostaglandin synthesis inhibition and the action of vasopressin: studies in man and rat, Am.J.Physiol. 232: F529 (1977).

48. H.J. Kramer, A. Bäcker, S. Hinzen, R. Düsing, Effects of inhibition of prostaglandin-synthesis on renal electrolyte excretion and concentrating ability in healthy man, Prostaglandins Med. 1:341 (1978).

AMINOGLYCOSIDE NEPHROTOXICITY : MECHANISM AND PREVENTION

Marc E. De Broe, Rubén A. Giuliano and Gert A. Verpooten

Department of Nephrology-Hypertension
University Hospital Antwerpen
Antwerpen, Belgium

INTRODUCTION

Nephrotoxicity limits the clinical utility of aminoglycosides (Lietman, 1985). Therefore, the identification of factors associated with a greater incidence of renal damage is critical. These factors can be classified in those related to the drug and its administration and those related to the clinical condition of the patient (Table 1).

Table 1. Risk factors for aminoglycoside nephrotoxicity.

DRUG-RELATED	PATIENT-RELATED
- Dose	- Age
- Duration of treatment	- Initial creatinine clearance
- Dosage regimen	- Prior renal insufficiency
- Prior aminoglycoside treatment	- Hepatic insufficiency
- Choice of drug	- Volume depletion
- Coadministration with diuretics, cisplatin, cyclosporin, etc.	- Electrolyte disturbance
	- Critically ill patient

In this paper, insights into the renal handling and the mechanism of nephrotoxicity of these drugs are reviewed. It is intended to help the clinician to better define the drug- and patient-related conditions which increase the risk of nephrotoxicity and this way, contribute to the design of measures for the prevention of this common cause of acute renal dysfunction.

RENAL HANDLING OF AMINOGLYCOSIDES

Aminoglycosides are highly charged, polycationic, hydrophilic drugs which cross biological membranes poorly or not at all. They distribute in the vascular and interstitial space (extracellular). They are not metabolized and are eliminated unchanged almost entirely by the kidneys (Lietman, 1985). Aminoglycosides are filtered by the glomerulus at a rate almost equal to water. After entering the luminal fluid of the proximal renal tubule, a small but toxicologically important portion of the filtered drug is reabsorbed and stored in the lysosomes of proximal tubular cells, where they may exert, in a concentration dependent manner, their primary toxic effects.

From extracellular to intracellular compartment

The transport of these drugs into proximal tubular cells involves interaction with acidic, negatively charged phospholipid binding sites (mainly phosphatidylinositol) at the level of the brush border membrane. This phospholipidic binding site appears to be a common anionic binding site which is competitively shared by aminoacids, cationic polypeptides, proteins and the aminoglycosides (Just and Habermann, 1977; Josepovitz et al., 1982). After charge mediated binding, the drug is taken up into the cell in small invaginations of the cell membrane, a mechanism called 'carrier mediated pinocytosis' (Collier et al. 1979). This mechanism is predominant for drug entry into the proximal tubular cells, however, other processes such as basolateral uptake have been suggested, although there is no compelling evidence to demonstrate a significant contribution of the latter mechanism to the total tissue accumulation of drug in vivo. 'Bulk fluid phase pinocytosis' has been found to be far less efficient than the parent uptake mechanism which involves binding to the membrane. Passive diffusion of the aminoglycosides through the cell membrane is a highly improbable mechanism for drug absorption because of the cationic and hydrophilic nature of these drugs (Kaloyanides and Pastoriza-Munoz, 1980). Within one hour after injection, the drug on the luminal side of the proximal tubular cell is translocated into apical cytoplasmic vacuoles (Silverblatt and Kuehn, 1979) (Figure 1).

Lysosomal storage

There is definite and unambiguous evidence that short after administration, aminoglycosides are present inside lysosomes of proximal tubular cells. This storage has been demonstrated by cell fractionation, autoradiography at ultrastructural level and more recently by immunofluorescence (Silverblatt and Kuehn, 1979; Wedeen et al., 1983). Small pinocytic vesicles generated from the brush border membrane and containing the aminoglycoside and other endocytosed material, fuse one to each other while migrating into the cell. Thereafter, these vacuoles quickly coalesce with lysosomes, sequestering the pinocytosed molecules inside those organelles. This transport mechanism has been questioned in experiments using freeze-dry autoradiography and immunofluorescence at light microscopical level (Wedeen et al., 1983). With these techniques it was shown that intracellular gentamicin is diffuse within the cytoplasma of proximal tubular cells over the first 6 hours after administration and before it becomes firmly bound and sequestered inside lysosomes. However, the methodologies used do not permit identification or examination of the fate of endocytic vacuoles.
In contrast to water and other small molecules (below 200 Dalton), intralysosomal aminoglycosides are not able to escape from these organelles in view of their relatively high molecular weight (450 Dalton), their cationic nature and their strong binding to the acidic phospholipids inside lysosomes favoured by the intraorganelle pH (4-5).
Since pinocytosis is a continuing phenomenon these drugs tend to accumulate extensively inside lysosomes in spite of the small amount of filtered drug which is actually taken up and stored in the renal cells. This is illustrated in the following example: at a steady-state gentamicin serum concentration of 5 μg/ml obtained by continuous infusion in a rat of 240 g, the renal cortex concentration is 30 μg/g after one hour (Giuliano et al., 1986a). Assuming the rat renal cortex is 0.8 g, the total cortical gentamicin is 24 μg under these conditions. The gentamicin load to the kidneys is 5 μg/ml x 93 % non-protein bound x 2 ml/min clearance x 60 min = 558 μg. The fraction of

the filtered load stored in the kidneys is therefore 24/558 (4.3%). Since lysosomes represent 3% of the cortical mass, and assuming that the drugs reach the lysosomes shortly after administration and that the whole bulk of intracellular aminoglycoside is located inside the lysosomes, the concentration of gentamicin within these organelles should therefore reach a value of 30/0.03 = 1000 μg/ml after one hour infusion, i.e. 2 mM concentration, a value 200-fold higher than the serum concentration. Thus the small fraction of the glomerular filtered drug which is taken up in proximal tubular cells is stored in one particular intracellular compartment resulting in 'huge' drug concentrations. In view of this observation and the fact that cortical concentrations of aminoglycosides are cumulative during treatment, it is not surprising that even at clinical dosage and therapeutic serum concentrations these drugs may cause toxicity.

Release from proximal tubular cells

Aminoglycosides are present in the kidney cortex long after they become undetectable in serum. However, there is a persistent release of the drug from their storage sites in the proximal tubular cells. A tissue half-life of more than 100 hours has been reported for gentamicin (Fabre et al., 1976; Giuliano et al., 1984). The pattern for drug release is dependent on the renal cortical concentration of drug achieved. In the absence of tissue damage, elimination is smooth and follows first-order kinetics. In contrast, if tissue necrosis is present drug release is abrupt since it follows the extrusion of cell debris containing the accumulated aminoglycoside into the tubular lumen and urine.

MECHANISM OF CELLULAR TOXICITY

Biochemical and morphological studies have identified the lysosomes as the first organelles to show alterations during aminoglycoside treatment (De Broe et al., 1984). Once trapped in the lysosomes of proximal tubular cells aminoglycosides inhibit lysosomal phospholipases and sphyngomyelinase (Laurent et al., 1982). In parallel with enzyme inhibition, undigested phospholipids originating from the turnover of cellular membranes accumulate in lysosomes. The overall result is a lysosomal phospholipidosis due to a non-specific accumulation of polar phospholipids in myeloid bodies (Kosek et al., 1974). This disorder is one of the earliest cellular alterations during treatment with these drugs, even at low, therapeutic doses (Tulkens et al., 1984). 'Acute' experiments in rats consisting in loading of the renal cortex tissue with various amounts of gentamicin, permitted the identification of a direct correlation between the dose of aminoglycoside, the renal cortical drug concentration achieved, the severity, the evolution and the recovery of the early cellular alterations (Giuliano et al., 1984). Acute loading of the renal tissue with aminoglycosides allowed also the identification of a threshold, expressed in cortical drug concentration, below which there is regression of the drug-induced biochemical and morphological changes in the absence of any sign of cell necrosis or regeneration. Above that threshold, the lysosomal phospholipidosis progresses and the overloaded lysosomes continue to swell even in the absence of any further drug administration. This may result in loss of integrity of the restricting membranes of the organelles and release of high amounts of aminoglycosides, lysosomal enzymes and phospholipids into the cytosol (Figure 2). At that stage, extralysosomal aminoglycosides are able to gain access and injure other organelles and disturb their functional integrity which may lead to cell death. Overt cell necrosis and regeneration is readily apparent. As a consequence, clogging of certain tubular segments by necrotic cells and cell debris, increased intratubular pressure and decrease of glomerular filtration rate may ensue, accompanied by drug release from the tissue following aberrant kinetics. Tubular cell regeneration is coexistent with tubular necrosis (Houghton et al., 1976) allowing recovery of the drug-induced damage. If the rate of cell regeneration overcomes that of necrosis, progressive deterioration of the renal function is avoided.

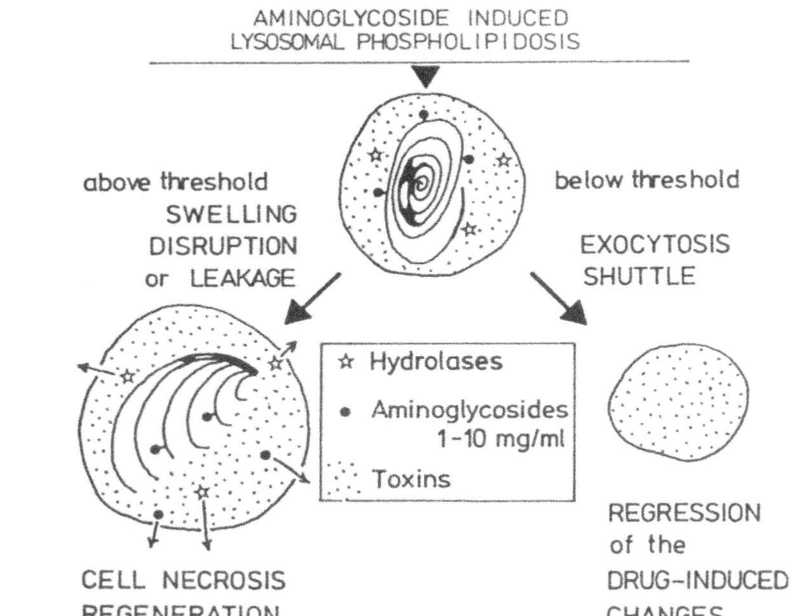

Figure 1. Renal handling of aminoglycosides. A. Glomerular filtration and and binding to membrane of the proximal tubular cell. B. Internalization and lysosomal sequestration of aminoglycosides.

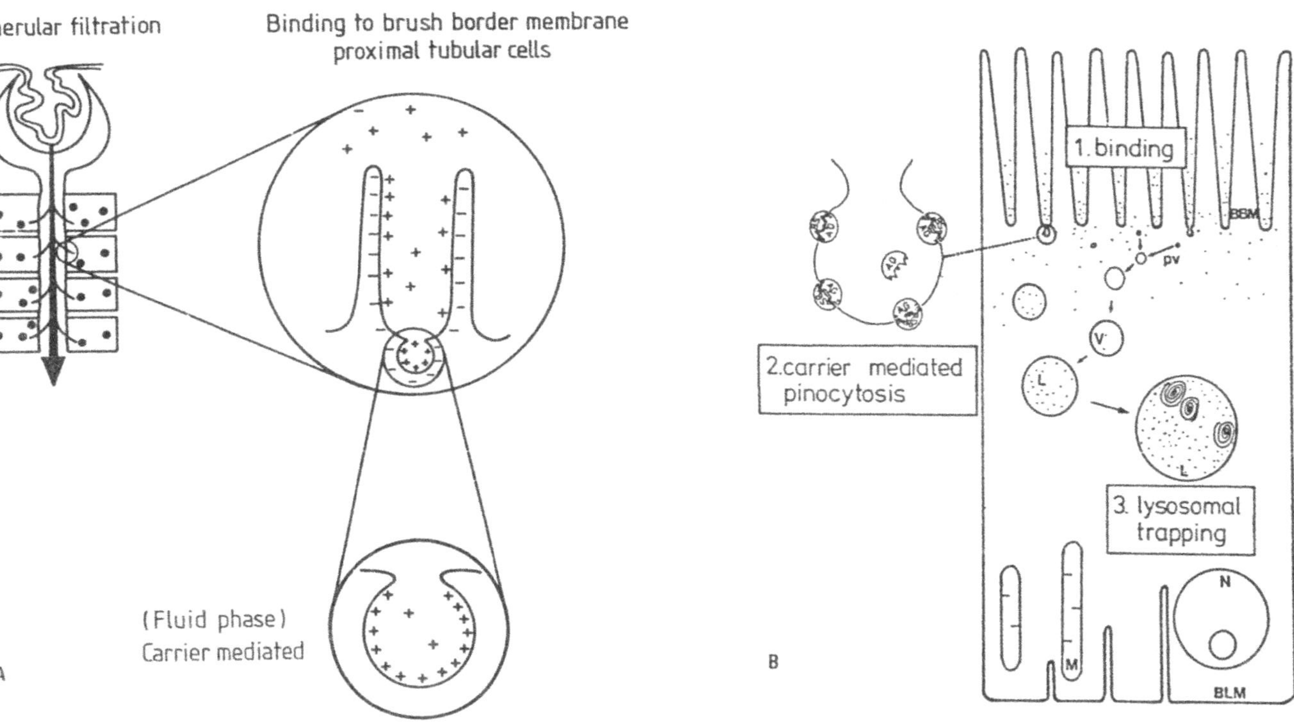

Figure 2. Evolution of the aminoglycoside-induced lysosomal phospholipidosis. It is dependent in part on the extent of drug accumulated inside the lysosomes. The round figures represent lysosomes.

DEFINITION OF NEPHROTOXICITY

There is no consensus in the definition of aminoglycoside-induced nephrotoxicity. This phenomenon is overestimated when relying on sensitive parameters of altered renal tubular function. Indeed, increases in urinary excretion of proximal tubular enzymes and β_2 microglobuline do not mean necessarily nephrotoxicity. Competition of β_2 microglobuline and the cationic aminoglycosides for the same binding site at the level of the proximal tubular brush boder is well documented. Increases in urinary excretion of those products may well be considered as early manifestations of the effect of aminoglycosides on the kidney. On the other hand, nephrotoxicity defined in terms of decreased glomerular filtration may lead to an underestimation of the occurrence of renal injury, although such a definition appears to be more useful from the clinical point of view. Aminoglycoside-induced nephrotoxicity, defined as a decrease in glomerular filtration rate and reflected in a rise in serum creatinine, appears to develop within days or weeks after the start of therapy and may become evident even after therapy has been discontinued (Lietman, 1985). There are two forms of aminoglycoside-induced acute renal failure, one frequently observed which consists of a slight, brief, increase in serum creatinine levels, and another one, more exceptional, which is a non-oliguric form of severe acute renal failure which may require dialysis. Most investigators agree that both forms are transient and, in most cases, reversible in a relatively short period of time. In fact, permanent renal failute attributed primarily or solely to the adverse effects of aminoglycosides, has never been definitely proven (Kleinknecht, 1985). Thus, prognosis is good compared to acute renal failure of other causes. However, renal insufficiency due to the treatment with aminoglycosides represents an additional complication for severely ill patients which may prolong hospitalization and increase the economic burden.

DRUG RELATED RISK FACTORS FOR NEPHROTOXICITY: PREVENTION

A great deal of knowledge gained on the renal handling and mechanism of nephrotoxicity can be now oriented to provide a rational basis for a better understanding of the nephrotoxicity and to identify those risk factors which can be prevented, influenced or exploited by the clinician. The nephrotoxicity of aminoglycosides is determined by two major variables: a) the amount of drug accumulation in the renal cortex, and b) the intrinsic potential of the drug to cause damage to subcellular structures (Kaloyanides and Pastoriza-Munoz, 1980). The extent of drug accumulation is thus intimately related to the onset and pathogenesis of aminoglycoside-induced nephrotoxicity, in the context that, any factor increasing the renal uptake of aminoglycosides is a risk factor for nephrotoxicity. Renal aminoglycoside concentrations are cumulative over treatment, however, a great variety of factors do exert an influence on their extent and evolution.

Duration of treatment

The duration of exposure of the brush border membrane of proximal tubular cells to these drugs is a critical factor for the nephrotoxic process since it determines the extent of drug uptake. Persistent exposure results undoubtedly in increased renal drug levels. This explains why despite maintenance of therapeutic serum drug concentrations, prolonged administration is a risk factor for nephrotoxicity. Although a safe duration of therapy has not been clearly identified, a treatment with aminoglycosides should not exceed two weeks (De Broe, 1985).

Choice of dosage regimen

This is another important determinant of the extent of cortical drug concentrations. Several groups have shown that the severity of experimental

nephrotoxicity of gentamicin is greater when the total daily dose is divided or given by continuous infusion, rather than when it is given as a single bolus (Reiner et al., 1978; Powel et al., 1983). The rationale for this important observation may be found in a recent comparative study of renal cortical uptake-storage kinetics of different aminoglycosides (Giuliano et al., 1986a). In the rat, steady-state elevations of serum gentamicin and netilmicin were associated with nonlinear increase in renal cortical levels, strongly suggesting saturable uptake. Cortical uptake of tobramycin, however, was linearly related to serum levels. Amikacin showed also in the rat, a mixed kinetic pattern for cortical accumulation, i.e. a linear pattern at high serum concentrations and saturation kinetics at low serum concentrations. In other words, for gentamicin and netilmicin, renal cortical uptake is less 'efficient' at high serum concentrations than the uptake observed at low serum concentrations. The renal uptake kinetic pattern for these two aminoglycosides permits prediction of a pronounced effect of dosage regimen on the amount of drug accumulation in the cortex. Indeed, the fraction of drug taken up by the proximal tubular cells is higher when the same amount of drug is given by continuous infusion (low persistent serum levels) than by intermittent or single injection(s) (high momentary serum levels which overcome the saturation limits of the uptake mechanism).
Available data show that cortical drug levels are 2-3 fold higher in the kidneys of rats treated with 10 mg/kg/day gentamicin by infusion than when the same dose was given by single daily injections (Giuliano et al., 1986b). On the other hand, cortical uptake of tobramycin in the rat was independent of the dosage schedule used as expected from the linear uptake kinetics of this aminoglycoside which implies that the fraction of drug taken up at low and high serum levels is proportional. Continuous infusion of amikacin in the rat resulted in somewhat higher cortical levels than did intermittent injections, but the differences between regimens were less remarkable than in the case of gentamicin. Indeed, the higher fractional uptake rate of amikacin at low serum levels compared to that at high serum levels, explains the effect of dosage schedule on the accumulation of this aminoglycoside.
A recent trial in humans found a critical effect of dosage schedule on renal uptake of gentamicin and netilmicin. The study was carried out in renal cancer patients with normal renal function (serum creatinine: .9-1.2 mg/dl and proteinuria lower than 300 mg/24 hrs) and submitted to nephrectomy. Prior to surgery the patients received gentamicin (4.5 mg/kg) or netilmicin (5 mg/kg) either in one single injection (given 24 hrs before surgery) or over a 1-day continuous infusion (Figure 4) (Verpooten et al., 1988). The single injection schedule resulted in 30-50% lower cortical drug levels for netilmicin and gentamicin respectively, compared to the administration of the same amount of drug by continuos infusion. From these studies may be intuitively concluded that continuous infusion is a risk factor for nephrotoxicity since it yields higher tissue aminoglycoside levels. On the other hand, dosage schedules resulting in low tissue levels may help prevent clinical nephrotoxicity. From the point of view of bactericidal effects, whether aminoglycosides should be given by single daily injections or by more frequent or continuous admistration necessitates confirmation. There is evidence, however, that once-daily dose therapy provides as efficient or higher antibacterial effect compared to more frequent or continuous administration. Indeed, aminoglycosides exhibit concentration dependent killing of gram negative bacteria and prolonged post-antibiotic effects (Blaser et al., 1985; Craig and Vogelman, 1987). In view of reduced cortical uptake and subsequent lower risk for nephrotoxicity, once-daily therapy is preferable if the same or better antibacterial effect could be clearly demonstrated compared to currently used strategies.

Choice of drug

An impressive number of comparative studies of aminoglycoside nephrotoxicity in humans is available (Whelton, 1985). It is difficult to draw

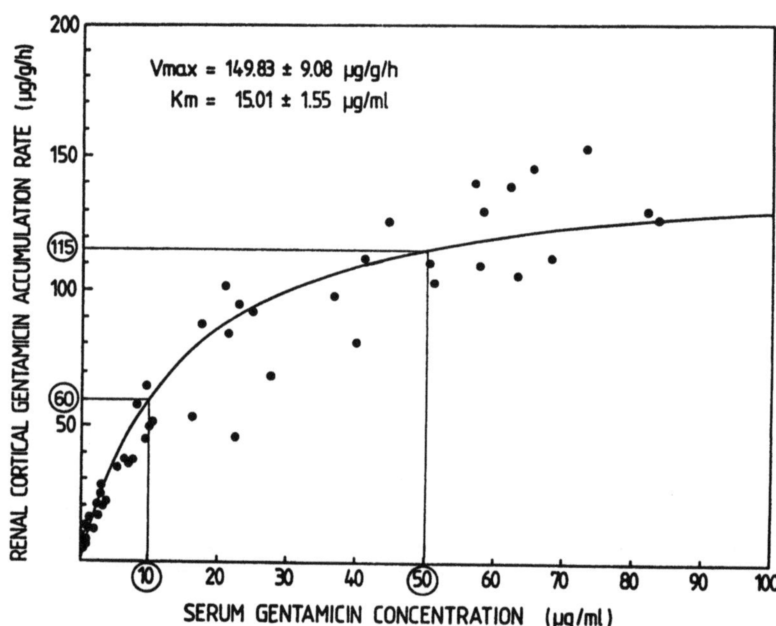

Figure 3. Relationships between increasing steady-state serum levels and renal cortical concentrations. Renal uptake of the aminoglycoside is saturable. A 5-fold rise in serum levels results in an almost 2-fold increase in renal drug levels. This kinetic pattern explains why high momentary peak levels as obtained after a single injection of a daily dose results in reduced cortical concentrations compared with administration of the same total dose as a continuous infusion which yields a low presistent serum level.

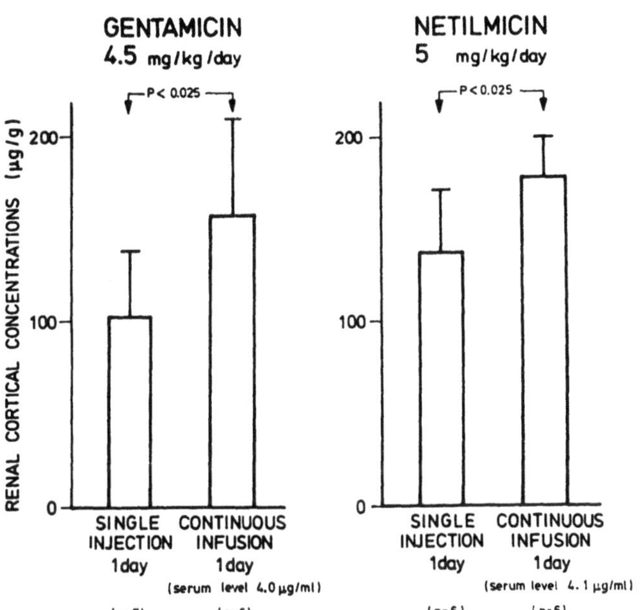

Figure 4. Influence of dosage schedule on the renal cortical accumulation of gentamicin and netilmicin in the human kidney. Continuous infusion, a schedule which yields low and persistent serum levels results, for both aminoglycosides, in higher drug concentration in the renal cortex after a 24 hrs treatment.

firm conclusions from these studies because of the multiple clinical variables and because most of the studies failed to achieve critical methodological standards for comparative drug trials. It is clear, however, that all aminoglycosides are nephrotoxic for the human kidney and the mechanism is very likely the same for all members of the group. In a prospective controlled randomized comparative short-term study in humans using clinical doses, gentamicin, tobramycin and netilmicin could not be distinguished on the basis of cortical drug accumulation, lysosomal overloading and effect on lysosomal phospholipases. Using the recommended clinical doses, amikacin induces significantly less lysosomal overloading and no loss of phospholipase activity. These data suggest that amikacin might be a lesser nephrotoxic aminoglycoside than gentamicin or tobramycin, when used in strictly comparable clinical conditions (De Broe et al., 1983; De Broe et al., 1984).

PATIENT RELATED RISK FACTORS FOR NEPHROTOXICITY. PREVENTION

Age

There are at least two reasons why advanced age has been suggested as a risk factor for aminoglycoside nephrotoxicity. Age goes along with a decreased renal function and an important decline of the regenerative response to drug-induced cell injury which is essential in keeping primary alterations below a critical threshold. In this context, older patients or animals are more susceptible to nephrotoxicity than are younger ones (De Broe, 1985).

Initial creatinine clearance

The initial creatinine clearance undoutedly relates to the capability of the kidney to take up and accumulate aminoglycosides from the luminal fluid. Moore et al. (1984) have shown that patients with a high initial creatinine clearance are at higher risk for the development of nephrotoxicity.

Prior renal insufficiency

Higher serum levels and protracted elimination caused by preexisting or developing renal failure will result in a greater or longer exposure of the remaining filtering nephrons to aminoglycoside, precipitating them to tubular lesions or necrosis. However, patients with pre-existing renal disease do not appear to be at high risk for the induction of further renal impairment when treated with aminoglycosides. This is the conclusion of two well designed prospective studies (Smith et al., 1978; Reyman et al., 1979) which appear to contradict impressions gained from poorly controlled retrospective studies and isolated case reports. Indeed, the widespread use of adjustment of the administration of aminoglycosides by reducing the dose and/or by extending the interval between doses may have contributed to this apparent lack of risk in renal failure patients. Moreover, it was shown experimentally that chronic renal failure rats accumulate less aminoglycosides than normal rats at comparable serum levels (Verpooten et al., 1986; Pattyn et al., 1988). Renal insufficiency is a clear risk factor if dosage is not carefully adjusted.

Hepatic insufficiency

A prospective clinical study has shown that liver disease was associated with the development of nephrotoxicity. Hepatic insufficiency leading to intra-renal vasoconstriction, reduced renal blood flow and stimulation of the renin-angiotensin system are proposed pathophysiological mechanisms(Moore et al., 1984).

MONITORING OF AMINOGLYCOSIDE THERAPY

There are two rationales for the monitoring of serum aminoglycoside levels: a therapeutic and a toxicological one. The routine and/or irrational use of recommended dosage regimens without serum concentration monitoring will result in widely variable serum concentrations and may unnecessarily predispose the patient to a higher risk of failure of treatment and/or toxicity. Therefore, monitoring of serum aminoglycoside levels during therapy is a prudent guide to ascertain safety and efficacy of treatment. Early in the therapy (after 2-3 doses) serum drug monitoring is required for possible dose correction in subsequent dosing. Dosing is best calculated and/or adapted taking into consideration the glomerular filtration rate of the individual patient (nomograms and formulas are available for the matter) For critically ill patients monitoring should be performed to ensure adequate therapeutic concentrations. Due to the over-emphasized importance of nephrotoxicity during aminoglycoside treatment underdosing rather than overdosing became a common prescribing error. Aminoglycosides and creatinine are both good markers of glomerular filtration rate, therefore, it is possible to rely on the simple and inexpensive serum creatinine determinations combined with a limited number of serum aminoglycoside levels for monitoring drug efficacy and toxicity.

CONCLUSIONS

As soon as treatment with aminoglycosides starts, the renal proximal tubular cells take up and accumulate small but toxicologically important fractions of the administered drug. A lysosomal phospholipidosis follows drug uptake and is the earliest alterations observed in those cells.
Drug accumulation is intimately related to the development of nephrotoxicity and further to acute renal failure. The higher the extent of tissue drug accumulation, the higher the risk for nephrotoxicity. Measures reducing cortical uptake-accumulation help prevent nephrotoxicity.
Correct duration of treatment and choice of drug and dosage schedule are critical factors determinant of the extent of drug accumulated. Once-daily therapy with gentamicin and netilmicin is potentially less nephrotoxic in view of reduced resultant cortical concentrations.
Age is a risk factor since it goes along with a decrease in renal function and a declined capacity for cell regeneration after aminoglycoside-induced injury. Correct adjustment of dosage to actual renal function may prevent high levels of renal drug accumulation.
Insight into the renal handling, mechanism of nephrotoxicity and the identification of risk factors enable the clinician to reduce drastically the prevalence and degree of renal damage induced by aminoglycosides.

REFERENCES

Blaser, J., Stone, B.B. and Zinner, S.H. 1985. Efficacy of intermittent versus continuous administration of netilmicin in a two-compartment model. Antimicrob. Agents Chemother. 27: 343-349.

Collier, V.V., Lietman, P.S. and Mitch, W.E. 1979. Evidence of luminal uptake of gentamicin in the perfused rat kidney. J. Pharmacol. Exp. Ther. 210: 247-251.

Craig, W.A. and Vogelman, B. 1987. The postantibiotic effect. Ann. Intern. Med. 106: 900-902.

De Broe, M.E., Paulus, G.J., Verpooten, G.A., Giuliano, R.A., Roels, F. and Tulkens, P.M. 1983. In "Proceedings of the 13th. International Congress of Chemotherapy : Side effects of antibiotics". August 28-September 2, 1983, SE 8.4/1, part 86. Spitzy, K.H. and Karrer, K, eds., 86/11-86/23.

De Broe, M.E., Paulus, G.J., Verpooten, G.A., Roels, F., Buyssens, N., Wedeen, R.P. 1984. Early effects of gentamicin, tobramycin, and amikacin on the human kidney. Kidney Int. 25: 643-652.
De Broe, M.E. 1985. Prevention of aminoglycoside nephrotoxicity. In: Proceedings of the European Dialysis and Transplantation Association-European Renal Association. Davison, A.M., and Guillow, P.J., eds., Baillière Tindall Pub., London, Vol 22: 959-973.
Fabre, J., Rudhart, M., Blanchard, P. and Regamey, C. 1976. Persistence of sisomicin and gentamicin in renal cortex and medulla compared with other organs and serum of rats. Kidney Int. 10: 444-449.
Giuliano, R.A., Paulus, G.J., Verpooten, G.A., Pattyn, V.M., Pollet, D.E., Nouwen, E.J., Laurent, G., Carlier, M.B., Maldague, P., Tulkens, P.M. and De Broe, M.E. 1984. Recovery of cortical phospholipidosis and necrosis after acute gentamicin loading in rats. Kidney Int 26: 838-847.
Giuliano, R.A., Verpooten, G.A., Verbist, L., Wedeen, R.P. and De Broe M.E. 1986 a. In vivo uptake kinetics of aminoglycosides in the kidney cortex of rats. J. Pharmacol. Exp. Ther. 236: 470-475.
Giuliano, R.A., Verpooten, G.A. and De Broe, M.E. 1986 b. The effect of dosing strategy on kidney cortical accumulation of aminoglycosides. Am. J. Kidney Dis. 8: 297-303.
Houghton, D.C., Hartnett, M.L., Campbell-Boswell, M., Porter, G. and Bennett, W. 1976. A light and electron microscopic analysis of gentamicin nephrotoxicity in rats. Am. J. Pathol. 82: 589-612.
Josepovitz, C., Pastoriza-Munoz, E., Timmerman, D., Scott, M., Feldman, S. and Kaloyanides, G.J. 1982. Inhibition of gentamicin uptake in rat renal cortex in vivo by aminoglycosides and organic polycations. J. Pharm. Exp. Ther. 233: 314-321.
Just, M. and Habermann, E. 1977. The renal handling of polybasic drugs. 2. In vitro studies with brush border and lysosomal preparations. Naunyn-Schmiedeberg's Arch. Pharmacol. 300: 67-76.
Kaloyanides, G.J. and Pastoriza-Munoz, E. 1980. Aminoglycoside nephrotoxicity. Kidney Int. 18: 571-582.
Kleinknecht, D., Landais, P. and Goldfard, B. 1985. Drug-associated acute renal failure. A prospective multicenter report. In: Proceedings of the European Dialysis and Transplantation Association - European Renal Association. Davison, A.M. and Guillou, P.J. eds. Baillière Tindall Pub. London 22: 1002-1007.
Kosek, J.C., Mazz, R.I. and Cousins, M.J. 1974. Nephrotoxicity of gentamicin. Lab. Invest. 30: 48-57.
Laurent, G., Carlier, M.B., Rollman, B., Van Hoof, F. and Tulkens, P.M. 1982. Mechanism of aminoglycoside-induced lysosomal phospholipidosis : in vitro and in vivo studies with gentamicin and amikacin. Biochem. Pharmacol. 31: 3861-3870.
Lietman, P.S. 1985. Aminoglycosides and spectinomycin : aminocyclitols. In: Principles and practice of infectious diseases. 2nd Edition. Part I: Basic principles in the diagnosis and management of infectious diseases. Mandel, G.L., Douglas Jr, R.G. and Bennett, J.E., eds. John Wiley and Sons, New York, Chichester: 192-206.
Moore, R.D., Smith, C.R., Lipsky, J.J., Mellitis E.D., and Lietman, P.S. 1984. Risk factors for nephrotoxicity in patients treated with aminoglycosides. Ann. Intern. Med. 100: 352-357.
Pattyn, V.M., Verpooten, G.A., Giuliano, R.A., Zheng, F.L. and De Broe, M.D. 1987. Effect of hyperfiltration, proteinuria and diabetes mellitus on the uptake kinetics of gentamicin in the kidney cortex of rats. J. Pharmacol. Exp. Ther. 244: 694-698.
Powel, S.H., Thompson, W.L., Luthe, M.A., Stern, R.C., Grossniklaus, D.A., Bloxham, D.D., Groden, D.L., Jacobs, M.R., Discenna, A.O., Cash, H.A. and Klinger, J.D. 1983. Once daily vs. continuous aminoglycoside dosing : efficacy and toxicity in animal and clinical studies of gentamicin, netilmicin and tobramycin. J. Infect. Dis. 147: 918-932.

Reiner, N.E., Bloxham, D.D., and Thompson, W.L. 1978. Nephrotoxicity of gentamicin and tobramycin given once daily or continuously in dogs. J. Antimicrob. Chemother. 4 (Suppl.A): 85-101.

Reymann, M.T., Bradac, J.A. and Cobbs, C.G. 1979. Correlation of aminoglycoside dosages with serum concentrations during therapy of serious gram negative bacillary disease. Antimicrob. Agents Chemother. 16: 353-365.

Silverblatt, F. and Kuehn, C. 1979. Autoradiography of gentamicin uptake by the rat proximal tubular cell. Kidney Int. 15: 335-345.

Smith, C.R., Maxwell, R.R. and Edwards, C.Q. 1978. Nephrotoxicity induced by gentamicin and amikacin. John Hopkins Med. J. 142: 85-90.

Tulkens, P.M., De Broe, M.E., Maldague, P. and Heuson-Stiennon, J.A. 1984. Lysosomal alterations in aminoglycoside-induced acute renal failure. In: Acute Renal Failure: correlations between morphology and function. Solez, K., and Whelton, A., eds. Marcel Dekker, Pub., New York: 299-327.

Verpooten, G.A., Giuliano, R.A., Pattyn, V.M., Scharpé, S.L. and De Broe, M.E. 1986. Renal cortical uptake kinetics of gentamicin in rats with impaired renal function. Am. J. Kidney Dis. 8: 304-307.

Verpooten, G.A., Giuliano, R.A., Verbist, L., Eestermans, G. and De Broe, M.E. 1988. A once-daily dosage schedule decreases the accumulation of gentamicin and netilmicin in the renal cortex of humans. Submitted.

Wedeen, R.P., Batuman, V., Cheeks, E.M., Marquet, E. and Sobel, H. 1983. Transport of gentamicin in rat proximal tubule. Lab. Invest. 48: 212-223.

Whelton, A. 1985. Therapeutic initiative for avoidance of aminoglycoside toxicity. J. Clin. Pharmacol. 25: 67-81.

THE NATURAL COURSE OF GOLD AND PENICILLAMINE NEPHROPATHY: A LONGTERM STUDY OF 54 PATIENTS

Clive L. Hall

Consultant Physician and Nephrologist

Royal United Hospital, Combe Park, Bath, BA1 3NG

SUMMARY

To elucidate the natural course of gold and penicillamine nephropathy and to facilitate appropriate clinical management 54 patients with rheumatoid arthritis who developed proteinuria during treatment with intramuscular gold thiomalate (21) or oral D penicillamine (33) were studied in detail throughout the whole of their renal illnesses. Renal biopsy was performed and creatinine clearance and proteinuria were measured serially for a median period of 60 months (range 16 - 130 months) in the gold treated and 74 months (range 13 - 158 months) in the penicillamine treated patients.

During gold (penicillamine) treatment 48% (43%), 71% (82%) and 86% (91%) of patients had presented with proteinuria by 6, 12 and 24 months of treatment. After stopping gold (penicillamine) treatment proteinuria reached a median maximum of 2.1 g/day (4.2 g/day) at 2 months (1 month) before resolving spontaneously so that by 6, 12 and 18 months 38% (36%), 62% (64%) and 76% (88%) of patients were free of proteinuria. The median initial and most recent creatinine clearances of the gold (penicillamine) treated patients were 77 ml/min (80 ml/min) and 59 ml/min (78 ml/min) respectively and no patients died from or needed treatment for chronic renal failure. HLA B8 and/or DR3 alloantigens were identified in 64% of the gold treated and 56% of the penicillamine treated patients. In the gold (penicillamine) treated patients renal biopsy revealed membranous glomerulonephritis (GN) in 72% (88%), an immune complex mesangial glomerulonephritis in 10% (6%), minimal change nephropathy in 10% (6%) and no significant glomerular abnormalities in 8% (0%).

The study has demonstrated the close similarity between gold and penicillamine nephropathy. It has also demonstrated that some 75% of cases develop during the first year of treatment, the proteinuria resolves completely when treatment is withdrawn, progressive deterioration of renal function is most uncommon, corticosteroid therapy is unnecessary and several different types of glomerulonephritis are associated with gold and penicillamine treatment.

INTRODUCTION

Gold & penicillamine have been accepted as effective second line treatment for rheumatoid arthritis but complications are common and include renal damage in 2-20% of patients. (1-3) This presents as proteinuria of widely varying severity (0.3-39.0 g/day) with the nephrotic syndrome in 16-70% of cases and causes otherwise successful treatment to be stopped. (1,4-10) Gold nephropathy has been observed at all ages (2-73 years) and with all gold preparations whether given parenterally or orally. (1,4) It may develop at any time from 2 weeks (total dose 10 mg) to 6 years (6000 mg) after the start of gold treatment (5,11-13) and occurs particularly in patients with sero negative rheumatoid arthritis (11,13,14). During penicillamine treatment the peak incidence occurs in the second 6 months of treatment (3,6-10) but proteinuria may develop at any time from 6 weeks to 5 years after the start of treatment. (8,10) In some patients the proteinuria resolves spontaneously or decreases to less than 0.5 g/day within 12 months of stopping gold or penicillamine treatment (6,7,10,13,15,16,17) but in other patients proteinuria in excess of 1 g/day persists (6,10,13,18,19) or responds only to high doses of corticosteroids (5,13,15,17,20,21,22) and no long term studies have been reported. Limited data indicate that renal function is usually normal or only slightly impaired (6,8,13,17,21) although severe impairment has been reported (16,20) and serial and long term measurements have not been made. Recent immunogenetic and metabolic studies have indicated that gold and penicillamine nephropathy are more likely to occur in patients positive for the HLA-B8 or HLA-DR3 antigens (23,24) or who have a low sulphoxidative capacity for carbocysteine. (25,26) Renal biopsy has usually shown membranous GN (6,10,13,17,18,20, 21) but not invariably so (1,6,11,16,21) and in patients with persisting proteinuria biopsies performed 12 months or more after stopping treatment have shown extensive immune deposits (6,10) and caused concern that progressive renal disease may develop. (1,6)

Current knowledge of gold and penicillamine nephropathy is based on reports of small series of patients none of which have contained the serial clinical data that are required for an understanding of the natural course of the diseases. To provide these essential data 21 patients with gold nephropathy and 33 patients with penicillamine nephropathy have been studied in detail and throughout the whole of their renal illnesses.

PATIENTS AND METHODS

Between August 1973 and October 1984 54 patients with rheumatoid arthritis who had not previously had proteinuria were referred with proteinuria that had developed during gold or penicillamine treatment. All patients fulfilled the American Rheumatism Association's criteria for the diagnosis of rheumatoid arthritis and in 46 circulating IgM rheumatoid factor was present. Twenty-one patients (10 men and 11 women) received sodium aurothiomalate intramuscularly as a standard regime of a 10 mgm test dose followed by 50 mgm at weekly intervals until a satisfactory clinical response was acheived when the 50 mgm injections were given at monthly intervals to maintain the remission. Thirty-three patients (11 men and 22 women) were receiving oral D-penicillamine treatment. Between 1973 and 1976 the penicillamine was given at a starting dose of 250 mg/day increasing by 250 mg/day at monthly intervals to 1000 mg/day taken in divided doses. From 1977 onwards a flexible low dose regime was used starting at 125 mg/day increasing gradually at monthly intervals to find the lowest clinically effective dose, frequently 375-500 mg/day which was then continued.

Before each injection of gold and at 1-2 monthly intervals during penicillamine treatment the urine was tested for protein (Labstix, Ames). When appreciable proteinuria was detected (> 0.3 g/l) the decision concerning nephrological referral was made by the rheumatological specialist responsible for the patient. After referral the gold or penicillamine treatment was stopped immediately and 24 hour urinary protein excretion and creatinine clearance were measured. Intravenous urography and percutaneous renal biopsy were carried out on all patients and the tissue obtained was processed by conventional methods and examined by light, immunofluorescence and electron microscopy permitting causes of proteinuria other than gold and penicillamine nephropathy (amyloid, vasculitis, systemic lupus erythematosus, analgesic nephropathy etc) to be excluded. Each patient was followed up at intervals of 1-3 months until the proteinuria had resolved and 1-2 yearly thereafter with measurements of the 24 hour creatinine clearance and urinary protein excretion. The results of the study are presented as the median value, the 25th and 75th centiles (q1 and q3 respectively) and, when indicated, the range to indicate the wide dispersion and non-parametric distribution of the data.

RESULTS

Table I shows details of the patients and their treatment. The renal biopsies were performed 2 months (q1=1, q3=5; range 0.1-29 months) after treatment had been stopped.

Table I - Clinical details of patients studied

	GOLD n=21		Penicillamine n=33	
	Median	q1-q3	Median	q1-q3
Rheumatoid factor (IU)	384	112-1024	596	240-1280
Age of onset of RA (years)	49	40-57	45	36-50
Time between diagnosis of RA and start of treatment (months)	42	11-86.5	75	34-153
Time between start of treatment and onset of proteinuria (months)	7	4-17.5	8	5-11
Total dose of gold received (mg) Dose of penicillamine (mg/day)	930	693-1895	625	438-1000
% of patients positive for HLA B8 HLA DR3	45.5 36.4		55.5 44.4	

Table II shows the time of onset of proteinuria (between 2 weeks and 74 months) after the start of treatment. With both gold and penicillamine treatment the peak incidence occurred between 4 and 6 months of treatment when 38% and 36% respectively of all cases presented. Overall by 6,12 and 24 months of gold (penicillamine) treatment 48% (43%), 71% (82%) and 86% (91%) of patients had presented.

Table II - Time of onset of proteinuria during treatment with gold and penicillamine

	Gold			Penicillamine		
Months of Treatment	No patients developing Proteinuria	% of total	Cumulative %	No patients developing Proteinuria	% of total	Cumulative %
1 2 3	1 1 0	9.5	9.5	0 2 0	6.1	6.1
4 5 6	4 2 2	38.1	47.6	1 6 5	36.4	42.5
7 8 9	1 1 1	14.3	61.9	1 2 3	18.2	60.7
10 11 12	0 1 1	9.5	71.4	3 4 0	21.2	81.9
16 17 18	0 1 1	9.5	81.0	1 1	6.0	87.9
20				1	3.0	91
23	1	4.8	85.7			
31	1	4.8	90.5			
39	2	9.5	100.0			
40				1	3.0	94
46				1	3.0	97
74				1	3.0	100

The severity of the proteinuria varied greatly (0.3-3.9 g/day) and was not associated with the duration or dose of treatment received. Table III shows the median initial and maximum measurements of proteinuria. In 10 (48%) gold treated patients and 15 (45%) penicillamine treated patients the initial proteinuria was also the maximum whilst in the remainder the proteinuria increased for 1-13 months after treatment was stopped. The nephrotic syndrome developed in 8 (38%) gold treated and 20 (61%) penicillamine treated patients and persisted for a median period of 4 months (range 1-18 months) but was controlled with a diet high in protein and low in salt and by treatment with diuretics.

Table III - initial and maximum measurements of proteinuria

	Gold		Penicillamine	
	Median	q1-q3	Median	q1-q3
Initial g/day	1.7	0.9-3.1	3.7	1.6-7.3
Maximum *g/day	2.1	1.1-4.1	4.2	1.8-7.7
Time of Maximum Proteinuria *(months)	2	1-6	1	0.1-3

* after stopping treatment

In all but 1 patient, who developed a fatal carcinoma of the renal pelvis, the proteinuria resolved completely. (fig 1)

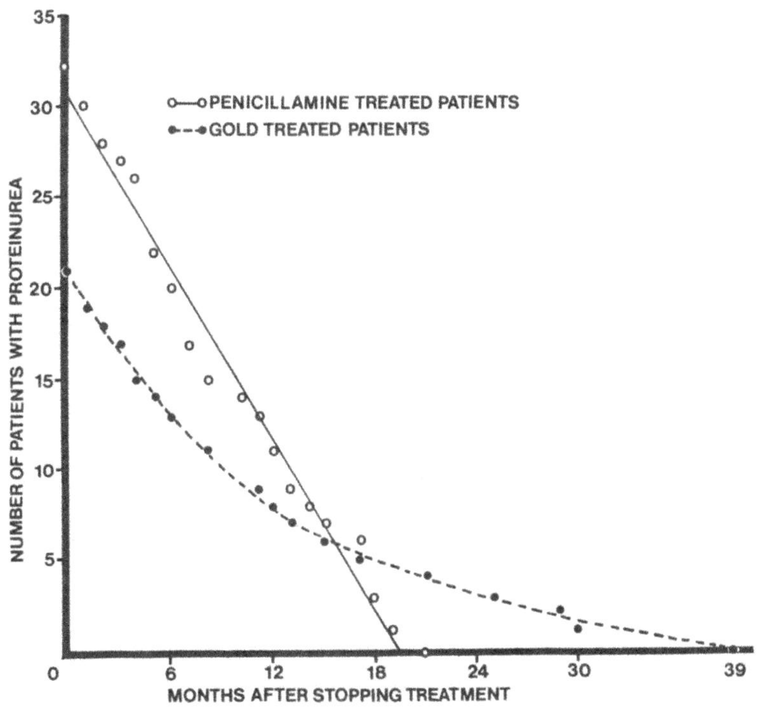

Fig 1 Resolution of proteinuria after stopping treatment

The median duration of the proteinuria in the gold treated patients was 11 months (q1=4, q3=19; range 1-39 months) and in the penicillamine treated patients 8 months (q1=5, q3=15; range 1-21 months). At 12 and 18 months after stopping treatment the proteinuria had resolved in 38% (36%), 62% (64%) amd 76% (88%) respectively of the gold (penicillamine) treated patients.

The median initial and latest measurements of creatinine clearance in the gold treated patients were 77 ml/min (q1=60, q3=108 ml/min), and 59 ml/min (q1=39, q3=85 ml/min), with a median interval of 60 months (q1=39, q3=85 ml/min) and in the penicillamine treated patients 80 ml/min (q1=61, q3=107 ml/min) and 78 ml/min (q1=62, q3=106 ml/min) with a median interval of 74 months (q1=43, q3=112 months) and the changes were not statistically significant. Table IV shows the initial creatinine clearances and those measured in the first and second 6 months and within 2 year intervals thereafter. Only 5 (24%) gold treated patients and 9 (27%) penicillamine treated patients had initial creatinine clearances of less than 60 ml/min. In all the gold treated and 29 of the 33 penicillamine treated patients the creatinine clearances improved during the follow-up period. In 2 penicillamine treated patients the creatinine clearance remained impaired but stable (40 and 57 ml/min) however in a further 2 patients renal function deteriorated progressively to 16 and 20 ml/min due to factors other than penicillamine nephropathy including rheumatoid vasculitis, malignant hypertension and refractory cardiac failure. No patients died from or needed treatment for chronic renal failure.

Table IV - Serial creatinine clearance measurements after stopping treatment

	Gold		Penicillamine	
Time	Median	q1-q3	Median	q1-q3
0	77	60-108	80	61-107
1-6	74	52-110	92	60-108
7-12	82	69-104	90	62-119
13-36	89	62-112	81	57-105
37-60	78	50-102	74	42-92
61-84	64	39-90	80	54-96
85-108	80	47-82	74	67-97
> 109			91	74-114

Tissue typing was performed in 29 patients. In the gold (penicillamine) treated patients the HLA B8 alloantigen was detected in 45% (56%), DR3 in 36% (44%) and DR4 in 36% (39%). Overall 64% of the gold treated and 56% of the penicillamine treated patients were positive for HLA B8 or DR3 or both.

Adequate renal biopsy speciments were obtained from all patients. In 15 (72%) gold treated and 29 (88%) penicillamine treated patients histological changes characteristic of membranous GN were present in the capillary loops with granular deposits of IgG and complement on immunofluorescence and subepithelial electron dense deposits on electron microscopy. On light microscopy, however, epimembranous "spikes" were seen in only 4 (19%) of the gold treated and 5 (15%) of the penicillamine treated patients and the most common abnormality was an increase in mesangial cells and matrix. Of the remaining 10 biopsies, 5 (2 gold and 3 penicillamine) showed mesangial electron dense deposits indicating an immune complex mesangial GN, 3 (2 gold and 1 penicillamine) showed extensive fusion of epithelial cell foot processes which, in the absence of other significant ultrastructural abnormalities, indicated a minimal change nephropathy and in 2 (gold treated) no glomerular abnormalities were detected suggesting a tubular cause for the proteinuria.

DISCUSSION

This long term study of gold and penicillamine nephropathy has identified the clinical features that comprise their natural course and has revealed their very close similarity. Gold and penicillamine nephropathy occur in patients with rheumatoid arthritis of all ages and in both sexes. The suggestions that gold nephropathy occurs predominantly in patients who are sero negative (11,13,14) and that proteinuria is uncommon during the first 6 months of penicillamine treatment (3) are not supported by the present data or several previous reports. (12,15,19,20,21) While confirming that proteinuria may develop at anytime during gold or penicillamine treatment (1) this study has shown that with both drugs the peak incidence occurs between 4 and 6 months after the start of treatment and that 70-80% present within the first year. It has been reported that the incidence of proteinuria during penicillamine treatment may be reduced by a low dose regime (125-500 mg/day). (3,27,28) However the present results indicate that there remains a significant incidence of proteinuria even with low dosage penicillamine treatment as eight (24%) patients were receiving 125-375 mg of penicillamine daily when proteinuria developed and a further eight were receiving 500 mg/day. No clinical variables have been found that accurately predict the development of gold and penicillamine nephropathy. (1) The association with the HLA alloantigens B8 and DR3 is only partial and tissue typing is too complex and expensive for routine use. (23,24) The possible association with a low sulphoxidative capacity for carbocysteine(25,26) requires prospective evaluation to determine its prognostic accuracy and the tests' technical complexity may limit any widespread clinical application. Thus regular analysis of urine with a reagent stick during treatment with gold or penicillamine remains the best clinical means of detecting nephropathy.

The present study confirms previous reports that the severity and duration of the proteinuria vary greatly and do not correlate with the duration or dose of treatment received. (5,6,7,8,9,13,16,17,19) In all but one patient, who developed a fatal carcinoma of the renal pelvis, the proteinuria resolved completely after treatment was stopped although in occasional patients it increased for 7-13 months and persisted for some 21 to 39 months. These data indicate that reports of apparently irreversible proteinuria and a progressive renal lesion due to gold or penicillamine treatment were premature and due to an inadequate follow-up period. (5,6,10,13,17,18,21)

The creatinine clearance measurements reported in this study are the first long-term serial measurements of renal function in gold and penicillamine nephropathy. They indicate that, with the exception of the very rare penicillamine induced crescentic glomerulonephritis (29,30) which was not seen in the 11 years of the study, progressive renal impairment that can be attributed primarily to gold or penicillamine nephropathy either does not occur or is very uncommon. Even when renal function was significantly impaired at presentation improvement occurred and was maintained in nearly all cases when the gold or penicillamine treatment was stopped. The two penicillamine treated patients with severely reduced renal function which continued to deteriorate when treatment was stopped both had other major factors contributing to their renal impairment.

These results show that, in patients with proteinuria, treatment with gold or penicillamine should be stopped and renal function and proteinuria monitored at intervals of 1-3 months until the proteinuria has resolved. The nephrotic syndrome that develops in one third of the gold treated and two thirds of the penicillamine treated patients can be controlled with a diet high in protein and low in salt and by treatment with diuretics. Treatment with high doses of corticosteroids which has been used previously (5,13,17,19,21,22) is not indicated as it is unnecessary and potentially hazardous and there is no evidence that it shortens the duration of the proteinuria or leads to the more rapid or more complete resolution of the renal lesion. Referral for renal biopsy is necessary only if nephrotic range proteinuria (> 3 g/day) persists for more than 1 year, if less severe proteinuria persists for more than 2 years, if renal function deteriorates appreciably or if there is concern that a second disease (usually amyloid) may be present. In the occasional patient with aggresive rheumatoid disease that has been controlled by gold or penicillamine therapy when all other second line agents have been ineffective or not tolerated, it may be appropriate to continue the gold treatment using auranofin (31) or the penicillamine in reduced dosage (3,32) provided that the proteinuria and creatinine clearance are monitored carefully. If nephrotic range proteinuria or deteriorating renal function occur the gold or penicillamine treatment should be discontinued immediately. (1)

Membranous GN is the renal lesion most commonly associated with gold and penicillamine treatment (5,6,7,8,9,10,11,12,13,18,20) and was seen in 71% and 88% respectively of patients in the present series. However other renal lesions occur and minimal change nephropathy and an immune complex mesangial GN were observed in association with both gold and penicillamine treatment in the present study. In addition there are reports of renal tubular lesions (1) due to gold treatment and IgA nephropathy (A G MacIver personal communication) and crescentic GN (24,30) due to penicillamine treatment. Thus gold and penicillamine nephropathy both encompass several types of renal damage due to different pathogenic mechanisms. In patients with rheumatoid arthritis not receiving gold or penicillamine treatment there is an increased incidence of both membranous GN (21,32) and mesangial changes (1,11,19) due to the deposition of immune complexes in specific regions of the glomerulus. Treatment with gold or penicillamine may modify the recipients immune system to enhance the persistance and deposition of existing 'rheumatoid' immune complexes causing an increased incidence of membranous GN and potentiating the mesangial GN of rheumatoid arthritis. (1) Gold treatment by a direct nephrotoxic action, may cause tubular proteinuria and the release of the renal tubular epithelial antigen which may be of particular importance in the immunopathogenesis of membranous GN. (1,14) Penicillamine is a potent hapten (33) and by this mechanism may release renal tubular epithelial antigen and glomerular basement membrane antigens leading to membranous GN and (very rarely) to Goodpastures syndrome respectively. (1) Both drugs modify lymphocyte function and may predispose to T cell mediated glomerular injury and minimal change nephropathy. (34) Thus treatment with gold and penicillamine may cause renal damage by mechanisms that are not a primary part of rheumatoid disease as well as by potentiating existing immune abnormalities. As treatment with gold and penicillamine are effective and widely used for active and progressive rheumatoid disease gold and penicillamine nephropathy will continue to occur and a detailed knowledge of the natural course of the conditions is essential for the correct management of affected patients.

ACKNOWLEDGEMENTS

The author wishes to acknowledge that much of the data presented herein is reproduced by the kind permission of the British Medical Journal - Br. Med. J. 295:745 (1987) and 296:1083 (1988).

REFERENCES

1. C. L. Hall. Gold and D penicillamine induced renal glomerular disease, *in* "The Kidney in Rheumatic Disease", P A Bacon and N M Hadler, eds London: Butterworths, (1982)
2. A. T. Day, T. R. Golding, P. N. Lee and A. D. Butterworth, Penicillamine in rheumatoid disease, a long term study. Br. Med. J. i: 180 (1974)
3. H. F. H. Hill. Treatment of rheumatoid arthritis with penicillamine. Semin Arthritis Rheum; 6:631 (1977)
4. W. A. Katz, R. C. Blodget and R. G. Pietruska, Proteinuria in gold treated rheumatoid arthritis, Ann Intern Med; 101:176 (1984)
5. D. S. Silverberg, E. G. Kidd, T. H. Schnitka and R. A. Ulan, Gold nephropathy: a clinical and pathological study. Arthritis Rheum; 13:812 (1970)
6. P. A. Bacon, C. R. Tribe, J. C. MacKenzie, J. Verrier-Jones, R. H. Cumming and B. Amer, Penicillamine nephropathy in rheumatoid arthritis. Q. J. Med; 45:661 (1976)
7. F. E. Dische, D. R. Swinson, E. D. B. Hamilton and V. Parsons, Immunopathology of penicillamine induced glomerular disease. J Rheumatol; 3:145 (1976)
8. A. M. Davison, A. T. Day, J. R. Golding and D. Thomson, Effect of penicillamine on the kidney. Proc. R. Soc. Med; 70 (Suppl 3); 109 (1977)
9. J. D. Kirby, P. A. Dieppe, E. C. Huskisson and B. Smith, D-penicillamine and immune complex deposition. Ann. Rheum. Dis; 38:344 (1979)
10. G. H. Nield, H. U. Gartner and A. Bohle, Penicillamine induced membranous glomerulonephritis. Lancet; 1:1201 (1975)
11. T. S. Tornroth and B. Skrifvars, Gold nephropathy: prototype of membranous glomerulonephritis. Am. J. Pathol; 75:573 (1974)
12. D. T. Davies, J. Dowling and J. Xipell, Gold nephropathy. Pathology; 9:281 (1977)
13. B. Skrifvars, T. S, Tornroth and G. N. Tallquist, Gold induced immune complex nephritis in seronegative rheumatoid arthritis. Ann. Rheum. Dis; 36:549 (1977)
14. B. Skrifvars, Hypothesis for the pathogenesis of sodium aurothiomalate induced immune complex nephritis. Scand. J. Rheumatol; 8:113 (1979)
15. S. W. Strunk and M. Ziff, Ultrastructural studies of the passage of gold thiomalate across the renal glomerular capillary wall. Arthritis Rheum; 13:39 (1970)

16. I. Watanabe, F. C. Whittier, J. Moore and F. E. Cuppage, Gold nephropathy: Ultrastructural, fluorescence, and micoanalytic studies of two patients. Arch Pathol Lab Med; 100:632 (1976)
17. G. W. Viol, T. A. Minielly and T. Bistricki, Gold nephropathy: tissue analysis by x-ray fluorescent spectroscopy. Arch Pathol Lab Med; 101:6 (1977)
18. J. H. Ross, F. McGinty and D. G. Brewer, Penicillamine nephropathy. Nephron; 26:184 (1980)
19. T. C. Lee, J. Dushkin, E. J. Eyring, E. P. Engelman and J. Hopper, Renal lesions associated with gold therapy: light and electron microscopic studies. Arthritis Rheum; 8:1 (1965)
20. H. R. Burger, J. Briner and M. A. Spycher, Affullige Haufung membrander Glomerulonephritiden nach Goldtheraple bel chronischer Polyarthritiseine Nebenwirkune eines neun Pripartates? Schweis Med Wochenschr 1979; 109:423 (1979)
21. B. Samuals, J. C. Lee, E. P Engelman and J. Hopper, Membranous nephropathy in patients with rheumatoid arthritis; relationship to gold therapy. Medicine 57:319 (1977)
22. A. D. Stephens, The management of cystinuria. Proc. Roy. Soc. Med. 70 (suppl 3); 24 (1977)
23. P. A. Wooley, T. Griffin, G. S. Panayi, J. R. Batchelor, K. T. Welsh and T. J. Gibson, HLA-DR Antigens and toxic reactions to sodium aurothiomate and D-penicillamine in patients with rheumatoid arthritis. N. Engl. J. Med; 303:300 (1980)
24. R. Speerstra, P. Reekers, L. B. van der Putte, J. R. van den Brouche, J. J. Rasker and D. J. de Rooi, HLA-DR antigens and proteinuria induced by aurothioglucose and D-penicillamine in patients with rheumatoid arthritis. J. Rheumatol. 10:448 (1983)
25. R. Madhok, H. A. Cappell and R. Waring, Does sulphoxidation state predict gold toxicity in rheumatoid arthritis? Br. Med. J; 294:483 (1987)
26. R. Ayesh, C. S. Mitchell, R. H. Waring, R. H. Witherington, M. H. Witherington, M. H. Siefert and R. L. Smith, Toxicity and sulphoxidation capacity in rheumatoid arthritic patients. Brit. J. Rheumatol; 26:197 (1987)
27. J. R. Golding, A. T. Day, M. R. Tomkinson, R. M. Brown, M V. Hassan, and S. R. Longstaff, Rheumatoid arthritis treated with small doses of penicillamine. Proc. Soc. Med. 70 (Suppl 3); 130 (1977)
28. H. F. H. HIll, A. G. S. Hill, A. T. Day, R. M. Brown, J. R. Golding and W. H. Lyle, Maintenance dose of penicillamine in rheumatoid arthritis : a comparison between standard and response related flexible regimes. Ann. Rheum. Dis 38:429 (1979)
29. T. Gibson, H. C. Barry and C. Ogg, Goodpastures syndrome and D-penicillamine. Ann. Intern. Med; 84:100 (1976)
30. J. N. McCormack, P, Wood and D. Bell, Penicillamine induced Goodpastures syndrome in "Penicillamine in rheumatoid disease", E. Munthe, ed, Fabritius and Sonner, Oslo (1977)
31. S. Tosi, M Cagnoli, M Murelli, K Messina and B. Columbo, Injectable gold dermatitis and proteinuria; retreatment with auranofin. Int J Clin Pharm Res; 5:265 (1985)
32. E. Honkanen, T. Tornroth, E. Petterson and B Skrifvars, Membranous glomerulonephritis in rheumatoid arthritis not related to gold or D-penicillamine therapy. Clin. Nephrol; 27:87 (1987)
33. I. A. Jaffe, Penicillamine in rheumatoid arthritis : clinical pharmacological & biochemical properties. Scand. J. Rheumatol 8 (Suppl 28): 58 (1979)
34 H. W. Schnaper and A. M. Robson, The nephrotic syndrome, in "Diseases of the Kidney", R. W. Schrier and C. W Gottschalk, eds, Little Brown and Co, Boston/Toronto (1988)

EFFECTS OF CONTRAST MEDIA ON RENAL HEMODYNAMICS AND TUBULAR FUNCTION: COMPARISON BETWEEN DIATRIZOATE AND IOPAMIDOL

Carlo Donadio, Gianfranco Tramonti, Roberto Giordani, Amalia Lucchetti, Andrea Calderazzi x, Paola Sbragia x, and Claudio Bianchi

Centro Nefrologico "Clara Monasterio Gentili", Clinica Medica 2, University of Pisa
x Istituto di Radiologia, University of Pisa, Italy

The administration of iodinated radiologic contrast media (CM) is the third cause of acute renal failure: about 12% of the cases in hospitalized patients (1,2).

Pre-existing renal disease, myeloma, diabetes, hypertension, heart failure, hepatic failure, dehydration, age>60 years and recent administration of CM are considered risk factors. Risk factors increase incidence and severity of renal injury after CM (3).

Different ionic or nonionic CM are available for intravenous administration. Ionic CM have a higher ratio between osmolality and iodine content than nonionic CM. Hyperosmolality of CM has been claimed as an important factor in renal damage (4). The proximal tubule is the main target of the nephron for CM. The tubular damage of CM could be due to osmolality or other chemical properties either directly or via alterations of renal hemodynamics (5,6).

The aim of this study is to evaluate the effects on renal hemodynamics and tubular function of IV administration of two different CM: diatrizoate meglumine (a high osmolality ionic CM), and iopamidol (a lower osmolality nonionic CM).

MATERIALS AND METHODS

Patients

Thirty-nine adult patients (20 females, 19 males), requiring radiological examinations with IV administration of iodinated CM, participated in this study. Thirty-six patients were investigated with intravenous urography (18 with diatrizoate, 18 with iopamidol) and three patients with computed body tomography (1 with diatrizoate and 2 with iopamidol). Their main clinical data were as follows:

- age 22-74 years, mean 49.6;
- body weight 45-110 kg, mean 71.6;
- systolic blood pressure 105-180 mmHg, mean 135.1;
- diastolic blood pressure 65-107 mmHg, mean 83.8;
- creatinine clearance 52-160 ml/min, mean 101.2.

None of the patients had been examined with CM in the month preceding the study. No nephrotoxic drug was administered in the period of the study. Three patients (one examined with diatrizoate and two with iopamidol) had type II diabetes. All patients were normally hydrated.

Patients were assigned to diatrizoate (n=19) or to iopamidol group (n=20) in a randomized fashion.

Contrast media

Diatrizoate meglumine (Angiografin 65% - Schering SpA Milano, Italy):

- osmolality 1,500 mOsm/kg;
- contrast medium concentration 650 g/l;
- iodine concentration 306 g/l;
- administered dose of CM 0.2-1.4 g/kg body weight, mean 0.78.

Iopamidol (Iopamiro 300 - Bracco Industria Chimica Spa Milano, Italy):

- osmolality 616 mOsm/kg;
- contrast medium concentration 612 g/l;
- iodine concentration 300 g/l;
- administered dose of CM 0.2-1.4 g/kg body weight, mean 0.76.

Methods

Different parameters of renal function were measured twice in the week preceding the administration of CM and 1, 3, and 5 days after the examination.

Urine: output (urine collected in the twelve night hours, 34 pts), specific gravity (26 pts), protein concentration (35 pts).

Plasma: creatinine (35 pts), urea (35 pts), uric acid (31 pts), sodium (34 pts), potassium (31 pts), calcium (34 pts), phosphorus (32 pts).

Clearances: creatinine (32 pts), urea (32 pts), uric acid (27 pts), sodium (23 pts), potassium (26 pts), calcium (26 pts), phosphorus (25 pts).

Renal hemodynamics: glomerular filtration rate (GFR) (32 pts) and effective renal plasma flow (ERPF) (27 pts) were measured once in the basal period and after 3 to 5 days from CM administration. The measurement of GFR and ERPF was performed by means of the noninvasive bladder cumulative method, using diethylene-triamine-pentaacetic acid labelled with 99mTc and 131I-hippuran, respectively (7,8).

Enzymuria: urinary enzyme activities of alanine aminopeptidase (AAP) (30 pts), gamma-glutamyltransferase (GGT) (31 pts), N-acetyl-beta-D-glucosaminidase (NAG) (28 pts) and lysozyme (LZM) (28 pts) were measured twice in the week preceding the administration of CM and 1, 3, and 5 days after (9-12).

Statistical analysis: paired Student t test was used to analyze data. A p value <0.05 was considered statistically significant.

RESULTS

The main renal effects of diatrizoate and iopamidol are reported in Table 1 and 2 respectively.

Urine. A slight decrease of urine output was observed one day after the administration of diatrizoate. Urine specific gravity remained stable with both CM. A minimal, but statistically significant, increase of urinary concentration of proteins was observed with iopamidol.

Plasma. Plasma creatinine, urea, uric acid, sodium, potassium, calcium and phosphorus were almost unmodified with both CM.

Clearances. After the administration of diatrizoate, a slight decrease in clearances of creatinine, urea, sodium, potassium, calcium and phosphorus was observed on the first day. The effect on urea, sodium and calcium clearances was statistically significant. On the third day potassium and phosphorus clearances were still lower than basal values. Uric acid clearance was modestly but constantly increased. A more evident increase of uric acid clearance occurred on the first day after iopamidol. No other variation in clearance values was observed with this CM.

Renal hemodynamics. Mean values of GFR showed a minimal decrease with diatrizoate, while ERPF was unchanged. As a consequence FF decreased. Mean values of GFR, ERPF and FF did not change after administration of iopamidol. Nevertheless, in one patient (74 years, no other risk factor) GFR and ERPF showed a clinically relevant decrease after iopamidol (from 89 to 46 ml/min and from 391 to 250 ml/min, respectively).

Enzymuria. The major effect of both CM was a relevant increase of urinary enzyme activities. On the first day, the increase of brush border enzymes AAP and GGT was maximum with both CM and statistically significant. In particular, AAP doubled in 13/15 pts examined with diatrizoate and in 8/15 with iopamidol; GGT doubled in 9/15 pts with diatrizoate and in 8/16 with iopamidol. Urinary enzyme activities returned to basal values within the fifth day with diatrizoate and on the third day with iopamidol. Lysosomal enzyme NAG doubled in 8/12 pts with diatrizoate and in 3/16 with iopamidol. Nevertheless, such an increase was not statistically significant. Finally, urinary excretion of lysozyme (a low mw protein filtered by the glomerulus and reabsorbed by the proximal tubule) doubled in 5/12 pts examined with diatrizoate and in 8/16 with iopamidol; this increase was statistically significant only with iopamidol.

Table 1. RENAL EFFECTS OF DIATRIZOATE (mean±SD; * $p<0.05$, ** $p<0.01$)

	n	Before	1st	3rd	5th day
URINE					
output (ml/12 hrs)	17	1058±589	809±359*	891±366	1021±431
specific gravity	15	1.015±0.003	1.015±0.006	1.015±0.006	1.015±0.005
proteins (mg/dl)	18	22±37	22±39	20±31	21±40
PLASMA					
creatinine (mg/dl)	18	1.01±0.27	1.03±0.30	1.04±0.31	1.01±0.29
urea (mg/dl)	18	35.6±5.1	36.6±7.8	34.2±6.1	34.1±7.0
uric acid (mg/dl)	16	5.5±1.5	5.4±1.1	5.1±1.1	5.0±1.1
sodium (mEq/l)	17	139.9±2.4	139.7±3.4	139.7±2.4	139.8±3.0
potassium (mEq/l)	15	3.8±0.5	3.8±0.5	3.8±0.5	3.9±0.6
calcium (mEq/l)	18	4.7±0.3	4.7±0.3	4.8±0.2	4.7±0.3
phosphorus (mEq/l)	16	2.2±0.4	2.3±0.7	2.2±0.3	2.2±0.3
CLEARANCES					
creatinine (ml/min)	15	108.2±28.1	97.7±26.0	108.3±33.2	107.6±29.4
urea (ml/min)	15	44.4±12.3	39.6±13.1*	44.4±16.6	45.8±13.5
uric acid (ml/min)	14	6.7±2.6	7.1±3.0	7.4±3.9	7.4±4.2
sodium (ml/min)	8	0.81±0.41	0.47±0.23*	0.76±0.50	0.71±0.55
potassium (ml/min)	12	7.3±3.4	6.1±2.3	6.1±3.0	6.7±4.1
calcium (ml/min)	13	1.25±0.83	0.86±0.56*	1.28±0.82	1.54±1.23
phosphorus (ml/min)	13	11.9±6.6	10.0±7.5	10.5±5.4	12.3±9.6
RENAL HEMODYNAMICS					
GFR (ml/min)	16	67.5±20.1		62.2±20.6	
ERPF (ml/min)	13	344.6±121.1		337.5±106.4	
FF (%)	13	20.4±7.2		18.6±4.9	
URINARY ENZYME ACTIVITIES					
AAP (U/g creat)	15	3.9±3.5	9.2±8.3**	6.6±8.6	3.9±3.0
GGT (U/g creat)	15	48.7±25.1	132.1±94.4**	70.6±97.4	45.6±19.0
NAG (μM/hr/g creat)	12	26.0±12.4	44.4±40.8	28.7±15.6	33.9±19.9
LZM (mg/g creat)	12	0.20±0.24	0.28±0.34	0.13±0.17	0.11±0.15

Both CM produced a more evident increase of the brush border enzymes AAP and GGT than that of NAG and LZM. The increase of urinary enzyme activities does not seem to have a predictive value for renal function damage. In fact, only in a few cases the increase of urinary enzymes was followed by the decrease of creatinine clearance, GFR or ERPF.

No correlation was found between the dose of CM infused and any of the observed renal effects.

Table 2. RENAL EFFECTS OF IOPAMIDOL (mean±SD; *p<0.05, **p<0.01)

	n	Before	1st	3rd	5th day
URINE					
output (ml/12 hrs)	17	855±235	776±354	807±291	794±261
specific gravity	11	1.015±0.005	1.017±0.009	1.014±0.004	1.013±0.004
proteins (mg/dl)	17	11±20	14±23**	16±35	16±27
PLASMA					
creatinine (mg/dl)	17	0.91±0.25	0.96±0.28	0.97±0.33	0.95±0.27
urea (mg/dl)	17	36.8±7.0	35.5±9.9	35.4±7.4	36.4±9.8
uric acid (mg/dl)	15	4.5±1.0	4.4±1.6	4.4±1.1	4.3±1.3
sodium (mEq/l)	17	140.5±4.2	140.8±4.0	141.2±4.4	139.9±3.0
potassium (mEq/l)	16	4.1±0.3	4.1±0.3	4.2±0.3	4.1±0.3
calcium (mEq/l)	16	4.6±0.4	4.7±0.3	4.7±0.3	4.7±0.4
phosphorus (mEq/l)	16	2.2±0.4	2.1±0.3	2.3±0.6	2.2±0.3
CLEARANCES					
creatinine (ml/min)	17	100.8±25.4	107.1±30.6	98.6±33.5	94.4±24.6
urea (ml/min)	17	39.2±12.3	40.6±15.1	39.0±11.4	35.4±10.3
uric acid (ml/min)	13	7.0±2.1	8.9±3.1	7.0±1.9	7.5±3.1
sodium (ml/min)	15	0.60±0.28	0.59±0.35	0.61±0.33	0.59±0.32
potassium (ml/min)	14	7.2±2.4	6.9±1.7	6.9±2.3	6.6±2.0
calcium (ml/min)	13	1.26±0.72	1.27±0.64	1.24±0.69	1.12±0.60
phosphorus (ml/min)	12	12.9±4.3	14.0±6.7	14.1±5.8	10.9±3.1
RENAL HEMODYNAMICS					
GFR (ml/min)	16	70.6±23.4		71.4±27.6	
ERPF (ml/min)	14	316.7±118.7		317.5±105.5	
FF (%)	14	22.4±6.2		21.5±6.2	
URINARY ENZYME ACTIVITIES					
AAP (U/g creat)	15	3.6±2.4	6.6±3.7**	3.6±2.7	3.0±1.4
GGT (U/g creat)	16	41.1±10.7	86.4±53.4**	39.4±12.1	37.3±13.8
NAG (μM/hr/g creat)	16	53.7±50.9	72.3±96.4	48.4±47.6	51.4±54.3
LZM (mg/g creat)	16	0.33±0.48	0.56±0.61*	0.50±0.79	0.37±0.43

DISCUSSION

The occurence of acute renal failure after administration of CM is well recognized. However, few prospective studies evaluated the effects of CM on renal function (mostly determined only as creatinine clearance). Recently, the effects of CM on proximal tubule has been studied by measuring urinary enzymes (sometimes only one enzyme was determined). The results reported appear conflicting (13-23).

A lower nephrotoxicity of nonionic low-osmolal CM has been claimed by some authors, mainly on the basis of urinary enzyme activities, but not confirmed by others (17-19, 22-24).

Up to now there has been no prospective study evaluating both renal hemodynamics (GFR and ERPF) and tubular effects (enzymuria) of ionic and nonionic CM.

Our results demonstrate a slight effect of diatrizoate on glomerular function as demonstrated by the decrease of mean values of GFR, creatinine and urea clearances. This effect was not observed in patients examined with iopamidol, except in one case who showed a relevant decrease of GFR and ERPF.

CM affect the proximal tubule, as indicated by the increase of urinary enzyme activities observed in most patients with both CM and by the reduction of clearances of sodium and calcium (induced by diatrizoate). A marked increase of enzymuria, mainly brush border enzymes, occurred frequently. The observed increase of urinary enzymes does not necessarily indicate a clinically relevant renal damage, but does suggest a transient dysfunction of proximal tubule. In fact, increased enzymuria was completely reversible in a few days. Furthermore, enzymuria does not seem to have a predictive value for the impairment of renal function. It is noteworthy that AAP and GGT increased more than the lysosomal enzyme NAG, thus suggesting a prevalent brush border involvement.

In conclusion, diatrizoate meglumine can determine a slight impairment of glomerular function. Both diatrizoate and iopamidol can induce a reversible tubular dysfunction, as demonstrated by the increase of enzymuria. The observed glomerular and tubular effects of CM have generally no clinical relevance.

Acknowledgments

This work was supported in part by a research fund from Ministero Pubblica Istruzione, Italy.

Mr. Joseph Franceschina is gratefully acknowledged for his valuable help in the preparation of this paper.

REFERENCES

1. S.H. Hou, D.A. Bushinsky, J.B. Wish, J.J. Cohen, and J.T. Harrington, Hospital-acquired renal insufficiency: a prospective study, Am. J. Med. 74: 243 (1983).
2. D. Kleinknecht, P. Landais, and B. Goldfarb, Les insuffisances rénales aiguës associées à des médicaments ou à des produits de contraste iodés. Résultats d'une enquête coopérative multicentrique de la Société de néphrologie, Néphrologie 7: 41 (1986).
3. R.O. Berkseth, and C.M. Kjellstrand, Radiologic contrast-induced

nephropathy, Med. Clin. North Am. 68: 351 (1984).
4. J.B. Forrest, S.S. Howards, and J.Y. Gillenwater, Osmotic effects of intravenous contrast agents on renal function, J. Urol. 125: 147 (1981).
5. R.W. Katzberg, R.C. Pabico, T.W. Morris, K. Hayakawa, B.A. McKenna, B.J. Panner, J.A. Ventura, and H.W. Fischer, Effects of contrast media on renal function and subcellular morphology in the dog, Invest. Radiol. 21: 64 (1986).
6. H.D. Humes, D.A. Hunt, and M.D. White, Direct toxic effect of the radiocontrast agent diatrizoate on renal proximal tubular cells, Am. J. Physiol. 21: F246 (1987).
7. C. Bianchi, Noninvasive methods for the measurement of renal function, in: "Renal function tests. Clinical Laboratory procedures and diagnosis", C.G. Duarte, ed., p. 65, Little, Brown, Boston (1980).
8. C. Bianchi, C. Donadio, and G. Tramonti, Noninvasive methods for the measurement of total renal function, Nephron 28: 53 (1981).
9. J.E. Peters, I. Schneider, and R.J. Haschen, Bestimmung der 1-Alanyl-Peptidhydrolase (Alanyl-Aminopeptidase, Aminosäure-Arylamidase) im menschlichen Harn, Clin. Chim. Acta 36: 289 (1972).
10. G. Szasz, Gamma-Glutamyltranspeptidase-Aktivität im Urin, Z. klin. Chem. klin. Biochem. 8: 1 (1970).
11. L.J. Merle, M.M. Reindenberg, M.T. Camacho, B.R. Jones, and D.E. Drayer, Renal injury in patients with rheumatoid arthritis treated with gold, Clin. Pharmacol. Ther. 28: 216 (1980).
12. D.J. Prockop, and W.D. Davidson, A study of urinary and serum lysozyme in patients with renal disease, New Engl. J. Med. 270: 269 (1964).
13. N. Milman, and P. Gottlieb, Renal function after high-dose urography in patients with chronic renal insufficiency, Clin. Nephrol. 7: 250 (1977).
14. T. Shafi, S.Y. Chou, J.G. Porush, and W.B. Shapiro, Infusion intravenous pyelography and renal function. Effects in patients with chronic renal insufficiency, Arch. Intern. Med. 138: 1218 (1978).
15. A. Rahimi, R.P.S. Edmondson, and N.F. Jones, Effect of radiocontrast media on kidney of patients with renal disease, Br. Med. J. 282: 1194 (1981).
16. J.L. Teruel, R. Marcén, J.M. Onaindía, A. Serrano, C. Quereda, and J. Ortuño, Renal function impairment caused by intravenous urography, Arch. Intern. Med. 141: 1271 (1981).
17. G.A. Khoury, J.C. Hopper, Z. Varghese, K. Farrington, R. Dick, J.D. Irving, P. Sweny, O.N. Fernando, and J.F. Moorhead, Nephrotoxicity of ionic and non-ionic contrast material in digital vascular imaging and selective renal arteriography, Br. J. Radiol. 56: 631 (1983).
18. M.E. Gale, A.H. Robbins, R.J. Hamburger, and W.C. Widrich, Renal toxicity of contrast agents: iopamidol, iothalamate, and diatrizoate, Am. J. Roentgenol. 142: 333 (1984).
19. J.E. Scherberich, W. Mondorf, F.W. Falkenberg, D. Pierard, and W. Schoeppe, Monitoring drugs nephrotoxicity. Quantitative estimation of human kidney brush border antigens in urine as a specific marker of tubular damage, Contrib. Nephrol. 42: 81 (1984).
20. W.M. Thompson, W.L.Jr. Foster, R.A. Halvorsen, N.R. Dunnick, A.J.

Rommel, and M. Bates, Iopamidol: new, nonionic contrast agent for excretory urography, Am. J. Roentgenol. 142: 329 (1984).

21. H.J. Smith, K. Levorstad, K.J. Berg, K. Rootwelt, and K. Sveen, High dose urography with renal failure. A double blind investigation of iohexol and metrizoate, Acta Radiol. Diagn. 26: 213 (1985).
22. G. Cavaliere, G. D'Arrigo, G. D'Amico, P. Bernasconi, G. Schiavina, L. Dellafiore, and D. Vergnaghi, Tubular nephrotoxicity after intravenous urography with ionic high-osmolal and nonionic low-osmolal contrast media in patients with chronic renal insufficiency, Nephron 46: 128 (1987).
23. C. Donadio, G. Tramonti, P. Lorusso, R. Giordani, A. Lucchetti, A. Calderazzi, C. Sbragia, P.L. Michelassi, and C. Bianchi, Effetti renali dei mezzi di contrasto: confronto tra diatrizoato di meglumina e iopamidolo (risultati preliminari), G. Ital. Nefrol. 4: 175 (1987).
24. S. Cedgard, H. Herlitz, K. Geterud, P. Attman, and M. Aurell, Acute renal insufficiency after administration of low-osmolar contrast media, Lancet ii: 1281 (1986).

NEPHROTOXICITY OF FUMARIC ACID MONOETHYLESTER (FA ME) *

M. Hohenegger[1], M.Vermes[1], A. Sadjak[2], G. Egger[2], S. Supanz[2], and U. Erhart[2]

[1] Institute of General and Experimental Pathology, University of Vienna

[2] Institute of Functional Patho!ogy, University of Graz

1. INTRODUCTION

Fumaric acid monoethylester (FA ME) is used as a therapeutic agent against psoriasis.As there exists some clinical evidence for nephrotoxicity (2,9) the present investigations were performed.

In this study the effects of a high single dose of this compound on renal function are presented. In control experiments also disodium fumarate (DI NA F) and fumaric acid diethylester (FA DE) were employed. The main functions investigated were glomerular filtration rate (GFR) and urine concentration ability. In vivo and in vitro experiments were combined and it was attempted to find correlations with histological lesions.Rats were employed as experimental animals.

2. MATERIALS AND METHODS

<u>In all chapters of the following presentation all compounds administered to the animals and all absolute amounts of substances excreted by the kidneys are normalized for 1oo g body weight(b.wt.).</u>

2.1. General

Male Sprague - Dawley rats, weighing 25o ± 5o g (Animal Breeding Institute of the Medical Faculty of the University of Vienna) were employed. They were kept under conditions as described previously (8).

2.2. In vivo experiments

2.2.1. Application of substances

In the later afternoon the animals got one of the following substan -

* This work was supported by " Deutscher Psoriasisbund " , Hamburg FRG.

ces dissolved in 2.5 - 3.o ml phosphate buffer (o.o5 M, pH 7.4) in doses between 1o and 1oo mg per stomach tube:

Fumaric acid monoethylester (FA ME)
Fumaric acid diethylester (FA DE)
Disodium fumarate (DI NA F)

These substances were obtained by Fluka, Buchs Switzerland.
A control group received the buffer alone; sometimes equivalent amounts of sodium chloride were added.

Eight - 12 hours before and afterwards food was withdrawn. Tap water was always allowed if nothing else is reported.

2.2.2. Inulin clearance and histology

Forty - five minutes before application of the substances above, a retard tablet containing 3oo mg inulin was implanted on the neck in light ether anesthesia. By this procedure constant inulin plasma levels are achieved for about 48 hours (7). Twenty hours after application of the compounds the urines were collected for 4 hours. Before the collection period diuresis was induced by 2 x 3 ml o.45 % sodium chloride solution given orally. After the collection period blood samples were taken in heparinized test tubes after incision of one carotid artery in ether anesthesia. After killing the animals by cervical dislocation the kidneys were rapidly removed and prepared for histological investigation (staining with PAS or Sudan III, see ref. 12).

2.2.3. Circulatory parameters and plasma metabolites

FA ME and the other compounds were applied as above. Sixteen - 18 hours after, oxygen consumption of the conscious rats was measured by employing a diaferometer (8). In light ether anesthesia arterial systolic blood pressure was then recorded by Dopplers ultrasound technique (Model 8o2-A Doppler, Parks Electronics, USA). Immediately after this, heart frequency was determined by electrocardiography (Cardiostat 7o3, Siemens FRG).

In other rats treated in the same way instead of measuring circulatory parameters blood was taken by cardiac puncture in light ether anesthesia and collected in heparinized test tubes. In heparin plasma creatinine, urea, sodium, potassium, glucose , triglycerides and osmolality were determined.

2.2.4. Urinary excretion and urine composition

After application of the compounds in the afternoon as above one group of rats had free access to water. In the next morning, about 16 hours later, 2.5 ml of water were given additionally by stomach tube. Then, the urines were collected for 4 hours and analyzed for osmolality, sodium, potassium, glucose and protein.

In another group of rats water was withdrawn overnight and about 17 hours after application of the compounds urines were collected over a period of 5 hours under prolonged water deprivation. In these urines osmolality was determined.

In all urine samples the sediment was examined by microscopy.

2.3. In vitro experiments

2.3.1. General

Normal untreated rats were killed by cervical dislocation. Different organs were rapidly removed and tissue slices were prepared by employing a razor blade. The thickness of the slices was about o.5 mm. Diaphragma was used without any treatment.

All incubations were performed in a Warburg apparatus if nothing else is indicated. The incubation medium was isotonic Krebs phosphate buffer, pH 7.4, shaking frequency 1oo /min. As gas phase air was employed throughout. Incubation temperature was always 37o C.

2.3.1. Oxygen consumption

Slices of liver, kidney cortex, outer and inner medulla as well as pieces from diaphragma (about 3o - 1oo mg each) were incubated as above for 1 - 2 hours. FA ME or DI NA F were added to the medium in concentrations between 1o and 1oo mg/dl. One or 2 hours after, the slices were placed into the chamber of an YSI oxygen monitor, Yellow Springs Instruments USA. Oxygen consumption was measured by employing a Clark electrode. The composition of the medium was thereby not altered. The recordings of oxygen consumption were performed over periods of about 2o minutes.

2.3.2. Glycolysis

Slices of kidney inner medulla were incubated as above for 1 hour. To the medium 14o mg/dl glucose were added; FA ME concentrations were between 1o and 1oo mg/dl.At the end of the incubation lactate was measured in the medium.

2.4. Chemical measurements

Osmolality was measured by freezing point depression using a Fiske osmometer.

Sodium and potassium were measured by flame photometry. An apparatus of Radiometer, Copenhagen was employed.

Creatinine was measured colorimetrically; urea, glucose, lactate and triglycerides were determined enzymatically as described in our previous papers (4,5,6,8).

Inulin was measured according to Renschler (1o). For all these measurements chemicals of Boehringer Mannheim and Merck Darmstadt, FRG were used.

Urinary protein concentration was measured according to Bradford (1) employing chemicals of Bio Rad, Richmond USA.

2.5. Statistics

From all experimental groups means ± standard deviations (SD) were calculated. The means were compared with t - tests.

3. RESULTS

3.1. General observations

The general state was reduced in about 25 % of the rats receiving 1oo mg FA ME 2o hours after application and later on. The time before no obvious signs of intoxication could be detetcted. Table 1 shows some measurements performed about 18 hours after 1oo mg FA ME. Whole body oxygen consumption and heart frequency are not significantly altered. There is a small increase of arterial systolic blood pressure.

Table 1. General observations in rats about 18 hours after oral application of different compounds (1oo mg). Number of measurements in ().

Compounds	Whole body oxygen consumption l/kg b.wt./24 hr	Arterial systolic pressure mm Hg	Heart frequency beats/min
Buffer alone	4o.5 ± 12.2 (8)	1o6 ± 18 (8)	385 ± 62 (4)
DI NA F	38.6 ± 5.1 (1o)	113 ± 21 (8)	443 ± 32 (3)
FA DE	39.6 ± 7.6 (6)	115 ± 22 (4)	39o ± 46 (4)
FA ME	36.5 ± 7.6 (12)	131 ± 18 (8)*	367 ± 39 (4)

* p < o.o5 vs. buffer.

3.2. Glomerular filtration rate (GFR)

Table 2 presents the results of GFR measurements. It can be seen that 1oo mg FA DE or DI NA F as well as 5o mg FA ME did not reduce GFR. On the other hand 1oo mg FA ME reduced inulin clearance by about 4o %.

Table 2. Inulin clearance in rats . Urine collection 2o - 24 hours after oral application of different compounds. Six measure - ments in each group.

Compounds		Inulin clearance ml/min/1oo g b.wt.	p vs. buffer
Buffer + 4o mg NaCl		1.27 ± o.o8	
DI NA F	1oo mg	1.13 ± o.o8	NS
FA DE	1oo mg	1.24 ± o.22	NS
FA ME	5o mg	1.15 ± o.12	NS
FA ME	1oo mg	o.69 ± o.o8	< o.o1

3.3 Plasma metabolites

According to table 3 plasma urea and creatinine concentrations are significantly elevated after 1oo mg FA ME only. Plasma osmolality, so - dium and potassium as well as glucose and triacylglycerol (data not shown in the table) remained within the normal range in animals of all groups.

3.4. Urinary excretion rates during water diuresis

From table 4 we see decreasing urine volume but increasing so - dium and potassium excretion after 1oo mg FA ME whereas glucose ex - cretion is not altered. Protein excretion shows a different behaviour. In 3 animals it was considerably augmented (see table) in 5 other rats , however, it remained within the normal range. In the urine sediments no pathologic cells and no abnormal counts of cells were found.

Table 3. Plasma metabolites 16 - 17 hours after oral application of different compounds (1oo mg). Number of measurements in ().

Compounds		Osmolality mOsm/kg	Sodium mMol/l	Potassium mMol/l	Urea mg/dl	Creatinine mg/dl
Buffer	(4)	288 ± 5.4	139 ± 6.7	4.8 ± o.5	32 ± 8	o.44 ± o.o6
DI NA F	(8)	289 ± 7.7	136 + 8.8	4.2 ± 1.3	37 ± 4	o.48 ± o.o8
FA DE	(4)	287 ± 3.3	135 ± 1.9	4.2 ± o.9	45 ± 13	o.54 ± o.o3
FA ME	(9)	291 ± 9.o	135 ± 6.1	4.3 ± 1.1	1o6 ± 43*	1.2o ± o.3o*

* $p < o.o1$ vs. buffer.

Table 4. Urinary excretion rates 16 - 2o hours after oral application of different compounds.Water load before collection period : 2.5 ml.

Compounds		Urine volume ml/4hr	Sodium mMol/4 hr	Potassium	Glucose mg/4 hr	Protein mg/4 hr
Buffer[1)]		2.3 ± o.5	18 ± 9	12 ± 8	1.1 ± o.22	o.47 ± o.14
DI NA F[2)]	1oo mg	2.4 ± o.5	46 ± 31	24 ± 22		o.51 ± o.17
FA DE[2)]	1oo mg	2.9 ± o.4	2o ± 12	56 ± 12		o.61 ± o.26
FA ME[1)]	25 mg	2.2 ± o.2	37 ± 8	21 ± 6	1.2 ± o.14	o.54 ± o.o7
FA ME[1)]	5o mg	2.3 ± o.3	3o ± 2	55 ± 26	1.4 ± o.o8	o.67 ± o.17
FA ME[3)]	1oo mg	1.7 ± o.8	83 ± 59	59 ± 12	1.2 ± o.27	1.12 ± 1.21*

1) n = 6; 2) n = 5; 3) n = 8. * In 3 animals 5.o, 8.o and 16.6 mg/4 hr, respectively.

3.5. Urinary excretion rates after water withdrawal overnight

Table 5 shows the effects of different oral doses of FA ME on urinary concentration ability. A significant decrease after 5o and 1oo mg can be observed. The other compounds had no influence on urine concentration under this condition (details not shown). Normal urine sediments were observed in this type of experiment, too.

3.6. Lactate production by kidney inner medulla in vitro

Table 5 further shows the results of some measurements of lactate production from glucose by slices of inner medulla under the influence of FA ME in the incubation medium. Ten mg/dl of this compound decreased lactate formation already significantly. The concentration of 25 mg/dl reduced lactate formation further; with 5o and 1oo mg/dl, respectively, no additional decrease occured.

Table 5. Influence of FA ME on urine osmolality after water deprivation overnight and on lactate production from glucose by kidney inner medulla of rats. Number of experiments in ().

In vivo			In vitro		
Oral doses of FA ME mg		Urine osmolality[1)] mOsm/kg	FA ME in incubation medium mg/dl		Lactate formation from glucose [2)] μMol/g wet wt./h
0	(3)	34o8 ± 952	0	(12)	32.7 ± 5.5
1o	(3)	2779 ± 222	1o	(6)	26.o ± 3.o**
25	(3)	1864 ± 348	25	(6)	17.o ± o.5**
5o	(3)	1135 ± 4o9*	5o	(6)	18.o ± o.6**
1oo	(5)	8o5 ± 34**	1oo	(6)	16.5 ± 2.2**

[1)] Urine collection: 9 a.m. - 1 p.m. [2)] 14o mg/dl incubation medium.
* $p < o.o5$ vs. controls; ** $p < o.o1$ vs. controls.

3.7. Oxygen consumption in vitro

As demonstrated in table 6 FA ME had no influence on oxygen consumption of different tissues in vitro. The negative results of experiments with lower concentrations are not shown.

Table 6. Oxygen consumption of tissue slices (ml/g wet wt./h). Influence of DI NA F and FA ME, respectively, in the incubation medium (1oo mg/dl each).

Tissue	Buffer alone*	DI NA F *	FA ME **
Diaphragma	o.48 ± o.23	o.41 ± o.12	o.37 ± o.15
Liver	o.77 ± o.25	o.59 ± o.19	o.53 ± o.27
Kidney			
Cortex	o.97 ± o.24	o.92 ± o.23	1.oo ± o.54
Outer med.	1.12 ± o.22	1.76 ± o.65	1.13 ± o.54
Inner med.	o.74 ± o.32	o.82 ± o.32	o.67 ± o.22

* n = 5; ** n = 1o. For all means: $p > o.o5$ vs. buffer.

3.8 Histology

In control rats nephrons revealed no abnormal aspect. Pycnotic nuclei and hyalinization of glomerular capillaries rarely occured. There was no difference between kidneys of controls and those from rats treated with DI NA F, 5o or 1oo mg, respectively.
Following 5o mg of FA ME pycnotic nuclei and hyalinization occured more frequently than in controls. The interlobular veins were congested. In such areas also interstitial bleedings and destruction of proximal

tubules could be observed. The higher dose of 1oo mg FA ME induced lesions as above but considerably more severe and more frequent. The vasa afferentia, however, were generally intact even in glomeruli showing hyalinizytion and shrinking. Less severe lesions were found after application of corresponding doses of FA DE.

4. DISCUSSION

4.1. General

During oral and local therapy of psoriasis with FA ME over several days or few weeks increase of serum creatinine and pathologic urine sediment have been observed in several patients (2,9). The doses applied per day were about 5o - 1oo times lower than the single doses given to our rats. In mice a total dose of 6.9 g /kg b.wt. given over a period of 8 days was lethal for all animals investigated (3). This dose is several times higher than the single dose applied in our rat experiments (5o or 1oo mg/ 1oo g b.wt.). In the mice kidneys (3) some minor flattening of tubular epithelium has been reported but in the heart diffuse necrotic areas occured. This is in contrast to our histological findings in rat kidneys although species differences and acute toxicity in our study and subacute toxicity in mice experiments have to be considered.Histological investigations of tissues other than kidneys were beyond the scope of our experimental design.
In our experiments, however, functional and morphological alterations are not always in accordance.

4.2. Correlations between histological and functional data

A single oral dose of 1oo mg FA ME reduced GFR by about 4o %. This is not caused by systemic vascular alterations as arterial blood pressure and whole body oxygen consumption were not reduced. There is ,however, good accordance with glomerular lesions observed by microscopy.
Similar lesions, less severe and less frequent, as observed after 5o mg FA ME as well as after 6o and 1oo mg FA DE, are not reflected by corresponding functional data like GFR and plasma levels of creatinine or urea. Tubular lesions as observed after 1oo mg FA ME are not always correlated with urine composition. Only 3 from 8 rats, treated in this way, showed pronounced proteinuria. Interstitial bleedings in kidney cortex did obviously not induce hematuria which was absent in all urinary sediments investigated. Besides of reduced GFR, loss of concentration ability after water deprivation was the most prominent finding in FA ME intoxication. This defect correlates well with reduced lactate production from glucose by the inner medulla. Glycolysis in turn is assumed to be an important metabolic pathway for energy turnover in this tissue (11). On the other hand kidney inner medulla did not show any microscopic lesions even following the high dose of 1oo mg FA ME.

4.3. Final considerations

Nephrotoxicity of considerable degree was found after FA ME only. Comparable doses of fumarate provoked no toxic effects and FA DE in equivalent doses induced no functional anomalities and much less morphologic changes than FA ME. Thus, the association of fumaric acid with one ethyl group seems to be essential for nephrotoxicity. The reason for this is not clear yet. General toxicity of FA ME as shown on lymphocytes is supposed to be inhibition of DNA and protein synthesis (3). Similar investigations on cells of the kidney and other organs are, however, lacking.

5. SUMMARY

The nephrotoxic actions of high single oral doses of fumaric acid monoethylester (FA ME) have been investigated in the rat. Fifty mg of this substance produced morphologic lesions of the glomeruli without reducing GFR. Following 1oo mg, the lesions were more pronounced and GFR was diminished by about 4o %. Despite of hemorrhages in kidney cortex the urines did not contain erythrocytes. Urinary protein was augmented in single cases only. Fifty to 1oo mg FA ME induced a marked concentration defect after water deprivation. In parallel FA ME reduced lactate pro - duction from glucose by kidney inner medulla in vitro. After in vivo application, however, no morphologic lesions were found in this zone of the kidney. FA ME had no effect on oxygen consumption of kidney slices despite of proximal tubular lesions observed histologically after 1oo mg orally. Thus, 1oo mg of FA ME have distinct nephrotoxic effects in the rat.

REFERENCES

1. Bradford M.M.: A rapid and sensitive method for the quantitation of microgram quantities of protein utilizing the principle of protein dye binding. Anal.Biochem. 72,248-254,1976.
2. Dubiel W., Happle R.: Behandlungsversuch mit Fumarsäuremonoäthyl - ester bei Psoriasis vulgaris. Z.Hautkrankh. 47,545-55o,1972.
3. Hagedorn M., Kalkoff K.W., Kiefer G., Baron D., Hug J., Petres J.: Fumarsäuremonoäthylester: Wirkung auf DNA Synthese und erste tier - experimentelle Befunde. Arch.Derm.Res. 254,67-73,1975.
4. Hohenegger M., Vermes M., Esposito R., Giordano C.: Effect of some uremic toxins on oxygen consumption of rats in vivo and in vitro. Nephron 48,154-158,1988.
5. Holzer F., Hohenegger M.: Sodium and potassium adaptation in the conscious rat. Pharmacology 1o,76-81,1973.
6. Hörl W., Echsel H., Hohenegger M.: The key role of sex dependency on kidney citrate metabolism in the rat. Res.Exp.Med. 185,69-75,1985.
7. Korsatko W., Sadjak A., Gall P., Supanz S.: Entwicklung kombinierter Inulin - PAH Retardimplantationstabletten zur Bestimmung der Clearance an wachen Ratten. Die Pharmazie 43,324-327,1987.
8. Om P., Hohenegger M.: Energy metabolism in acute uremic rats. Nephron 25,249-253,198o.
9. Raab W.: Psoriasis Behandlung mit Fumarsäure und Fumarsäureestern. Z.Hautkrankh. 59,671-679,1984.
1o. Renschler D.: Die enzymatischen Methoden zur Bestimmung von Inulin. Klin.Wschr. 41,615-618,1961.
11. Ruiz-Guinazu A., Pehling G., Rumrich G., Ullrich K.J.: Glucose- und Milchsäurekonzentration an der Spitze des vasculären Gegenstrom-systems im Nierenmark. Pflügers Arch.Ges.Physiol. 274,311-317,1961.
12. Sadjak A.,Egger G., Kink E., Korsatko W.: Functional and morphological changes in the rat kidney after long term adrenaline appli - cation. Exp.Pathol. 25,27-33,1984.

For correspondence:
Prof.M.Hohenegger
Laxenburgerstrasse 39
A-11oo Wien
Austria

CYCLOSPORIN AND RENAL INJURY

R. Maiorca, F. Scolari, S. Savoldi, S. Sandrini, P. Scaini, and L. Cristinelli

Institute of Nephrology, University and Spedali Civili, Brescia, Italy

Ciclosporin (Cs) introduction as a new immunosuppressive drug has led to a significant improvement in graft and patient survival in organ transplantation (1-5) and has opened new perspectives in the treatment of autoimmune diseases and steroid-resistant nephrotic syndrome (6-8).

Despite the results initially observed in animal models (9), the use of immunosuppressive doses of the drug in man is associated with the appearance of nephrotoxicity, as Calne et al. first pointed out (10). The acute occurrence of this untoward effect is characterized by a delayed graft function or a transient dose-dependent decline in glomerular filtration rate (GFR) and by changes in tubular function (1-4). Moreover, a Cs-induced chronic nephrotoxicity, with a histological picture of arteriolar lesions and interstitial fibrosis, has been described (4, 11, 12).

PHYSIOPATHOLOGY

Cs-induced nephrotoxicity, because of its incidence and importance, has been the subject of many experimental and clinical investigations, aimed at clarifying its pathophysiological mechanism. However, the pathogenesis of renal damage has not been completely clarified yet, and results from animal experiments cannot always be extended to man. In fact, the different animal models present resistance to the nephrotoxic effect of Cs, which is species-related and appears only when elevated, supraimmunosuppressive doses of the drug are employed (13,14). Moreover, while acute nephrotoxicity seems easy to reproduce, an adequate model of Cs-induced chronic nephrotoxicity does not exist, so far. This is likely due to the incapacity of reproducing the characteristic arteriolar lesions described by Mihatsch et al. in man (15). Most experimental studies have been carried out in rats, presenting Cs pharmacokinetic profiles similar to those observed in man and an elevated glomerular filtration surface (13): this partly accounts for the need of very high doses of drug in order to obtain renal functional changes similar to those in man. These studies have led to divergent opinions on the physiopathologic mechanisms responsible for the occurrence of nephrotoxicity.

While in the first studies Cs-toxicity was considered the result of tubular toxic lesions, more recently the attention has been drawn on the Cs-induced intrarenal hemodynamic changes. A selective increase in the renal vascular resistances with marked reduction of the renal blood flow, following both acute infusion and chronic administration of Cs in rats, has been reported (13,16). Micropuncture studies have showed a reduction of glomerular plasma flow (QA), of glomerular ultrafiltration coefficient (Kf), and of single nephron glomerular filtration rate (SNGFR) (17,18). In rats treated with Cs for 7-14 days, English et al. (19) described a progressive decrease of lumen diameter in the glomerular afferent arteriole, providing an anatomic correlate of these changes. Intrarenal hemodynamic variations have been proved to induce functional damage in humans as well. In normal subjects, acute Cs infusion increased renal vascular resistances and decreased renal plasma flow and GFR. Dopamine treatment prevented this vasoconstriction (20). Heart transplant patients treated with Cs presented a significantly reduced renal perfusion index in comparison with patients on conventional therapy (4, 21). Moreover, conversion from Cs to Azathioprine (Aza) in renal transplant patients was associated with a significant reduction in renal vascular resistances (22).

Causes of this impairment of glomerular dynamics following Cs-therapy are still matter of debate. As angiotensin is known to induce renal vasoconstriction and Kf reduction, the role of the renin-angiotensin system (RAS) has been extensively investigated. In laboratory animals, Cs was found to stimulate RAS, both in vitro and in vivo (23, 24). However, a clearcut relationship between RAS activation and renal vasoconstriction has not been demonstrated. Renal denervation and pharmacological blockade with alfa-adrenergic antagonists were found to determine a protective effect on Cs-treated rats (16), suggesting a renal sympathetic nervous system-mediated vasoconstriction. In an experimental model Captopril minimized the renal effects of Cs (17). On the other hand, pretreatment of animals with angiotensin I-converting enzyme inhibitor did not prevent the fall in RBF (16). In humans, as documented both in renal and in heart transplant patients (21, 25), Cs seems to induce RAS suppression. Myers et al. recently hypothesized a partial block in the intrarenal conversion of the prohormone to active renin (21).

Changes in the synthesis of prostaglandins (PGs), hormonal system also involved in the maintenance of intrarenal circulatory homeostasis, are regarded as contradictory. Some Authors report a suppression of the PGs intrarenal synthesis either directly (26) or by inhibition of prostacyclin synthesis factor (PSF)(27). Murray et al. , instead, point out an increase in urinary 6-keto-PGF1- excretion after acute and chronic Cs administration, and an exacerbation of the vasoconstrictor effects of the drug, following cyclo-oxigenase inhibitors (16). An increase in urinary levels of TxB2 has been recently documented in Cs-treated rats (28), suggesting an imbalance in vasoconstrictor and vasodilatory PGs production to account for changes in glomerular hemodynamics. The pathogenetic role of renal PGs seems to be supported by the protective effect exerted by misoprostol, a PGE1 analog, on intrarenal hemodynamic changes (29). Data reported in humans are equally conflicting and inconclusive. Inhibition of PGs synthesis (30) and increase in TxA2/PGI2 ratio (31) were reported in renal transplant patients. An imbalance in PGs synthesis could account for not only hemodynamic changes but also the finding of glomerular capillary thrombosis; this histological picture, recalling thrombotic microangiopathy, has been described both in rabbit and in man treated with Cs. However, no change in the renal production of PGs and TxA2 (32) was found after conversion from Cs to Aza, even though a significant improvement of RBF was present.

Finally, in sensitized lymphocytes, Cs is known to bind to Calmodulin, an intracellular calcium binding protein (33). This binding could induce a change in the intracellular distribution of calcium, determining a contraction in vasal smooth muscular cells. A possible role of this mechanism is suggested by the protective action of calcium channel blockers on intrarenal, Cs-induced, hemodynamic changes. The protective role of these drugs is particulary valuable in preventing the acute renal failure resulting from the combination of Cs toxicity and ischemic damage.

The prevailing role of hemodynamic changes, however, cannot rule out the involvement of Cs-induced tubular lesions in the pathogenesis of functional impairment. Several studies have documented cellular vacuolization, due to dilation of endoplasmic reticulum, and inclusion bodies, corresponding to autolysosomes and giant mitochondria (14,15). In particular, in rats treated with high doses of Cs, Whiting et al. (14) observed the appearance of tubular damage associated with enzymuria and reduced renal function. According to the authors, the impaired reabsorption of the proximal tubule and the increased distal sodium delivery might induce, through the RAS stimulation, an activation of the tubulo-glomerular feedback mechanism, resulting in decreased GFR. However, in the experimental studies GFR reduction was found to be associated with an increase in the fractionary sodium reabsorption (35) and was not found to be associated with significant changes in tubular function (15, 19). Tubular toxicity, on the contrary, correlates with the highest doses of the drug (15). From these studies, renal vasculature results to be the major target of Cs, which is able to induce a mared intrarenal vasoconstriction.

CLINICAL PICTURE

Three main clinical syndromes are commonly attributed to the use of Cs:

- acute nephrotoxicity,
- delayed allograft function,
- chronic nephrotoxicity.

ACUTE NEPHROTOXICITY

It is defined by the occurrence of decreased GFR, which is reversible after a reduction in CS dose. In renal transplant patients, acute nephrotoxicity is the major cause of graft impairment. In the first clinical trials, in which high doses of Cs were used, a high incidence of acute nephrotoxicity, in the range of 70-80% (35,37), was observed; moreover, nephrotoxicity resulted untreatable in a significant number of patients, who has to be shifted to conventional therapy (35, 38, 39). More flexible therapeutic protocils, guided by monitoring of circulating levels, allowed a reduction in frequency and severity of this untoward effect, and it is more recently reported in 26-35% of the renal transplant patients (40,41). In our experience, 103 consecutive renal transplant patients were treated with CS and low dose steroids. Cs dosage was adjusted in order to maintain blood trough levels of 200-500 ng/ml. Actuarial cumulative incidence of acute nephrotoxicity, referred to as 25% incrase in serum creatinine levels, was of 21, 23, 26% at 6, 12, 24 months respectively.

Cs acute nephrotoxicity is not confined to renal transplantation alone. In heart transplant patients, who have healthy native kidneys, a significant reduction of the glomerular filtration rate and an increased incidence of acute renal filure (4) was observed after introduction of Cs therapy. Similar findings were reported in liver transplantation (5). In bone marrow transplant patients, CS treatment significantly enhanced the incidence of renal impairment following the use, frequent in these patients, of nephrotoxic drugs (42). Finally, transient and reversible worsening in renal function has been documented in 60% of patients treated with CS because of autoimmune disease (7).

A major risk of acute nephrotoxicity may result from maintenance of high circulating drug levels (40,43-45). Significantly higher Cs blood levels are seen when renal impairment is due to acute nephrotoxicity rather than to rejection (46). In heart transplant patients, Meyers et al. observed a significant reduction in glomerular filtration rate (4); however, as Kahan et al. outline, plasma Cs levels were steadily maintained within a toxic range of 300-350 ng/ml (47).

In a preliminary study on 33 renal transplant patients we observed a significant correlation between Cs blood levels and acute nephrotoxicity episodes, occurring only when whole blood trough levels exceeded 500 ng/ml (48). We examined the occurrence of 27 episodes of acute nephrotoxicity detected in 25 patients in 103 consecutive renal transplants. Cs blood levels were 905±393ng/ml at diagnosis and 357±112 ng/ml after recovery ($p<.001$), obtained through a marked reduction of the drug dosage (from 9.3±4.1 to 5.7±3.5 mg/kg; $p<.001$).

Relationship between circulating Cs levels and acute nephrotoxicity is due to individual variability in drug absorption, metabolism and clearance. The role of different Cs pharmacokinetic profiles in determining clinical complications has been confirmed by pre-transplant studies in which a lower Cs clearance in patients who subsequently developed nephrotoxicity (49) was documented. Besides, the use of drugs competing with Cs liver metabolism, such as ketoconazole and erythromycin, determines high circulating Cs levels, enhancing the risk of acute nephrotoxicity (50, 51). The reduction of drug clearance observed in hepatic dysfunction represents a similar condition (52).

Some Authors have not confirmed the relationship between Cs circulating levels and acute nephrotoxicity (53, 54). Namely, levels that are toxic in some patients may be well tolerated by others (55) and, on the other hand, acute nephrotoxicity may ensue despite circulating levels thought to be in the therapeutic range (56). These data suggest individual susceptibility to the toxic effect of Cs. Furthermore, renal tissue may be sensitized to Cs toxicity by additional lesions (acute tubular necrosis - ATN, and/or rejection) or by administration of drugs causing synergistic nephrotoxicity (aminoglycosides, amphotericin B, methotrexate, sulfonamides, vancomycin, non-steroidal antiinflammatory drugs) (57, 58).

In renal transplantation, problems of differential diagnosis between nephrotoxicity and acute rejection may arise. No clinical, biochemical, immunologic or histopathologic criteria enable us to establish this diagnosis with certainty. Therefore, diagnosis of acute nephrotoxicity is one of exclusion, and subsequent to the improvement of renal function after reduction of Cs dose. Several clinical parameters can be of help in making the correct diagnosis. Acute rejection is suggested by a rapid decline of renal function, associated with a decreased urine output, increased body weight, and appearance of fever (59, 60). Moreover, acute nephrotoxicity may occur at any time during follow-up, whilst the incidence of acute rejection is much higher in early post-transplant period (59). As already reported, monitoring of circulating Cs levels is considered helpful by most Authors: high levels significantly correlate with acute nephrotoxicity episodes rather than with acute rejection (47, 58-60). Hayry and von Willebrand (61) introduced fine needle aspiration biopsy to detect interstitial mononuclear infiltrate or morphological changes in tubular cells induced by either immunological events or Cs toxicity. Besides, the use of indirect immunofluorescence and immunoperoxidase techniques allowed the Authors to demonstrate Cs deposits in tubular cells in the course of acute clinical nephrotoxicity (62). In our series we confirmed the fine needle technique to be of help, although it is affected by false positive and false negative findings (63); on the contrary, we could not find any relationship between Cs deposits, revealed by immunoperoxidase, and clinical episodes of nephrotoxicity, casting doubts on the clinical value of these findings (64).

Renal biopsy, therefore, represents the most reliable diagnostic tool (65, 66). As morphological patterns of acute rejection have not been changed by Cs (67), the finding of arteritis, glomerulitis, diffuse interstitial infiltrate and interstitial edema provides a highly reliable diagnosis of acute rejection. The finding of tubular lesions characterized by inclusion bodies and isometric vacuolization of epithelial tubular cells and microcalcifications is a more tipical though unspecific expression of Cs toxicity (12, 57). Peritubular capillary congestion, in addition to signs of toxic tubulopathy, has been described by Mihatsch et al. (12, 57). It must be stressed that clinical acute nephrotoxicity may be accompanied by a morphological picture of substantial normality (57).

DELAYED ALLOGRAFT FUNCTION

The onset of acute renal failure (ARF), sustained by a histolological picture of acute tubular necrosis (ATN), is rather frequent in the immediate post-operative course of renal transplantation (1, 36, 54) and can account for a worsening long term graft prognosis (41). Recovery from oligoanuria can be delayed by Cs and also by the coadministration of nephrotoxic drugs or contrast media and by a superimposed, misdiagnosed acute rejection. Moreover, the presence of ATN sensitizes renal tissue to Cs toxicity which may occur even whithout high circulating levels of drug and may thereby be underestimated (57). Post-transplant ATN may consequently result in a complex picture of interactive nephrotoxicity.

Many factors, leading to ischemic damage, contribute to the genesis of post-transplant ATN: donor hypotension, warm and cold ischemia, perfusion modatilities, anastomosis time and recipient hypovolemia. In experimental models ARF can be induced by combined ischemic damage and toxic effect of Cs (68). In renal transplantation, particularly from cadaveric donor, Cs use could therefore make the onset of ATN more likely or delay its recovery. In the early phase of the Multicentre European trial, Cs was not employed in presence of post-transplant oligoanuria, to avoid combining ishemic and toxic damages (69). This approach has now been set aside by all tranplant centers. In the Canadian Multicenter trial, ATN incidence was found to be higher, though not statistically different, in patients treated with Cs (52%) than in those treated with conventional therapy (39%)(1). Najarian et al. observed post-transplant ATN in 31% of patients treated with Cs and in 30% of those treated with Aza(36). However, Cs treated patients experienced a significantly more prolonged oligoanuria (15.8±18 vs 7.4±3 days; $p<.02$). A high incidence of post-transplant ATN (72% on CS, 68% on Aza), probably due to the long exposure of kidneys to warm and cold ischemia was recently reported by Australian Authors (54). Recovery from ARF required much more time in Cs-treated patients (25.5 vs 11.2 days; $p=.007$). Moreover, 25% of Cs-treated patients with post-transplant ATN improved their renal function only after shifting to conventional therapy; one patient recovered renal function 82 days after transplantation. These data support the role of Cs in potentiating ischemic damage; this is also confirmed by the increased incidence of ARF requiring dialysis observed in heart transplantation after Cs introduction (70). A histologic picture of diffuse interstitial fibrosis was described in patients with renal transplant and prolonged oligoanuria (67) and in patients with heart transplant and protracted ARF (71). The deleterious Cs effect in prolonging oligoanuria is likely to be mediated not only by the direct tubular toxicity, but also by Cs ability to increase renal vascular resistances when ARF recovery is associated with progressive increase in RBF.

We could not observe any difference in the incidence of post-transplant ATN between 59 Cs-treated patients (34%) and 99 Aza-treated patients (43%; historical control). Moreover, no difference was observed in the duration of oligoanuria (10.7± 8.4 in Aza-group; 10.6± 5.1 in Cs-treated patients). Our present policy, regarding the last 31 .patients, of inducing volume expansion of the recipients in the preoperatory phase, and of infusing, pre- and post-operatively, dopamine or calcium channel blockers associated with the careful monitoring of circulating Cs levels, has allowed us to significantly reduce the incidence of post-transplant ATN to16%.

CHRONIC NEPHROTOXICITY

While acute nephrotoxicity is a well defined clinical and physiopathological picture, characters and modalities related to the onset of Cs-induced chronic renal damage are still matter of controversy. Assessment of Cs role in inducing chronic renal damage has been delayed by the fact that most studies have been carried out in renal transplant patients, in whom it was difficult to exclude the concomitant existence of chronic rejection; moreover, the lack of an adequate animal model of chronic nephrotoxicity made every pathogenetic hypothesis merely speculative. A substantial contribution to the knowledge of chronic Cs-induced lesions has been provided by studies performed in patients with healthy native kidneys and heart transplant or autoimmune disease (21, 72, 73). In renal transplant, since the beginning, numerous clinical trials have documented that Cs use, despite a reduced incidence and severity of rejection, was associated with a significant and persistent increase in serum creatinine levels, attributing to Cs a direct role in the genesis of the renal functional impairment (1, 2, 36). Curtis et al. recently documented that renal vasoconstriction is reversible if Cs is withdrawn 8 months after starting therapy (22). Moreover, an improvement in renal function occurs when the drug is withdrawn within 6-12 months after the introduction of Cs-therapy, suggesting hemodynamic factors to account for Cs-induced reduction of glomerular filtration rate (74, 75). After a longer term of therapy, however, Cs may determine an irreversible chronic nephropathy. Myers et al. supported this hypothesis after observing in Cs-treated heart transplant patients the occurrence of progressive chronic nephropathy, clinically characterized by proteinuria and hypertension (21). The renal biopsy performed in 12 patients revealed arteriolar hyalinosis and a more typical picture of obliterative arteriolopathy presenting deposits of proteinaceous material in the necrotic arteriolar wall, similar to that described by Mihatsch et al. (57). In the areas proximal to the arteriolar lesions, a variable degree of interstitial fibrosis and tubular atrophy, mainly in a striped form, was detectable. Some glomeruli showed moderate ischemic and/or sclerotic lesions. Six control biopsies, carried out 6-24 months later, documented the progression of arteriolar hyalinosis and the worsening of the obliterative arteriolar lesion or its ex novo appearance. Five out of 73 patients experienced progression towards end-stage renal failure. Myers et al. (21) hypothesized long term Cs administration, for over 12 months of therapy, to determine, as a result of prolonged vasoconstriction, a progressive damage in renal microcirculation, with subsequent tubulointerstitial ischemic damage.

In renal transplant patients, long term Cs administration does not seem to induce such severe and progressive functional and morphological changes. Several Authors observed that renal function, though significantly reduced compared to that found in Aza-treated patients, was substantially stable after 24-36 months of follow-up (1, 3, 39, 76). Arteriolar and tubulointerstitial lesions have been detected by several histological evaluations. Thiru et al. (77) first documented interstitial fibrosis and tubular atrophy in a more severe degree in Cs-treated patients than in those on conventional therapy. Klintmalm et al. detected a variable degree of interstitial fibrosis in 96% of patients on Cs and in 77% of patients on Aza(11). The appearance and the degree of the lesion positively correlated with the cumulative drug dose during the first 6 months, and with the number of acute toxic episodes, suggesting that Cs contributes to the lesion. A clear progression of interstitial fibrosis was documented in only 3 out of 17 patients who underwent a control biopsy after 12 months. According to the Authors, in lack of severe vascular lesions, a chronic interstitial nephritis could account for the renal damage.

In association with striped interstitial fibrosis, Mihatsch et al. (57) described a Cs-associated arteriolopathy. This lesion is prevalent in arterioles and rarely extends to tha vascular pole of the glomerulus or to the glomerular tuft. The light microscopy picture is not specific: it is possible to detect severe arteriolar hyalinosis, arteriolar necrosis or intimal mucoid thickening, similar to the finding observed in the uremic hemolytic syndrome. Electron microscopy revealed protein deposits in the vascular wall and necrosis of the myocytes. In advanced phases the lesion may not be distinguished from hypertensive or diabetic arteriolopathy. A pathogenetic relationship between Cs-associated arteriolopathy and interstitial fibrosis was suggested by the significant correlation observed between severity of arteriolopathy and extension of interstitial fibrosis. The vascular lesion was detected in patients with the highest circulating levels in the first three months. Pathogenesis of Cs-associated arteriolopathy is unknown, but a mechanism similar to that operating in thrombotic microangiopathy is suggested. Sommer et al. recently provided support to this pathogenetic hypothesis (78). Arteriolopathy of the arcuate interlobular vessels, with intimal proliferation and thrombotic occlusion developed in 7.5% of 200 renal transplant patients treated with Cs. Some patients exhibited thrombocytopenia and microangiopathic hemolytic anemia, suggestive of a hemolytic uremic syndrome. In Authors' opinion Cs induces an alteration in the platelets-endothelium interaction, by inhibition of prostacyclin stimulating factor, as documented in rabbits treated with high doses of drug (79-81).

We evaluated the incidence of interstitial fibrosis and arteriolar hyalinosis in renal biopsies obtained 6 and 18 months after transplantation in 32 renal transplant recipients treated with low dose steroids and Cs (82). Cs dosage was established in order to achieve blood trough levels of 200-500 ng/ml. Interstitial fibrosis was present in 63% and 87% at 6 and 18 months respectively. Only two patients showed a severe degree of lesion at 18th month. Interstitial fibrosis was not found to be related to Cs cumulative dose or circulating levels. At 6th month, it was significantly correlated with the number of acute nephrotoxicity episodes, but the finding was not confirmed at 18 months. A mild degree of arteriolar hyalinosis was detected in 15% of patients at 6 months; at 18 months the lesion was present in 43% of patients in a mild or moderate degree. No relationship was found between arteriolar hyalinosis and number of acute nephrotoxicity and rejection episodes, Cs cumulative dose and circulating levels, ATN, warm and cold ischemia, hypertension, donor age; however, arteriolar hyalinosis frequently accompanied hypertension, post-transplant ATN and donor's older age. Finally, arteriolar hyalinosis was not related to the finding of interstitial fibrosis. No worsening of renal function was observed after a 24 month follow-up; mean serum creatinine was 1.35 ±.5 mg/dl at 6th month and 1.5±.5 mg/dl at 24th month. These data seem to confirm that with Cs, after 18 months of therapy, a certain degree of interstitial fibrosis is inevitable in most renal transplant patients. However, the lesion probably results from multiple factors. It seems that other pathogenetic factors are to be invoked in the appearance of arteriolar hyalinosis as well, as a causative role of the drug has not been proved. The adoption of a protocol apt to obtain blood levels within a therapeutic range, like that employed in our Centre, is likely to reduce the severity of the lesions related to chronic nephrotoxicity.

In renal transplantation, chronic damage induced by Cs is more moderate than in heart transplantation (21). The heavy incidence and severity of chronic nephrotoxicity observed in heart transplant patients may result from the use of elevated drug doses and from the maintainance of circulating Cs levels within a persistently toxic range, in the first post-transplant period. A predisposing role in determining renal damage may be played by chronic pre-transplant renal hypoperfusion (83). On the other hand, in renal transplantation, an underestimated chronic Cs toxic damage might be responsible for part of the late graft failure, generally attributed to chronic rejection.

Chronic tubulointerstitial lesions have recently been described in patients affected by autoimmune disease, treated with Cs. Palestine et al. (72) documented interstitial fibrosis and tubular atrophy in 17 patients treated by Cs for two years because of uveitis. These lesions were detectable even in patients presenting normal renal function at biopsy. Similar tubulointerstitial lesions, associated with arteriolar hyalinosis, have been confirmed by Svenson et al. (73) in a small group of patients treated with Cs, for various autoimmune diseases. In both these studies Cs was employed in doses ranging from 10 to 15 mg/kg. The evidence of histologic lesions due to chronic nephrotoxicity in patients with autoimmune disease supports the pathogenetic role of Cs. Since concomitant factors such as ischemic damage, acute or chronic rejection, hypoperfusion and use of nephrotoxic drugs are missing, the changes detectable in these patients can only be ascribed to Cs.

CONCLUSIONS

Animal models of Cs nephrotoxicity suggest that Cs impairment in renal function is consistent more with an ischemic glomerular process than with a direct toxic tubular effect of the drug; transition from acute hemodynamic changes to a chronic, progressive renal injury has not been documented in animals. In man, where Cs induces the same hemodynamic changes observed in the laboratory animals, chronic tubulointerstitial damage is probably a consequence of the Cs-associated arteriolopathy, a lesion not yet reproduced in experimental models.

The clinical use of Cs involves a balance between toxicity and efficacy. Nephrotoxicity can be reduced, but not avoided, by low Cs -dose and careful monitoring of circulating levels. In the organ transplantation field Cs administration is justified by the significant improvement obtained in patient and graft survivals. In autoimmunity Cs treatment should be reserved to life-threatening diseases, when conventional immunosuppression has failed.

REFERENCES

1. The Canadian Multicentre Transplant Study Group, A randomized clinical trial of Cyclosporin in cadaveric renal transplantation, N. Engl. J. Med. 309:809 (1983).
2. European Multicentre Trial Group, Cyclosporin in cadaveric renal transplantation: one year follow-up of a multicentre trial, Lancet 29:986 (1983).
3. R. M. Merion, D. J. G.White, S. Thiru, D. B.Evans, R. Y. Calne, Cyclosporine: five years experience in cadaveric renal transplantation, N. Engl. J. Med. 310:148 (1984).
4. B. D. Myers, J. Ross, L. Newtov, J. Luetscher, M. Perlroth, Cyclosporine-associated chronic nephropathy, N. Engl. J. Med. 311:699 (1983).
5. S. Iwatsuki, C. O. Esquivel, G. B. G. Klintmalm, R. D. Gordon, B. W. Shaw, T. E. Starzl, Nephrotoxicity of Cyclosporine in liver transplantation, Transplant. Proc. 17, 4 (Suppl.1):191 (1985).
6. A. Van Rijthoven, B. Dijkmans, H. S. Goei The, J. Hermans, Z. Montnor-Beckers, P. Jacobs, Cyclosporin treatment for rheumatoid arthritis: a placebo controlled, double blind, multicentre study, Ann. Rheumatic Diseases 45:726 (1986).
7. A. G. Palestine, R. B. Nussenblatt, C-C. Chan, Side effects of systemic Cyclosporine in patients not undergoing transplantation, Am. J. Med. 77:652 (1984).
8. A. Tejani, K. Butt, H. Trachtman, M. Suthanthiran, C. J. Rosenthal, R. Khawar, Cyclosporine A induced remission of relapsing nephrotic syndrome in children, Kidney International. 33:729 (1988).
9. A. W. Thomson, P. H. Whiting, I. D. Cameron, S. E. Lessels, J. G. Simpson, A toxicological study in rats receiving immunotherapeutic doses of Cyclosporin, Transplantation. 31:121 (1981).

10. R. Y. Calne, K. Rolles, S. Thiru, P. Mc Master, G. N. Craddock, Cyclosporin A initilly as the only immunosuppressant in 34 recipients of cadaveric organs: 32 kidneys, 2 pancreas and 2 livers, Lancet. 2:1033 (1979).
11. G. Klintmalm, S. O. Bohman, B. Sundelin, H. Wilczek, Interstitial fibrosis in renal allografts after 12 to 46 months of Cyclosporin treatment: beneficial effect of low doses in early post-transplantation period, Lancet. 27:950 (1984).
12. M. J. Mihatsch, G. Thiel, H. P. Spichtin, M. Oberholzer, F. P. Brunner, F. Harder, V. Olivieri, R. Bremer, B. Ryffel, E. Stocklin, J. Torhorst, F. Gudat, H. U. Zollinger, R. Loertscher, Morphological findings in kidney transplants after treatment with Cyclosporine, Transplant. Proc. 15, 4 (suppl.1):2821 (1983).
13. B. A. Sullivan, L. J. Hak, W. F. Finn, Cyclosporine nephrotoxicity: studies in laboratory animals, Transplant. Proc. 17,4 (suppl.1):145 (1985).
14. P. H. Whiting, A. W. Thomson, J. T. Blair, J. G. Simpson, Experimental Cyclosporin A nephrotoxicity, Br. J. Exp. Path. 63:88 (1982).
15. M. J. Mihatsch, B. Ryffel, M. Hermle, F. P. Brunner, G. Thiel, Morphology of Cyclosporine nephrotoxicity in the rat, Clin. Neph. 25 (suppl.1):2 (1986).
16. B. M. Murray, M. S. Paller, T. F. Ferris, Effect of Cyclosporine administration on renal hemodynamics in conscious rats, Kidney Int. 28:767 (1985).
17. E. J. G. Barros, M. A. Boim, H. Ajzen, O. L. Ramos, N. Schor, Glomerular Hemodynamics and hormonal participation on Cyclosporine nephrotoxicity, Kidney Inter. 32:19 (1987).
18. M. Sabbatini, C. Esposito, F. Uccello, A. Dal Canton, V. Andreucci, Effects of Cyclosporine on glomerular dynamics: micropuncture study in the rat, in Abstrats of The Second International Congress on Cyclosporine. Washington 1987:117 (1987).
19. J. English, A. Evan, C. D. Houghton, W. M. Bennett, Cyclosporine-induced acute renal disfunction in the rat, Transplantation. 44,1:135 (1987).
20. G. Conte, P. Napodano, L. De Nicola, G. Gigliotti, C. Libetta, P. Imperatore, A. Testa, V. Sepe, A. Dal Canton, V. Andreucci, Dopamine counteracts the acute renal effects of Cyclosporine in normal subjects in Abstracts of The Second International Congress on Cyclosporine. Washington 1987:121 (1987).
21. B. D. Myers, R. Sybley, L. Newton, S. J. Tomlanovich, C. Boshkos, E. Stinson, J. A. Luetscher, D. J. Whitney, D. Krasny, N. S. Coplon, M. G. Perlroth, The long-term course of Cyclosporine-associated chronic nephropathy, Kidney Int. 33:590 (1988).
22. Curtis J. J., Luke R. G., Dubovsky E., Diethelm A. G., Whelchel G. D., Jones P.: Cyclosporin in therapeutic doses increases renal allograft vascular resistance. Lancet 1986, 30:477
23. C. R. Baxter, G. C. Duggin, B. M. Hall, J. S. Horvath, D. J. Tiller, Stimulation of renin release from rat renal cortical slices by Cyclosporin A, Res. Commun. Chem. Pathol. Pharmacol. 43, 3:417 (1984).
24. N. Perico, A. Benigni, E. Bosco, M. Rossini, S. Orisio, F. Ghilardi, A. Piccinelli, G.Remuzzi, Acute Cyclosporine A Nephrotoxicity in rats: which role for renin-angiotensin system and glomerular prostaglandins?, Clin. Nephrol. 25 (suppl.1):83 (1986).
25. J. P. Bantle, K. A. Nath, D. E. Sutherland, J. S. Najarian, T. F. Ferris, Effects of Cyclosporine on the renin angiotensin aldosterone system and potassium excretion in renal transplant recipients, Arch. Int. Med. 145:505 (1985).
26. T. P. Fan, G. P. Lewis, Mechanism of Cyclosporine A-induced inhibition of prostacyclin synthesis by macrophases, Prostaglandins. 30: 735 (1985).
27. G. Neild, G. Rocchi, L. Imberti, Z. Brown, G. Remuzzi, D. G. Williams, Effect of Cyclosporine on prostacyclin synthesis by vascular tissue in rabbits, Transplant. Proc. 15 (suppl.1):2398 (1983).
28. A. Kawaguchi, M. N. Goldman, R. Shapiro, M. L. Foegh, P. W. Ramwell, R. R. Lower,

Increase in urinary thromboxane B2 in rats caused by Cyclosporine, Transplantation. 40:214 (1985).
29. M. S. Paller, Effects of the prostaglandin E1 analog misoprostol on Cyclosporine nephrotoxicity, in Abstracts of The Second International Congress on Cyclosporine. Washington 1987:32 (1987).
30. D. Adu, C. J. Lote, J. Michael, J. H. Turney, P. McMaster, Does Cyclosporine inhibit renal prostaglandin synthesis?, Proc. EDTA-ERA. 21:969 (1984).
31. T. Kho, K. Leunissen, J. Van Hooff, Cyclosporine and urinary prostaglandins, in Abstracts of The Second Internatinal Congrss on Cyclosporine. Washington 1987:36 (1987).
32. D. Jorkasky, P. Audet, S. Williams, R. Grossman, M. Conrad, Cyclosporine-induced nephrotixicity: role of prostaglandins, Transplant. Proc. 19, 1:1742 (1987).
33. P. M. Colombani, A. Robb, A. D. Hess, Cyclosporine A binding to calmodulin: a possible site of action on T lymphocytes, Science. 228:337 (1985).
34. K. A. Duggan, G. J. Macdonald, J. A. Charlesworth, B. A. Pussel, Verapamil prevents post transplant oliguric renal failure, Clin. Nephrol. 24, 6:289 (1985).
35. H. Dieperink, H. Starklint, P.P. Leyssac, Nephrotoxicity of Cyclosporine-an animal model: study of the Nephrotoxic effect of Cyclosporine on overal renal and tubular function in conscious rats, Transplant. Proc. 15 (suppl.1):520 (1983).
36. J. S. Najarian, D. S. Fryd, M. Strand, D. Canafax, N. L. Ascher, W. D. Payne, R. L. Simmons, D. E. R. Sutherland, A single institution, randomized, prospective trial of Cyclosporine versus Azathioprine-Antilymphocyte globulin for immunosuppression in renal allograft recipients, Ann. Surgery. 201,2:142 (1985).
37. B. D. Kahan Meeting report: the first international congress on Cyclosporine: Houston, Texas. Dial. Transplant. 12:620 (1983).
38. S. M. Flechner, C. T. Van Buren, R. Kerman, B. D. Kahan, The effect of conversion from Cyclosporine to Azathioprine immunosuppression for intractable nephrotoxicity, Transplant. Proc. 15 (suppl.1):653 (1983).
39. G. Thil, M. Mihatsch, J. Landmann, M. Hermle, F. P. Brunner, F. Harder, Is Cyclosporine A-induced nephrotoxicity in recipients of renal allografts progressive?, Transplant. Proc. 17,4 (suppl.1):169 (1985).
40. E. Irschik, H. Tilg, D. Niederwieser, G. Gastl, C. Huber, R. Margreiter, Cyclosporin blood levels do correlate with clinical complications, Lancet. September 22:692 (1984).
41. R. Pichlmayr, K. Wonigeit, B. Ringe, T. Block, R. Raab, B. Heigel, P. Neuhaus, Rejection and nephrotoxicity . Diagnostic problems with Cyclosporine in renal transplantation, Proc. EDTA-ERA, 21:947 (1984).
42. G. C. Yee, M. S. Kennedy, H. J. Deeg, T. M. Leonard, E. D. Thomas, R. Storb, Cyclosporine-associated renal dysfunction in marrow transplant recipients, Transplant. Proc. 17, 4 (suppl.1): 196 (1985).
43. G. Klintmalm, J. Sawe, O. Ringden, C. von Bahr, A. Magnusson, Cyclosporine plasma levels in renal transplant patients, Transplantation. 39, 2:132 (1985).
44. S. Drakopoulos, D. J. G. White, R. M. Merrion, S. Winter, R. Y. Calne, An assesment of the clinical value of monitoring Cyclosporine plasma levels, Transplant. Proc. 17:1258 (1985).
45. P. A. Keown, C. R. Stiller, A. C. Wallace, F. N. McKenzie, W. Wall, Cyclosporine nephrotoxicity: exploration of the risk factors and prognosis of the renal injury, Transplant. Proc. 17, 4 (suppl.1):247 (1985).
46. D. W. Holt, J. T. Marsden, A. Johnston, M. Bewick, D. H. Taube, Blood Cyclosporin concentrations and renal allograft dysfunction, Br. Med. J. 293:1057 (1986).
47. B. D. Kahan, C. T. Van Buren, C. A. Wideman, D. A. Cooley, O. H. Frazier, Nephrotoxicity of Cyclosporine, N. Engl. J. Med. 312, 1:48 (1985).
48. R. Maiorca, L. Cristinelli, F. Scolari, S. Sandrini, S. Savoldi, G. Brunori, E. Prati, L. Lojacono, D. Salerni, G. Tonini, Cyclosporine toxicity can be minimized by careful

monitoring of blood levels, Transplant. Proc. 17 (suppl.2):54 (1985).

49. S. Savoldi, B. D. Kahan, Relationship of Cyclosporine pharmacokinetic parameters to clinical events in human renal transplantation, Transplant. Proc. 18 (suppl.5):120 (1986).

50. C. W. B. Jensen, S. M. Flechner, C. T. Van Buren, O. H. Frazier, D. A. Cooley , M. I. Lorber, B. D. Kahan, Exacerbation of Cyclosporine toxicity by concomitant administration of erythromycin, Transplantation. 43:263 (1987).

51. R. M. Ferguson, D. E. R. Sutherland, R. L. Simmons, G. S. Najarian, Ketoconazole, Cyclosporin metabolism and renal transplantation, Lancet. 2: 882 (1982).

52. G. C. Yee, M. S. Kennedy, R. Storb, E. D. Thomas, Effect of hepatic dysfunction on oral Cyclosporine pharmacokinetics in marrow transplant patients, Blood. 64:1377 (1984).

53. L. D. Bowers, D. M. Canafax, J. Singh, R. Seifedlin, R. L. Simmons, J. S. Najarian, Studies of Cyclosporine blood levels: analysis, clinical utility, pharmacokinetics, metabolites, and chronopharmacology, Transplant. Proc. 18,(suppl.5):137 (1986).

54. B. M. Hall, D. J. Tiller, G. G. Duggin, J. S. Horvath, A. Farnsworth, J. May, J. R. Johnson, A. G. R. Sheil, Post-transplant acute renal failure in cadaver renal recipients treated with Cyclosporine, Kidney Int. 28: 178 (1985).

55. K. Wonigheit, P. F. Hoyer, G. Schumann, B. Ringe, A. Frei, R. Picklmayr, Experiences with a blood level-adjusted Cyclosporine regimen in kidney and liver allograft recipients, Trasplant. Proc. 18 (suppl.5):181 (1986).

56. B. D. Kahan, Individualization of Cyclosporine therapy using pharmacokinetic and pharmacodynamic parameters, Transplantation. 40,5:457 (1985).

57. M. J. Mihatsch, G. Thiel, V. Basler, B. Ryffel, J. Landman, J. von Overbeck, H. U. Zollinger, Morphological patterns in Cyclosporine-treated renal transplant recipients, Transplant. Proc., 17,4 (suppl.1):101 (1985).

58. B. D. Kahan, Clinical summation. An algorithm for the management of patients with Cyclosporine-induced renal dysfunction, Transplant. Proc. 17,4 (suppl.1):303 (1985).

59. G. Klintmalm, O. Ringden, C. G. Groth, Clinical and laboratory signs in nephrotoxicity and rejection in Cyclosporine-treated renal allograft recipients, Transplant. Proc. 15, 4 (suppl.1):2815 (1983).

60. D. Taube, G. Neild, P. Hobby, D. Holt, K. Welsh, J. S. Cameron, A comparison of the clinical, histopathologic, cytologic, and biochemical features of renal transplant rejection, Cyclosporine A nephrotoxicity, and stable renal function, Transplant. Proc., 17, 4 (suppl.1):179 (1985).

61. P. Hayry, E. von Willebrand, Transplant aspiration cytology, Transplantation. 38:7 (1984).

62. E. von Willebrand, P. Hayry, Cyclosporin-A deposits in renal allografts, Lancet. 2:189 (1983).

63. P. Scaini, S. Savoldi, M. Favret, E. Prati, A. Manganoni, G. Setti, L. Cristinelli, F. Scolari, R. Maiorca, E' evitabile la nefrotossicità acuta da Ciclosporina, Nefrologia, Dialisi, Trapianto, Wichtig Editore, Milano, Italy:272 (1984).

64. P. Scaini, R. Tardanico, M. Favret, F. Scolari, S Savoldi, G. C. Cancarini, E. Prati, S. Sandrini, G. Brunori, L. Cristinelli, Are Cyclosporin A deposits in renal allografts of clinical significance?, Proc. EDTA-ERA, 22:546 (1985).

65. R. K. Sibley, J. Rynasiewicz, R. M. Ferguson, D. Fryd, D. E. R. Sutherland, R. L. Simmons, J. S. Najarian, Morphology of Cyclosporine nephrotoxicity and acute rejection in patients immunosuppressed with Cyclosporine and prednisone, Surgery. 94:225 (1983).

66. G. H. Neild, D. H. Taube, R. B. Hatley, L. Bignardi, J. S. Cameron, D. G. Williams, C. S. Ogg, C. J. Rudge, Morphological differentiation between rejection and Cyclosporin nephrotoxicity in renal allografts, J. Clin. Pathol. 39: 152 (1986).

67. A. Farnsworth, B. M. Hall, A. B. P. Ng, G. G. Duggin, J. S. Horvath, A. G. R. Sheil, D.

J. Tiller, Renal biopsy morphology in renal transplantation, Am. J. Surg. Pathol. 8: 243 (1984).

68. B. C. Konf, L.C. Racuse, A. Whelton, K. Solez, Acute renal failure produced by combining Cyclosporine and brief renal ischemia in the Munich Wistar rat., Clin. Nephrol. 25(suppl.1):171 (1986).
69. European multicentre trial, Cyclosporin A as sole immunosuppressive agent in recipients of kidney allografts from cadaver donors, Lancet. 2:57 (1982).
70. S. Schuler, D. Thomas, R. Hetzer, Cyclosporine A-related nephrotoxicity after cardiac transplantation: the role of plasma renin activuty, Transplant. Proc. 19:3998 (1987).
71. B. D. Myers, Cyclosporine nephrotoxicity, Kidney Int. 30:964 (1986).
72. A. G. Palestine, H. A. Austin III, J. E. Balow, T. T. Antonovych, S. G. Sabnis, H. G. Preuss, R. B. Nussenblatt, Renal histopathologic alterations in patients treated with Cyclosporine for uveitis, N. Engl. J. Med. 314,20: 1293 (1986).
73. K. Svenson, S-O. Bohman, R. Hallgren, Renal interstitial fibrosis and vascular changes, Arch. Intern. Med. 146: 2007 (1986).
74. J. R. Chapman, D. Griffiths, N. G. L. Harding, P. J. Morris, Reversibility of Cyclosporin nephrotoxicity after three months' treatment, Lancet. 1:128 (1985).
75. B. von Graffenried, W. B. Harrison, Ciclosporin in autoimmune diseases. Side effects (with emphasis on renal dysfunction) and recommendations for use, in "Ciclosporin in autoimmne diseases", R. Schindler ed., Springer-Verlag, Berlin (1985).
76. F. Scolari, S. Sandrini, S. Savoldi, L. Cristinelli, B. Brunori, E. Prati, G. Sacchi, R. Tardanico, G. C. Cancarini, R. Maiorca, Is Cyclosporine-induced chronic nephrotoxicity inevitable?, Transplant. Proc. 19:1745 (1987).
77. S. Thiru, E. R. Maher, D. V. Hamilton, D. B. Evans, R. Y. Calne, Tubular changes in renal transplant recipients on Cyclosporine, Transpl. Proc. 15, 4 (suppl.1): 2846 (1983).
78. B. G. Sommer, J. T. Innes, R. M. Whitehurst, H. M. Sharma, R. M. Ferguson, Cyclosporine-associated renal arteriopathy resulting in loss of allograft function, Am. J. Surg. 149:756 (1985).
79. C. Leithner, H. Sinzinger, E. Pohanka, M. Schwarz, G. Kretschmer, G. Syre, Recurrence of haemolytic uraemic syndrome triggered by Cyclosporin A after renal transplantation, Lancet. 1:1470 (1982).
80. H. Shulman, G. Striker, H. J. Deeg, M. Kennedy, R. Storb, E. D. Thomas, Nephrotoxicity of Cyclosporin A after allogeneic marrow transplantation, N. Eng. J. Med. 305:1392 (1981).
81. G. H. Neild, R. Reuben, R. B. Hartley, J. S. Cameron, Glomerular thrombi in renal allografts associated with Cyclosporin treatment, J. Clin. Pathol., 38: 253 (1985).
82. S. Savoldi, F. Scolari, S. Sandrini, P. Scaini, G. Sacchi, R. Tardanico, C. Camerini, B. Salerni, G. Tonini, U. De Nobili, R. Maiorca, Ciclosporine chronic nephrotoxicity: hystological follow up at 6th and 18th month after renal transplantation, Transpl. Proc. (in press) (1988).
83. J. Goldstein, Y. Thoua, F. Wellens, J. L. Lecrerc, J. L. Vanherweghem, P. Vereerstraeten, G. Primo, C. Touissant, Cyclosporine nephropathy after heart and heart-lung transplantation, Proc. EDTA-ERA. 21:973 (1984).

CYCLOSPORIN A AND DRUG INTERACTION

R. Menta, S. David, and V. Cambi

Cattedra di Nefrologia
Università degli Studi di Parma
Via Gramsci 14, 43100 Parma, Italy

INTRODUCTION

Studies of drug interactions during Cyclosporin A (CyA) therapy are based mostly on spontaneous reports. Between 1985 and 1987 35 significant clinical manifestations arising from pharmacological interaction were published by three major medical journals. This work is a summary of clinical complications after combined use of CyA and several other drugs.

Because the interpretation of CyA pharmacokinetics is not clear, drug interactions have been divided into 4 groups.

TAB. 1

1. DRUGS DECREASING CYCLOSPORIN A IMMUNOSUPPRESSIVE EFFECTS BY REDUCING BLOOD LEVELS

2. DRUGS ENHANCING CYCLOSPORIN NEPHROTOXICITY BY INCREASING BLOOD LEVELS

3. DRUGS ENHANCING CYCLOSPORIN NEPHROTOXICITY WITHOUT INTERFERENCE WITH BLOOD LEVELS

4. DRUGS REDUCING CYCLOSPORIN NEPHROTOXICITY WITHOUT INTERFERENCE WITH BLOOD LEVELS

The study of drug interactions is an important means towards understanding CyA toxicity. Spontaneous reports of drug interactions are the best form of accurate post-marketing drug surveillance (1)(2) unless institutional centres exist (3).

CyA PHARMACOKINETICS AND METABOLISM

Oral administration of CyA induces tissue accumulation after 2 to 4 hours. The absorption is in the range 27-40% of the administered dose, with tissue concentration reaching a maximum after 8 hours. Concentrations 3 to 14 times greater than those found in the serum are reached in many tissues including skin, adipose tissue, liver and kidney. Moreover, between 50% and 90% of the CyA present in the tissues consists of the parent compound (4)(5). CyA is metabolized mostly by liver. The presence of hydroxilated and N-demethylated metabolites of CyA suggests an important role for the cytochrome P-450 (Cyt-P450) system. CyA can reduce self metabolism by a "suicide metabolite" (6). Generally, an increase in CyA metabolism is associated with a reduction in nephrotoxicity, while a reduction in the metabolism rate of the drug induces an increase in the blood levels with a mutual increase of nephrotoxicity. Urinary excretion of CyA is negligible: in the rabbit CyA has a clearance of 0.003 ml/min/Kg (7). In the dog cumulative urinary excretion of radiolabeled drug in the period up to 96 hors amounted to only 10% and 17% of the oral and intravenous doses, respectively (8).

INTERACTIONS

1. Drugs Reducing Cyclosporin Blood Levels with Reduction of Immunosuppressive Action

Reductions in CyA blood levels have been reported when drugs able to induce microsomal enzymes, particularly Cyt-P450 were administered during CyA therapy. This type of interaction induces manifestation of acute rejection episodes.

TAB. 2

RIFAMPICIN	9 - 10 - 11
PHENYTOIN	12
CARBAMAZEPINE	13
SULPHADIMIDINE	14
NAFCILLIN	15

Rifampicin induces a marked reduction in CyA blood levels. This reduction of levels is associated with acute rejection episodes. When Rifampicin was administered for TBC therapy before transplantation, acute rejection was particularly early - i.e. within the second day (19). This important interaction is mandatory for the post-transplant anti-tuberculosis therapy based on Isoniazid associated with pyrizinamide (9) or Pyridoxine (10). CyA-Rifampicin interaction is, however, more complex than simple enzymatic induction. During Aspergillus Fumigatus infections, in which Rifampicin and Amphotericine B have synergetic action, diphasic pattern of pharmacological interaction has been demonstrated (11). In the first phase the increase in CyA dosage (4 times the usual dosage = 30 mg/Kg/day) permitted CyA blood levels to reach the therapeutic window for 6 weeks. After this period, despite the fact that Amphotericine B partially counterbalanced the Rifampicin effects, CyA blood levels became undetectable. Drug interaction between CyA and Rifampicin is therefore not due simply to enzymatic induction, and is not fully explainable. Induction of microsomal enzymes explains the low blood level and reduction in immunosuppressive properties during CyA Phenytoin association in epileptic fits (12) as well as when carbamazepine is used for severe eye pain (13), Carbamazepine induced early (within 3 days) and strong reductions in CyA blood levels (1/10 of foregoing individual levels).

Sulphadimidine was preferred to Cotrimoxazole to prevent further compromise of renal function during Pneumocystis Carini infection (14). During Sulphadimidine administration two patients developed rejection episodes while their serum Cyclosporin concentration was unrecordable. This could reasonably be ascribed to interference on hepatic metabolism.

Subtherapeutic CyA concentrations during Nafcillin therapy in two separate administrations was documented as well. Increased CyA hepatic metabolism with associated reduction in immunosuppressive properties was suggested (15).

2. Drugs Increasing Cyclosporin A Blood Levels Leading to Nephrotoxicity

TAB. 3

ERYTHROMYCIN	17, 18, 19, 20
KETOCONAZOLE - ITROCONAZOLE	21, 22
STEROIDS	24, 25, 26
METHYLTESTOSTERONE - ORAL CONTRACEPTIVES	28, 29
DILTIAZEM	30, 31
NICARDIPINE	32
VERAPAMIL	33
RANITIDINE - CIMETIDINE	34, 35
COLCHICINE	39

Legionella and Mycoplasma infections are quite frequent in immunosuppressed patients, and prophilaxis and/or therapy with Erythromycin (E) is widely used, despite its well known interaction with CyA. An increase in CyA blood levels when E is added has been reported during renal transplantation (17) and during diabetes I (20).

Case report

A 40 year old man was submitted to cadaveric kidney transplant: pneumotorax was diagnosed on the 5th day after surgery, due to application of a subclavian catheter. Pleural effusion and lobar atelectasis was diagnosed. Body temperature was 38.5°C. To prevent pulmonary infections prophylactic antibiotic therapy was initiated with E 1 g four times a day, Tobramicine

100 mg/16 h, Cotrimoxazole 2 g twice a day. No reduction in CyA schedule was made. Table 4 shows the course of serum creatinine and CyA blood levels. Fortyeight hours after the beginning of antibiotic therapy, CyA blood levels exceeded 2000 ng/ml and serum creatinine reached 2.3 mg/dl. Two days later, because of objective improvement in lung findings, antibiotic therapy was stopped, and CyA blood levels remained high until the 13th day. Tobramycin was administered properly and for a short time, Cotrimoxazole was administered at low dosage, therefore the rise in serum creatinine was due to a rise in CyA blood levels.

The interactions between CyA and E are summarized in Table 5.

TAB. 4

CyA-E INTERACTION. VARIATION IN CyA BLOOD LEVELS AND SERUM CREATININE

Days post-TRX		CyA-emia (ng/ml)	Serum creatinine (mg/ml)
5	A.M.8	455	2
	P.M.8	889	
6	A.M.8	580	2
	P.M.8	958	
7	A.M.8	868	1.8
	P.M.8	2297	
8	A.M.8	1076	1.9
	P.M.8	1080	
9	A.M.8	1280	2.3
10	A.M.8	1680	1.7
11	A.M.8	1093	2.7
12	A.M.8	1048	2.0
13	A.M.8	549	1.4

TAB. 5

CyA/ERYTHROMYCIN INTERACTIONS

1 - NO TEMPORAL PEAK CHANGE IN CyA SERUM MAXIMUM LEVEL (unchanged at 4 hours after administration)

2 - SLOPE OF REGRESSION LINE OF 4-24 Hrs CyA BLOOD CONCENTRATION SIGNIFICANTLY LOWER WHEN ERYTHROMYCIN IS ADMINISTERED

3 - THROUGH LEVELS AT 24 Hrs SIGNIFICANTLY HIGHER WITH THAN WITHOUT ERYTHROMYCIN

4 - THE AREA UNDER CURVE (AUC) FROM 0 TO 24 Hrs INCREASED TO 156% OF THE CONTROL VALUES UNDER THE INFLUENCE OF ERYTHROMYCIN

5 - CyA HALF-LIFE SIGNIFICANTLY INCREASED BY ERYTHROMYCIN COTHERAPY

6 - THE AUC COMPARABLE TO CONTROL VALUES WOULD BE OBTAINED BY REDUCING TO 64% THE CYA DOSE ADMINISTERED TO ERYTHROMYCIN TREATED PATIENTS

Ketoconazole (21) and Itroconazole (22) could also influence CyA blood levels in some way and enhance nephrotoxicity. CyA blood levels increase 2 and 4 times, and serum creatinine rises from 30% to 220%. From the experimental point of view, Ketoconazole imitates the action of Cobaltus chloride, which is the standard inhibitor of Cyt-P450 adopted in pharmacological studies (23). A possible influence on CyA binding is also suspected.

CyA and steroids (S) interfere with each other. The association of CyA and methylprednisolone pulses therapy can complicate the diagnoses of acute rejection, especially in children, because it induces convulsions (26) and increases CyA blood levels (27). We studied the effects of methylprednisolone pulses in a group of patients (N= 5) submitted to kidney transplantation.

TAB. 6

INFLUENCE OF METHYLPREDNISOLONE PULSE THERAPY ON CyA BLOOD LEVELS

Pts.	Mean CyA blood levels pre-pulse therapy (ng/ml)	Mean CyA blood levels during pulse therapy (ng/ml)	%	p
M.A.	780 ± 5	836 ± 308	6	n.s.
R.M.	457 ± 180	632 ± 141	38	0.05
B.N.	573 ± 103	743 ± 333	30	0.05
M.P.	371 ± 41	561 ± 140	51	0.05
P.F.	824 ± 56	889 ± 136	8	n.s.
	601 ± 197	730 ± 134	27	n.s.

t-test

As shown in Table 6, only 3 over 5 patients had documented increases in CyA blood levels. Methylprednisolone (28) and Levonorgestrol (29) induced increased CyA blood levels and nephrotoxicity. Additional liver toxicity was also suspected. Due to hepatic metabolism of these drugs interaction with Cyt-P450 could be suggested.

Difficult to understand are the interactions between CyA and Calcium channel blockers. Diltiazem interferes with CyA metabolism and thus changes its nephrotoxic potential (30). However prevention of delayed graft function in cadaver kidney transplant by Diltiazem was reported, despite an average increase in CyA blood levels of about 80%. A protective effect by Calcium channel blockers against CyA induced vasoconstriction was suggested. Nicardipine, instead, increases CyA blood levels and enhances nephrotoxicity (32).

Case Report

A 33 year old woman with a positive anamnesis for hypertension was submitted to cadaveric kidney transplantation. She was oliguric for 15 days after surgical intervention: fine needle aspiration biopsy (FNAB) showed

CyA nephrotoxicity and CyA doses were tapered off to 8 mg/Kg/day on the 20th day. Renal function subsequently improved. The patient become hypertensive and Nifedipine (20 mg twice a day) was started. Because of untoward effects (headhache, facial erytema and leg edema) Nifedipine was stopped and Nicardipine was administered. CyA blood levels were however monitored four times daily for the known interactions. Thirtysix hours after the beginning of therapy CyA blood levels exceeded 2000 ng/ml. FNAB showed renewed microvacuolization and serum creatinine increased reaching 2.6 mg/dl despite a 20% reduction in CyA doses. Nicardipine was stopped and Betablockers administered. Nicardipine was administered 3 hours after CyA administration and peack levels were increased by 45%. Fifty days later she had a serum creatinine of 1.6 mg/dl.

Verapamil was said to interfere with CyA in vitro: however the main action was an enhanced immunosuppressive capacity (33). Antipeptic ulcer prophilaxis in patients submitted to transplantation is widely used. Cimetidine increases CyA blood levels and nephrotoxicity, while these effects have not been described for Ranitidine (34). However drug interaction is mainly rappresented by increased liver toxicity (36). Because liver toxicity is reported during both Ranitidine (37)(38) and CyA therapy, a doubt can arise in differential diagnosis.

Colchicine can increase CyA blood levels and toxicity.

Case Report

A 40 year old woman with gouty nephropathy was submitted to cadaveric kidney transplantation. Long lasting anuria complicated by CyA toxicity followed. After early conversion to triple therapy, kidney function improved, and serum creatinine reached 1.5 mg/dl. On the 56th day an acute gouty attack was diagnosed and Colchicine administered. 24 hours later CyA blood levels showed a six-fold increase. Daily urine output decreased and body weight increased: serum creatinine reached 2 mg/dl. Colchicine was stopped and rapid recovery of kidney function was observed. Colchicine induced the most pronounced increase in CyA blood levels (Tab. 7).

TAB. 7

CLINICAL AND LABORATORY DATA SHOWING THE ABRUPT INCREASE IN CyA LEVEL AFTER COLCHICINE ADMINISTRATION AND SUBSEQUENT RISE IN PLASMA CREATININE AND FALL IN URINARY OUTPUT

Days after trasplant	CyA blood level (ng/ml)	Serum creatinine (umol/l)	Daily urine output (ml)	BW (Kg)
56	266	133.0	1000	48.2
57	419	124.1	1250	48.4
58	1519	118.0	600	49.0
59	475	177.4	1250	48.5
60	175	150.8	1800	48.6
61	110	133.0	850	48.0

3. Drugs Enhancing Cyclosporin Nephrotoxicity without Interference with Blood Levels

The use of known nephrotoxic drugs could, of course, enhance CyA toxicity. A lot of reports on this subject have been published. Most of them concern the drugs in Table 8.

TAB. 8

ACYCLOVIR	40, 41
AMPHOTERICIN B	42
AMINOGLYCOSIDES - GENTAMICIN	43
CAPTOPRIL	45
FUROSEMIDE	46, 47
SULFAMETOXAZOLE TRIMETHOPRIM	49
MANNITOL	48

Acyclovir was said to induce additional nephrotoxicity because of intratubular deposition of drug cristalls (41); this report has not been confirmed by other authors (40).

During concomitant administration of CyA and Amphotericine B, in marrow transplant recipients, a doubling in serum creatinine levels was reported in 38% of the patients within 14-30 days (42).

An increase of incidence of acute tubular necrosis (ATN) in the post-transplant period (67% vs. 10%) was reported when perioperative Gentamicine prophilaxis was adopted (43) Experimental confirmation of additional nephrotoxicity was also reported (44) and clinically demonstrated. Diuretics are often used in the post-transplant period. When Furosemide was added to CyA therapy a significant worsening in kidney function accompanied by an increase in urinary enzymes of about 80% was observed. Experimental doubling of CyA blood level after 14 days of Furosemide therapy was demonstrated. This data was thought to be due to reduction of the activity of hepatic microsomial enzymes (300) reduction of Cyt-P450 and a 50% in demethilating activity) (45). An increase in serum alkaline phosphatase was also reported (46). Moreover, the association of the two drugs could enhance liver toxicity (47). Mannitol, too, is often used in the post-transplant period. Marked microvacuolization was reported thirty hours after mannitol infusion. Additional nephrotoxicity was said to be reversible. Clinical observation was experimentally confirmed (48). When Bactrim was added to CyA therapy an increase in serum creatinine was also reported during conventional therapy: Cotrimoxazole alone did not worsen kidney function, while Trimethoprin could increase CyA nephrotoxicity (49).

4. Drugs that Prevent CyA nephrotoxicity without Interfering with CyA Blood Levels

Pharmacological interaction studies have lead to the search for drugs that reduce nephrotoxicity without changing the immunosuppressive properties of CyA. Table 9 shows the most important drugs tested.

TAB. 9

AROCLOR 1254	50
CAPTOPRIL	51
DOPAMINE	52
HYDERGINE	53, 54
PG - PGE2	55, 56
PRAZOSINE	57
THEOPHILLINE	51

Aroclor 1254, an inducer of Cyt-P450, is one of the most promising ones. Experimental studies have shown a reduced nephrotoxicity without interference with immunosuppressive effectiveness. This approach is clearly better than the use of Phenobarbitone that causes several undesirable side-effects (50). A different approach to reverting an altered tubuloglomerular feed-back using ACE inhibitors (Captopril) or Theofilline, which block the adenosine receptors, has been attempted, but no significant improvement was obtained. This supports the hypothesis of direct tubular toxicity on the part of CyA (51).

Experimental evidence in rats has shown that Dopamine infusion reduces CyA nephrotoxicity, but Dobutamine does not (52).

The first report about Hydergine was also encouraging, but sebsequent studies did not show any benefit despite the use of several therapeutic schedules (starting from 3 to 8 mg/day) (53), (54). Synthetic Postaglandines (55) and PGE (56) have been demonstrated to revert CyA nephrotoxicity, but PGE2 has an effect on gastric absorption with a dangerous reduction in immunosuppressive action.

Chronic Prazosine administration has also been experimentally useful in treating nephrotoxicity; however, since renal denervation was also associated in the experimental model, these data are considered to be as an indirect demonstration of sympathic vasoconstriction rather than of the clinical efficacy of Prazosine (57).

DISCUSSION

Separate acute and chronic histopathologic findings during CyA nephrotoxicity were described (58)(59). The abundant data reported here, moreover, emphasize the difficulty of properly using CyA in clinical practice. Because the differential diagnosis between acute rejection and nephrotoxicity during the early post-transplant period is not simple, maximum attention must be given to sporadic therapy during these clinical phases. Clinical monitoring (CyA blood levels) must be accurate and is expensive. We do not know how important acute drug induced CyA nepthrotoxicity can be, or if drug interactions can affect long term graft survival. However, at present we can affirm that:

1) Hepatic metabolism is the most important factor in pharmacokinetic studies as demonstrated by the dramatic effects brought about by drugs that interfere with the Cyt-P450 system.
2) Up to now there are no drugs that can reduce CyA nephrotoxicity. Aroclor 1254 is the most promising drug.

At present, triple conversion therapy represents merely an attempt to reduce nephrotoxicity, but it carries with it the risk of acute and irreversible graft rejection.

ACKNOWLEDGMENT

The authors thank "Nephrology '80" for the combination given to the prepration of the manuscript.
channel blockers.

REFERENCES

(1) F. Aramburu, B. Begaud, J.C. Pere, S. Marcel and H. Albin, Role of Medicine Journals in Adverse Drugs Reaction Alerts, Lancet ii:550 (1985)
(2) J.C. Roujean, J.C. Guillaume, J. Revuz and R. Touraine: Reporting Adverse Drug Reaction, Lancet ii:1244 (1985)
(3) N. Moore, M.Biour, G. Paux, E. Loupi, B. Begaud, F. Boismare and R.J. Roxer, Adverse Drug Reaction Monitoring: Doing the French Way, Lancet ii: 1056 (1985)
(4) P.H. Whiting, M.D. Burke and A.W. Thomson, Drug Interaction with Cyclosporin. Implication from Animal Studies, Trans. Proc. XVIII, 6:56 (1986)
(5) W. Niederbenger, M. Lemarie, G. Maurer, K. Nussbaumer and O. Wagner, Distribution and Binding of Cyclosporin in Blood and Tissue, Trans. Proc. XV:2419 (1983)
(6) M.D. Burke and P.H. Whiting, The Role of Drug Metabolism in Cyclosporin A Nephrotoxicity, Cl. Nephrol. 25(S1):S111-S117 (1986)
(7) R.J. Caterson, G.G. Dugging, L. Critchley, C. Baxter, J.S. Horvat,B.M. Hall and D.J. Tiller, Renal Tubular Transort of Cyclosporin A and Associated Changes in Renal Function, Cl. Nephrol. 25(S1):S30 (1986)
(8) P.H. Whiting, A.W. Thompson and J.G. Simpson, Cyclosporin Toxicity, Metabolism and Drug Interaction. Implications from Animal Studies, Trans. Proc. XVII:134 (1985)
(9) R.A. Coward, A.T. Raftery and C.B. Brown, Cyclosporin and Anti-tubercolous Therapy, Lancet i:1342 (1985)
(10) W.A. Jurewicz, B.K. Gunson, T. Ismail, L. Angrisani and P. McMaster, Cyclosporin and Antitubercolous Therapy, Lancet i:1343 (1985)
(11) D.L. Modry, E.B. Stinson, P.E. Oyer, S.W. Jameson, J.C. Baldwin and N.E. Shuhway, Acute Rejection and Massive Cyclosporin Requirements in Heart Transplant Recipients Treated with Rifampicin, Transplantation 39:313 (1985)
(12) P.H. Whiting, Generalized epileptic Fits in Renal Transplant recipients Given Cyclosporin A, Br. Med. J. 1:162 (1985)
(13) P. Lele, P. Peterson, S. Tang, B. Jarrell and J.F. Burke, Cyclosporin and Tegretal - Another Drug Interaction, Kidney Int. 27:344 (1985)
(14) D.K. Jones; M. Hakim, J. Wallwork and T.W. Higenbottam, Serious Interaction between Cyclosporin A and Sulphamidine, Br. Med. J. 292:728 (1986)

(15) S.A. Veremis, M.S. Maddux, R. Pollak and M.F. Mozes, Subtherapeutic Cyclosporin Concentrations During Nafcillin Therapy, Transplantation 1:913 (1987)

(16) Cyclosporin a New Immunosuppressive Drug, Medical Letter 25:77(1985)

(17) R. Ptachinski, B. J. Carpenter, G.J. Burckart, R. Venkataramanan and J.T. Rosenthal, Effect of Erythromycin on Cyclosporin Levels, N. Engl. J. Med. 2:1416 (1985)

(18) D.E. Kohan, Possible Interaction between Cyclosporin and Erythromycin, N. Engl. J. Med. 1:448 (1986)

(19) P. Vereet Straeten, P. Thiry, P. Kinnaert and C. Toussaint, Influence of Erythromycin on Cyclosporin Pharmacokinetics, Transplantation S (July) 44:155 (1987)

(20) R. Martell, D. Heinrichs, C.R. Stiller, M. Jenner, P.A. Keown and J. Dupre, The Effects of Erythromycin in Patients treated with Cyclosporin, Ann. Int. Med. 104:660 (1986)

(21) H. Dieperink and J. Moller, Ketoconazole and Cyclosporin, Lancet 2:1217 (1987)

(22) J.T.C. Kwan, P.D. Foxall, D.G.C. Davidson, M.R. Bending and A.J. Eisinger, Interaction of Cyclosporin and Itraconazole, Lancet 2:282 (1987)

(23) M.D. Burke and P.H. Whiting, The Role of Drug Metabolism in Cyclosporin A Nephrotoxicity, Cl. Nephrol. 25:111 (1986)

(24) M.A. Boogaerts, P. Zachee and R.L. Verwilghen, Cyclosporin, Methilprednisolone and Convulsions, Lancet 2:1216 (1982)

(25) E. Langhoff, S. Madsen, H. Flachs, K. Olgaard, J. Ladefoged and E. Hvidberg, Inhibition of Prednisolone Metabolism by Cyclosporin in kidney Transplanted Patients, Transplantation 39:106 (1985)

(26) L. Oest, Effects of Cyclosporin on Prednisolone Metabolism, Lancet 2:451 (1984)

(27) G. Klintmalm and J. Säve, High Dose Methylprednisolone Increases Plasma Cyclosporin Levels in Renal Transplant Recipients, Lancet 1:731 (1984)

(28) B. Broch Moller and B. Ekelund, Toxicity of Cyclosporin During Treatment with Androgens, N. Engl. J. Med. 2:1416 (1985)

(29) G. Deray, P. Hoang, P. Cacoub, V. Assogba, P. Grippon and A. Baumelan, Oral Contraceptive Interaction with Cyclosporin, Lancet 1:158 (1987)

(30) J.M. Pochet and Y. Pirson, Cyclosporin-Diltazem Interaction, Lancet 1:979 (1986)

(31) K. Wagner and H.H. Neumayer, Prevention of Delayed Graft Function in Cadaver Kidney Transplants by Diltiazem, Lancet 2:1355 (1985)

(32) B. Bourbigot, J. Guiserix, J. Airiau, L. Bressolette, J.F. Morin and J. Cledes, Lancet 1:1447 (1986)

(33) A. Lindholm and S. Henricsson, Verapamil Inhibits Cyclosporin Metabolism, Lancet 1:1262 (1987)

(34) J. Zazgornick, J. Schneider. G. Gremmel, P. Balcke, H. Kopsa, K. Derfler and E. Minar, Ranitidine Does not Influence the Blood Cyclosporin Levels in Renal Transplant Patients (RTP) Kidney Int. 6:401 (1986)

(35) M. Jarowenko, C.T. Van Buren, W.G. Kramer, M.I. Lorber, S. Flechner and B. Kaham, Ranitidine, Cimetidine and the Cyclosporin-Treated Recipient, Transplantation 42:311 (1986)

(36) C. Hiesse, M. Cantarovich, C. Santelli, P. Francais, B. Charpentier, D. Fries and C. Buffet, Ranitidine Hepatotoxicity in Renal Transplant Patient, Lancet 1:1280 (1985)
(37) M.A. Souza Lima, Hepatitis Associated with Ranitidine, Ann. Int. Med. 101:207 (1984)
(38) M. Black, W.E. Scott and R. Kanter, Possible Ranitidine Nephrotoxicity, Ann. Int. Med. 101:208 (1984)
(39) R. Menta, E. Rossi, A. Guariglia, S. David and V. Cambi, Reversible Acute Cyclosporin Nephrotoxicity Induced by Colchicine Administration, Nephrol. Dial. Transplant. 2:380 (1987)
(40) P.C. Johonson, K. Kumor, M.S. Welsh, J. Woo and B. Kahan, Effects of Coadministration of Cyclosporin and Acyclovir on Renal Function of Renal Allograft Recipients, Transplantation 44:329 (1987)
(41) D. Brigden, A.E. Rosling and N.C. Woods, Renal Function after Acyclovir Intravenous Injection, Am. J. Med. 73:182 (1982)
(42) M.S. Kennedy, H.J. Deeg, M. Siegel, J.J. Crowley, R. Storb and E.D. Thomas, Acute Renal Toxicity with Combined Use of Amphotericin B and Cyclosporin after Marrow Transplantation, Transplantation 35:211 (1983)
(43) A. Termeer, A.J. Hoitsma and R.A.P. Koene, Severe Nephrotoxicity Caused by the Combined Use of Gentamicin and Cyclosporin in Renal Allograft Recipients Transplantation 42:221 (1986)
(44) P.H. Whiting, J.D. Simpson, R.J.C. Davidson and A.W. Thomson, The Toxic Effects of Combined Administration of Cyclosporin A and Gentamicin, Br. J. Exp. Pathol. 63:554 (1982)
(45) J.R. Mitchell, W.Z. Potter, J.A. Minson and D.J. Jollow, Hepatic Necrosis Caused by Frusemide, Nature 251:508 (1974)
(46) P.H. Whiting, C. Cunningham, A.W. Thomson and J.G. Simpson, Enhancement of High Dose Cyclosporin A Toxicity By Frusemide, Bioch. Pharm. 33:1074 (1984)
(47) S.S. Thorgeirsson, H.A. Sasame, J.R. Mitchell, D.J. Jallow and W.Z. Potter, Biochemical Changes after Hepatic Injury from Toxic Doses of Acetaminophen or Furosemide, Pharmacology 14:205 (1976)
(48) F.P. Brunner, M. Hermle, M.J. Mihatsch and G. Thiel, Mannitol Potentiates Cyclosporin Nephrotoxicity, Cl. Nephrol. 25:130 (1986)
(49) J. Thompson, D.H.K. Chalmers, A.G.W. Hunnisett, R.F.M. Wood and P.J. Morris, Nephrotoxicity of Trimethoprim and Cotrimoxazole in Renal Allograft Recipients Treated with Cyclosporin, Transplantation 36:204 (1982)
(50) C. Cunningham, P.H. Whiting, M.D. Burke, D.N. Wheatley and J.G. Simpson, Increasing the Hepatic Metabolism of Cyclosporin Abolishes Nephrotoxicity, Trans. Proc. XV:2713 (1983)
(51) J.F. Gerkens and A.J. Smith, Effect of Captopril and Theophylline Treatment on Cyclosporin-Induced Nephrotoxicity in Rats, Transplantation 40:214 (1985)
(52) T.L. Kho, K.M. Leunissen, G.A.K. Heidendhal, P. Lijnen, A. Amery and J.P. Van Hoff, Nephrotoxic Effect of Cyclosporin A can be Reversed by Dopamine Nephrol. Dial. Transplant. 1:140 (1986)
(53) T.L. Kho, R. Kengen, K.M.L. Leunissen, J. Teule and J.P. Van Hooff, Hydergine and Reversibility of Cyclosporin Nephrotoxicity, Lancet 2:394 (1986)

(54) R.B. Nussenblatt, H.A. Austin, A.G. Palestine and H.G. Preuss, Hydergine and Cyclosporin Nephrotoxicity, Lancet 1:1220 (1986)

(55) L. Makowka, W. Lopatin, T. Gilas, J. Falk, M.J. Phillips and R. Falk, Prevention of Cyclosporin Nephrotoxicity by Synthetic Prostaglandins

(56) B. Ryffel, P. Donatsch, P. Hiestand and M.J. Mihatsch, PGE2 Reduces Nephrotoxicity and Immunosuppression of Cyclosporin in Rats, Cl. Nephrol. 25:95 (1986)

(57) B.M. Murray and M.S. Paller, Beneficial Effects of Renal Denervation and Prazosin on GFR and Renal Blood Flow after Cyclosporin in Rats Cl. Nephrol. 25:37 (1986)

(58) R. Sibley, J. Rynasiewicz, R.M. Ferguson, D. Fryd, D.E.R. Sutherland, R.L. Simmons and J.S. Najarian, Morphology of Cyclosporin and Prednisone, Surgery 94:225 (1983)

(59) B.D. Meyers, J. Ross, L. Newton, J. Luetscher and M. Perlroth, Cyclosporin-Associated Cronic Nephropathy, N. Engl. J. Med. 311:699 (1984)

MAGNESIUM AFTER RENAL TRANSPLANTATION - COMPARISON BETWEEN CYCLOSPORINE A AND CONVENTIONAL IMMUNOSUPPRESSION

Wilhelm Kaiser, Georg Biesenbach, Engelbert Kramer, and Jan Zazgornik

II Medical Department (Head: Prof. J. Zazgornik)
General Hospital of Linz
Linz, Austria

INTRODUCTION

Neurotoxicity and hypertension are typical side-effects of cyclosporine A. In bone-marrow transplantation using cyclosporine A for immunosuppression the onset of neurotoxicity[1] and hypertension[2] had been correlated with hypomagnesemia. We therefore studied the differences in serum magnesium and urinary magnesium excretion in both cyclosporine and azathioprine/prednisone immunosuppressed renal transplant patients, respectively.

PATIENTS AND METHODS

In 23 renal transplant patients mean age of 37 (16-62) years immunosuppressed with cyclosporine A (CYA) in different combinations and 9 patients mean age of 41 (24-56) years with azathioprine/prednisone (AZA) we measured serum magnesium, renal magnesium excretion and fractional excretion of magnesium (FEmg). There were no differences in graft function in the investigated patients (creatinine clearance 61,8 ml/min in CYA and 61,3 ml/min in AZA. The mean time of graft function was 20,9 (7-43) months in CYA and 73,3 (24-158) months in AZA. Parameters were measured monthly for a 3 months period in 1986. This procedure was repeated one year later. From AZA one patient had to be dropped out because of graft failure. CYA consisted of 13 patients in 1986 and additional 10 patients in 1987 (see table 1). Patients with graft function less than 6 months, dysproteinemia, hyper- or hypocalcemia, serum creatinine more than 2,5 mg/dl or diuretics therapy were excluded from the study. Magnesium was estimated spectrophotometrically by methyl-thymol-blue (ACA, DuPont). Cyclosporine A was given twice daily, trough-levels were estimated by RIA. FEmg was calculated by the well-known formula FEmg = mg(urine)/mg(serum) x creatinine(serum)/ /creatinine(urine). Statistical calculations were done by unpaired Students t-test.

Table 1. Patients and immunosuppression

	CYA			AZA
Patients	n= 23			n= 9
Graft function	20,9 months (7-43)			73,3 months (24-158)
Serum creatinine	1,65 mg/dl (0,7-2,3)			1,7 mg/dl (1,0-2,3)
Clearance (creatinine)	61,8 ml/min (31-98)			61,3 ml/min (30-118)
Immunosuppression	Aza/Pr	CyA	CyA/Pr	CyA/Pr/Aza
(1986)	n= 9	n= 1	n= 9	n= 3
(1987)	n= 8	n= 1	n=13	n= 9

RESULTS (table 2, figures 1-3)

CYA showed lower serum magnesium levels (0,709 ∓ 0,08 mmol/l) than AZA (0,85 ∓ 0,10 mmol/l). This difference is of high statistical significance ($p < 0,001$). The lowest magnesium levels (0,671 ∓ 0,05 mmol/l) with simultaneous highest renal magnesium losses (148 ∓ 78 mg daily, FEmg = 8,0 ∓ 2,8 %) were associated with high cyclosporine trough-levels (> 600 ng/ml). Although trough-levels from 200-400 ng/ml and from 400-600 ng/ml are associated with significant lower magnesium levels in comparison to AZA, these 3 groups show the same renal magnesium losses (92 ∓ 53 mg daily, 80 ∓ 39 mg daily versus 98 ∓ 52 mg daily) and the same fractional excretion (6,0 ∓ 2,4 %, 6,1 ∓ 2,5 % versus 6,2 ∓ 1,6 %). These data indicate tubulotoxicity also in these cyclosporine groups, because intact tubular reabsorption would have to decrease magnesium excretion in hypomagnesemia.

Table 2. Results

	Serum mg (mmol/l)	FEmg (%)	Excretion of magnesium (mg/die)	Number of estimations
*AZA	0,850∓0,10	6,2 ∓ 1,6	98 ∓ 52	n = 51
*CYA (together)	0,709∓0,08	6,4 ∓ 2,5	93 ∓ 54	n =108
CyA/Az/Pr	0,708∓0,10	6,5 ∓ 3,1	90 ∓ 40	n = 36
CyA/Pr	0,711∓0,08	6,3 ∓ 2,3	93 ∓ 58	n = 66
Trough-levels (ng/ml)				
200-400	0,713∓0,09	6,0 ∓ 2,4	92 ∓ 53	n = 68
400-600	0,699∓0,08	6,1 ∓ 2,5	80 ∓ 39	n = 43
> 600	0,671∓0,05	8,0 ∓ 2,8	148 ∓ 78	n = 7

*$p < 0,001$

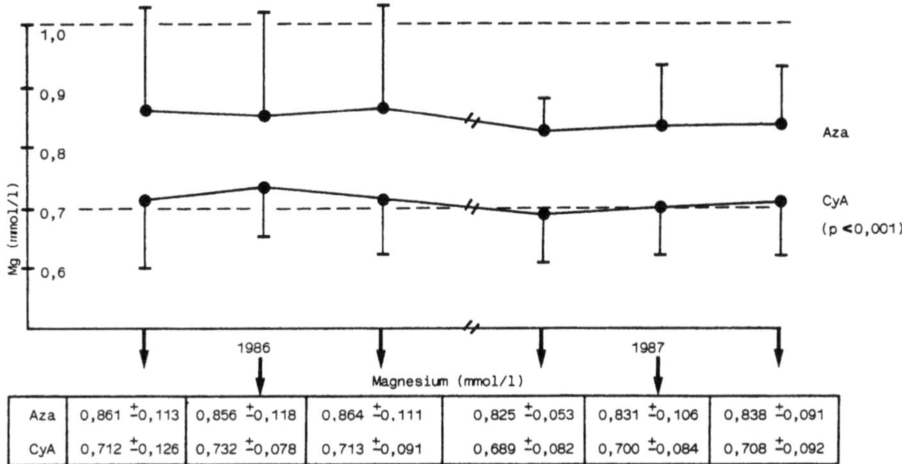

Magnesium (mmol/l)

Aza	0,861 ±0,113	0,856 ±0,118	0,864 ±0,111	0,825 ±0,053	0,831 ±0,106	0,838 ±0,091
CyA	0,712 ±0,126	0,732 ±0,078	0,713 ±0,091	0,689 ±0,082	0,700 ±0,084	0,708 ±0,092

Figure 1. At each time CYA showed lower serum magnesium levels than AZA ($p < 0,001$; mean values and standard deviations).

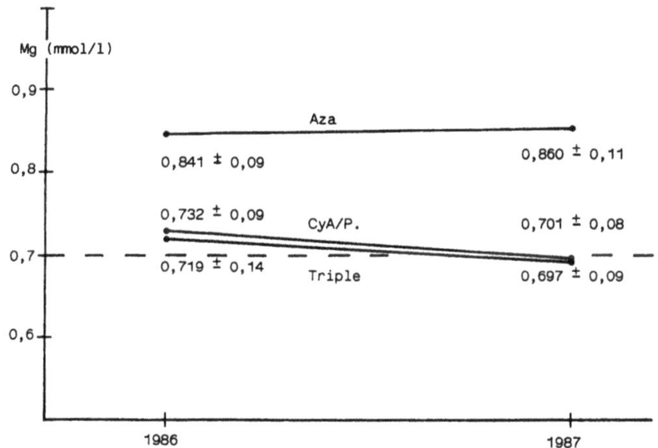

Figure 2. Serum magnesium concentration and immunosuppressive regime: azathioprine/prednisone (Aza), cyclosporine A/prednisone (CyA/P) and triple therapy (azathioprine/prednisone/cyclosporine)

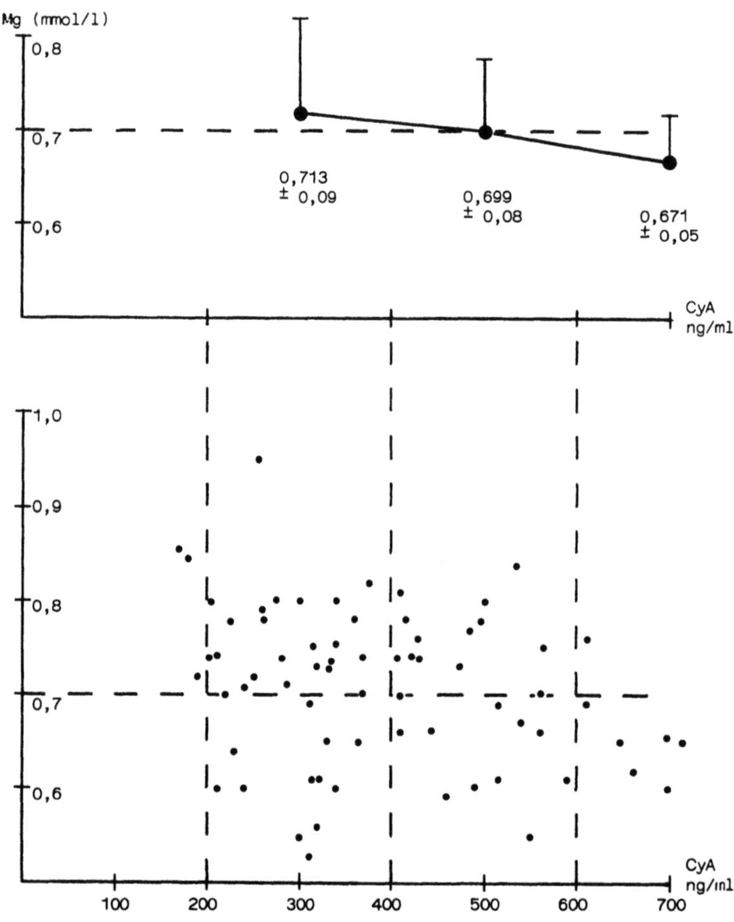

Figure 3. Serum magnesium concentration and cyclosporine trough-levels. The lowest magnesium levels are associated with trough-levels > 600 ng/ml.

DISCUSSION

Some side effects of cyclosporine A had been associated with hypomagnesemia in bone marrow transplantation[3] and in autoimmune diseases[4] due to renal magnesium wasting. All these reports concern intact kidneys and those results are in discussion. Some patients had had simultaneous therapy with aminoglycosids or amphotericin B, others had diarrhoe, low plasma protein concentrations or hypocalcemia or had parenteral nutrition with inadequate magnesium substitution[1,2].

Many disturbances of electrolyte regulation and acid-base metabolism after renal transplantation are reported. Tubular acidosis[5], hypo- and hyperkalemia[6], hypercalcemia[7] and hypophosphatemia[8] are known. Clinical data according hypomagnesemia are rare.

Bachem et al[9] compared magnesium levels in azathioprine/prednisone treated patients with a cyclosporine group during 3 weeks following renal transplantation. Patients with cyclosporine A showed significant lower magnesium levels (0,52 mmol/l) than patients with azathioprine/prednisone (0,79 mmol/l) in this early period of graft function. These findings were corroborated by intracellular estimations of magnesium in erythrocytes and lymphocytes.

Our results show persistent latent hypomagnesemia in cyclosporine group in long time follow-up. At each time of the study conventional treated patients had magnesium levels within normal range and were significantly higher ($p < 0,001$) than cyclosporine patients. There were no differences neither cyclosporine A/prednisone nor triple therapy with cyclosporine A/prednisone/azathioprine (figure 2). This indicates cyclosporine A to be responsible for latent hypomagnesemia.

Cyclosporine A treated patients showed the same renal magnesium losses as conventional treated patients (table 2). In our opinion cyclosporine A tubulotoxicity is responsible for this disorder in magnesium reabsorption. Intact tubular system would have to decrease magnesium excretion to a minimum in latent hypomagnesemia.

We could not find any statistical correlation to cyclosporine trough-level. The highest renal magnesium losses (148 ± 78 mg daily) and the highest fractional excretion of magnesium ($8,0 \pm 2,8$ %) were found in patients with trough-levels more than 600 ng/ml. This group simultaneously showed the lowest magnesium levels ($0,671 \pm 0,05$ mmol/l). This tendency is of no statistical significance, but there had been only 7 events of trough-levels > 600 ng/ml in our study.

We noticed 3 events of cyclosporine neurotoxicity. 2 of them were associated with very low magnesium levels (0,60 mmol/l and 0,61 mmol/l), both improved with substitution of magnesium and reduction of cyclosporine A.

Using cyclosporine A in renal transplantation magnesium showed be controlled sometimes, especially in neurotoxicity. We conclude that disturbances in magnesium regulation are part of cyclosporine's tubulotoxicity.

REFERENCES

1. B. C. Thompson, K. M. Sullivan, H. C. June, E. D. Thomas, Association between cyclosporine neurotoxicity and hypomagnesemia, Lancet II:1116 (1984).
2. C. H. June, C. B. Thompson, M. S. Kennedy, T. P. Loughran, H. J. Deeg, Correlation of hypomagnesemia with the onset of cyclosporine-associated hypertension in marrow transplant patients. Transplantation 41 (1):47 (1986)

3. C. H. June, C. B. Thompson, M. S. Kennedy, J. Nims, E. D. Thomas, Profound hypomagnesemia and renal magnesium wasting associated with the use of cyclosporine for marrow transplantation. Transplantation 39 (6):620 (1985).
4. A. G. Palestine, H. A. Austin, R. B. Nussenblatt, Cyclosporine-induced nephrotoxicity in patients with autoimmune uveitis. Transplant. Proc. 17 (4), Suppl. 1:209 (1985).
5. D. C. Battle, M. F. Mozes, J. Manaligod, A. L. Arruda, N. A. Kurtzman, The pathogenesis of hyperchloremic metabolic acidosis associated with kidney transplantation. Am. J. Med. 70:786 (1981).
6. R. A. De Fronzo, M. Goldberg, C. R. Cooke, C. Barker, R. A. Grossman, Z. Agus, Investigations into the mechanism of hyperkalemia following renal transplantation. Kidney Int. 11:357 (1977).
7. S. N. Chatterjee, R. M. Friedler, T. V. Berne, S. B. Oldham, F. R. Singer, S. G. Massry, Persistent hypercalcemia after successful renal transplantation. Nephron 17:1 (1971).
8. J. Zazgornik, F. Kokot, K. Fürst, P. Schmidt, J. Pietrek, H. Czembirek, H. Kopsa, P. Balcke, Elisabeth Paietta, Roentgenologic soft tissue and bone changes, parathyroid-hormone, 25-hydroxy-cholecalciferol, calcium-phosphorus concentrations in serum in dialyzed and renal transplant patients. Dialysis & Transplantation 8:389 (1979).
9. M. G. Bachem, B. Köhler, H. Bauer, B. Zanker, H. E. Franz, E. F. Pfeiffer, Cyclosporin A bedingter Magnesiummangel nach Nierentransplantation. Klin. Wochenschr. 64 (Suppl. V): 202 (1986).

A CASE OF RELAPSING RENAL MICROPOLYARTERITIS: A POSSIBLE ASSOCIATION WITH ASSUMPTION OF NON STEROIDAL ANTIINFLAMMATORY DRUGS (NSAID)

P. Stanziale, G. Fuiano, M.M. Balletta, V. Sepe, G.C. Marinelli, G. Colucci, and V.E. Andreucci

Chair of Nephrology, 2nd Faculty of Medicine Naples, Italy

The onset of renal micropolyarteritis has been associated with the administration of a number of drugs: penicillins, sulphonamides and phenytoin have been more frequently recorded. The relationship between NSAID and renal micropolyarteritis, although hypothesized in other reports (1) (2), is often difficult to demonstrate, because initial symptoms of vasculitis frequently include arthritis and or arthralgias: consequently many patients are given NSAID for relieving these symptoms, often *after* the onset of the disease.

By contrast, the present case strongly suggests that the assumption of NSAID may induce or, at least, precipitate a preexisting mild vasculitic syndrome.

CASE REPORT

A 56 y. o. previously healthy woman, developed arthralgias and myalgias; laboratory investigations showed elevated erithrosedimentation rate (ESR), moderate anemia (blood haemoglobin: 11.4 g/dl), normal renal function and normal urynalysis. Two months after, persisting myalgias and arthalgias (laboratory investigations being unchanged), the patient was given diclofenac for three weeks; because poor clinical improvement was obtained diclofenac was then replaced by naproxen, which was continued for about one month. After 20 days from the withdrawal, the patient developed "constitutional" simptoms (i.e. weakness, malaise, flulike symptoms), rashes and gross haematuria. For this reason the patient was referred to our Department.

Phisical examination showed bilateral leg oedema, mild spleen enlargement; chest x-ray showed a picture consistent with interstitial pneumonia. Laboratory investigations showed anaemia (blood haemoglobin: 5.7g/dl), leucocytosis (GB.: 15.000/mm^3), eosinophilia (29%), thrombocytosis (465.000 mm^3) and renal function impairment: plasma creatinine: 7.4 mg/dl; creatinine clearance: 9.7 ml/min, blood urea nitrogen: 210 mg/dl. Mild hypoalbuminemia was also present (2.2 g/dl); both alpha 2 globulins and gamma

Table 1. Laboratory findings

	Onset	Acute fase	Follow up	Relapse
Time to onset (months)		3	8	12
P Creatinine (mg/dl)	0.7	7.4	3.0	8.2
GFR (ml/min)	75	9.7	20	6.0
Blood Hb (g/dl)	11.4	6.7	8.2	5.1
B W C (/mm^3) (x1000)	7.5	15	7.4	12
Eosinophils (%WBC)	2	29	0	16
Thrombocytes (x1000)	377	492	240	350
IgG (mg/dl)	--	4332	1306	1848
IgE (U.I./ml)	--	>1000	--	465
Proteinuria (g/day)	0.2	3	0.8	3.7

globulins were elevated (15% and 33% of total proteins, respectively); serum immunogloblins were (mg/dl): IgG: 4332, IgA 297, IgM 155, IgE 1000 U.I./ml. C_3 was moderately reduced. Serum cryoglobulins, AntiDNA antibodies and antinuclear factors were also sought and resulted negative. Urinalysis showed heavy proteinuria (4 g/24 hours), haematuria (25-35 red blood cells per microscopic field) and granulous casts. Both kidneys presented normal size, as assessed by ultrasound investigation. Renal biopsy showed crescents in 30% of glomeruli, most presented fibrinoid necrosis and mesangial proliferation; interstitial infiltrates and tubular dilation and atrophy were also present. Immunohistochemical study, performed by direct immunofluorescence tecnique on frozen tissue, showed glomerular deposits of IgM, C_3 and fibrinogen and tubular and vascular deposits of IgE and IgA. Diffuse IgA deposits were seen in the interstitial tissue. A diagnosis of renal vasculitis was made and immunosuppressive therapy with methylprednisolone pulse therapy (300 mg i.v. x 3 consecutive days) associated with oral prednisone (initially 60 mg/day, gradually reduced to 8 mg/day) and dipiridamole (75 mg t.i.d.) was started. Steroids were continued for 8 months. Renal function gradually improved, plasma creatinine decreasing to 3.8 mg/dl after 1 month of therapy with Creatinine clearance: 18 ml/min, and remained steady for several months, (plasma creatinine averaging 3 mg/dl in different controls). Steroid therapy was withdrawal. However, after 2 months, the patient presented a relapse of arthritis, and developed again severe anaemia (blood Hb: 5.1g/dl), with eosinophilia (1920 eosinophils/mm^3); IgG were mildly elevated and serum complement factors normal; renal function worsened, plasma creatinine being 5.9 mg/dl at admission and peaking to 8.2 mg/dl.

Because patient did not give consent, a renal biopsy was not performed. Again the patient was treated with steroids, but without any improvement of renal function and haematologic parameters. The patient was started on regular dialytic treament.

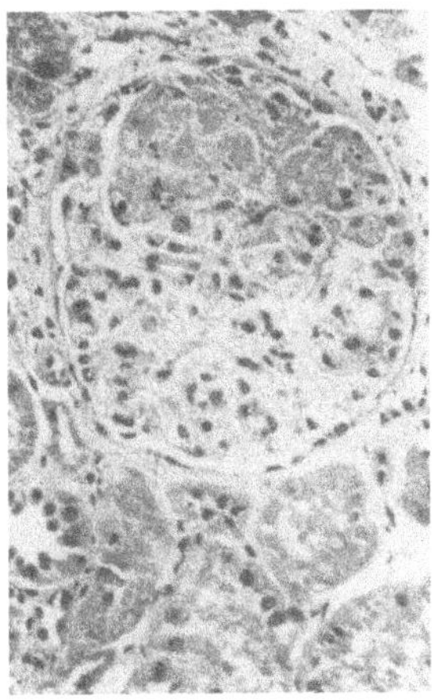

Fig 1. HE-400x; necrotic segmental and acellular area of glomerulus

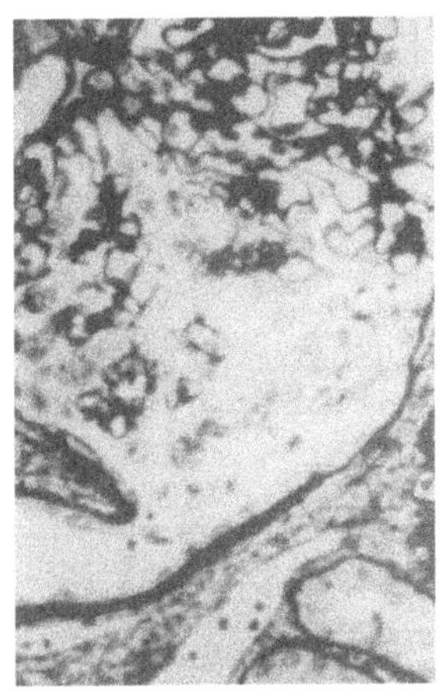

Fig 2. Silver methenamine -400x; segmental proliferation of parietal epitelial cells, forming epitelial crescent

DISCUSSION

Renal micropolyarteritis is a frequent cause of "glomerular" acute renal failure, as pointed out in recent studies (3-5). Although the possible association between NSAID and renal micropolyarteritis has been reported (1,2), the role of these drugs in inducing or in worsening the disease is unclear. In the present case the relationship between the assumption of diclofenac and naproxen and the acute phase of the disease has witnessed by the patient's history and by the observed histological and laboratory findings. In fact, the patients developed acute symptoms few weeks after the assumption of diclofenac and naproxen. The following findings confirm this association: a) increased serum IgE; b) eosinophilia; c) rashes; d) severe interstitial nephritis; e) IgE deposits in the vascular and tubular structures of the kidney. A role of allergic factors other then NSAID can be excluded on the basis of the clinical history. However, what should be pointed relevant only in aggravating a pre-existing vasculitic background. The second acute episode appears paradoxically to confirm this interpretation; in fact, only a mild allergic component was present and no significant improvement of renal function occurred despite the treatment with steroids.

In conclusion, our data suggest that micropolyarteritis may be rapidly aggravated by NSAID: for this reason, these drugs should be avoided when a sudden onset of arthralogias and arthritis is associated with other symptoms (e.g. rashes, weakness, respiratory symptoms) suggesting an underlying vasculitis.

REFERENCES

1. Serra A, Cameron JS,: Clinical and pathologic aspects of renal vasculitis. Seminars in Nephrology 5: 15-33,1985.
2. Leung ACT, Mc Lay A, Bobbie JW, Boulton Jones JM: Phenylbutazone-induced systemic vasculitis with crescentic glomerulonephritis. Arch Int Med 145: 685-687, 1985.
3. Savage COS, Winearls CG, Evans DJ, Rees AJ, Lockwood CM. Microscopic polyarteritis: presentation, pathology and prognosis. Quart J Med 56: 467-483, 1985.
4. Coward RA, Handy Nat, Shortland JS, Brown CB: Renal micropolyarteritis: a treatable condition. Nephrol Dial Transplant 1: 31-37, 1986.
5. Fuiano G, Cameron JS, Raftery M, Hartley BH, Williams DG, Ogg CS. Improved prognosis of renal microscopic polyarteritis in recent years. Nephrol Dial Transplant, 1988 (in press).

RANDOMIZED MULTI CENTER STUDY COMPARING NEPHROTOXICITY OF CEFTAZIDIME VERSUS THE COMBINATION OF PIPERACILLIN AND NETILMICIN WITH AND WITHOUT FUROSEMIDE

A. Werner Mondorf, Christina Bonsiepe and Wolfgang Mondorf

Zentrum der Inneren Medizin der Universitatskliniken Frankfurt

Theodor-Stern-Kai 7, D-6000 Frankfurt 70, FRG

INTRODUCTION

In human subjects, it is very difficult to correlate the extent of tissue damage and change in kidney function during administration of potentially nephrotoxic durgs (1-3). The rise of creatinine in the serum and the decrease of creatinine clearance are a late manifestation of renal nephrotoxicity (4). In early phases of renal nephrotoxicity, the so-called "creatinine blind phase", the release of several renal tissue enzymes can be used an markers of early tissue damage (5). Among those enzymes are: alanine-aminopeptidase (AAP), alkaline phosphatase (AP), gamma-glutamyl-transpeptidase (g-GT), n-acetyl-β-d-glucosaminidase (NAG) etc. (6). Previous clinical results did show that increasing elimiation of the brush border enzyme AAP always preceded changes of functional parameters (7). For assessment of tubular toxicity of drugs in clinical trials AAP determination in urine is useful because of the recognition of tubular alteration or injury in an early phase long before glomerular paramenters show definite changes. Effects of aminoglycosides in recommended dosages lead to an alteration of tubular cells with the release of increasing amounts of marker enzymes into urine according to the accumulation of the drug in the tubular cells (8). AAP elimination in urine is dependent on dose regimen and sex (9). During tubular alteration of the total amount of enzyme activity in tubular cells increase (10). Lesions of tubular cells are characterized by the appearance of aggregates of enzymes and membrane fragments in urine. In this stage the creatinine-clearance decrease. During tubular necrosis filaments and cytoskeleton appears in urine (6), e.g. under treatment with cis-paltinum (7). In volunteer studies we need such early phase paramenters, since it would not be ethical to continue the application of drugs up to the point when we recognize changes in serum creatinine or decreasing creatinine-clearance. For the following reasons we chose the AAP as an useful parameter for determination of toxic tubular alteration or damage.

1. Superficial localization of the AAP at the luminal side of the microvilli of the proximal tubule. A huge surface is densely covered with this enzyme.

This localization results in an early release of this enzyme caused by tubulo-toxic drugs.
2. Under normal conditions metabolic processes result in highly constant individual as well as interindividual daily release of this enzyme.
3. AAP has a high in vitro stability. It can be stored for weeks at +4°C and for month at -20°C when glycerol 1:10 is added (11).

MATERIAL AND METHOD

The present study deals with the evaluation of tubular toxicity in patients undergoing severe infections comparing piperacillin (PIP) in combination with netilmicin (NET) and ceftazidime (CAZ) as a single drug. The study was designed as a prospective open , randomized comparative multicenter study. A total of 100 patients participated in the study and 95 patients could be evaluated for nephrotoxicity (table 1).

Table 1

C E F T A Z I D I M E n = 49	2 x 2g / d
P I P E R A C I L L I N + N E T I L M I C I N n = 46	200 -300mg /kg / d 4 - 6mg /kg / d

Within a maximum of 10 days the patients were treated with the single drug CAZ or the combination of PIP plus NET. Urinalysis and AAP excretion in 24h urines as well as serum creatinine were determined. The kinetic activity of AAP measured in untreated urine specimens. L-alanine-p-nitrilide was used as the substrate (Merck, Darmstadt) for AAP in phosphate buffer at pH 7.6. In the test batch 0.2ml of a 1.66×10^{-2}M solution of l-alanine-p-nitranilide was used, into which 0.4ml untreated urine was pipetted and made up to a final volume of 2ml with 0.1M phosphate buffer, 1.4ml. The measurement was carried out in a 405nm photometer at 25°C. All enzyme activities as measured were converted to 24h excretion. For storage all samples were added glycerol (1:10) for preservation of the enzymes and afterwards deep-freezed at -20°C.

RESULT AND DISCUSSION

Characterization of group members

Basis data did not differ in both groups (table 2). Within both groups no difference of age could be seen. Male and female were nearly equally distributed. In both groups of patients general status of health was evaluated mostly as poor, especially in the PIP+NET group which showed a tendency towards poor status of health (figure 1). Severity of main infection did show that severe infections were slightly higher represented in the PIP+NET group (figure 2).

Table 2

C A Z	No of patients: 49	age: 66(mean)	male: 53%	female: 47%
P I P + N E T	" 46	" 63	" 59%	" 41%

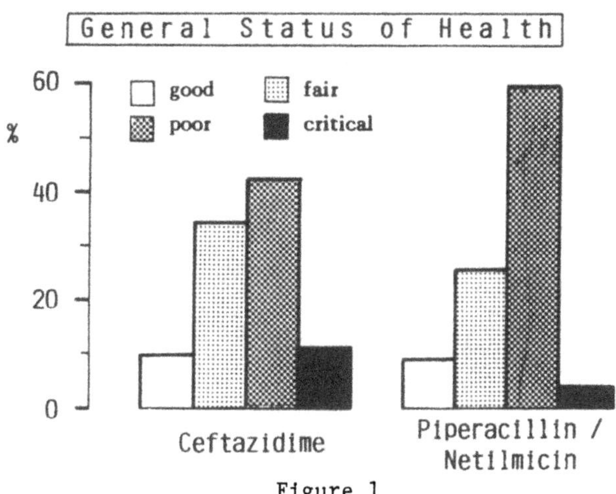

Figure 1

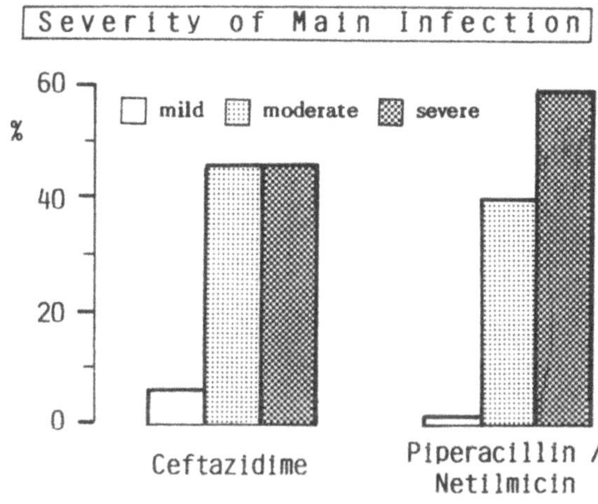

Figure 2

Behavior of AAP during treatment with different antibiotics

49 patients were treated with CAZ and 46 with the combination of PIP+NET. The behavior of AAP activity in 24h urine before (0), during (1-10), immediately post (ipost) and post treatment day(day) is demonstrated in Fig. 3. Comparing both treatment groups the AAP elimination showed marked differences. In the CAZ group the AAP excretion remained nearly constant with no significant change compared to pretreatment days. In contrast to this findings the treatment with PIP+NET resulted in a fourfold higher AAP-excretion in relation to the pretreatent days. Both groups had an equally onset of AAP-activity in 24h urine which was 3 to 5 times above normal (normal values of AAP for male ranges between 2.500 and 3.500mU/24h and for female between 1.500 and 2.500mU/24h (5).

Serum creatinine decreased in the CAZ grou, by an avergae of -8µmol/l and creatinine-clearance increased +10ml/min. In the PIP+NET group we found the opposite results. Serum creatinine increased +8µmol/l and creatinine-clearance decreased -5ml/min. (figure 4).

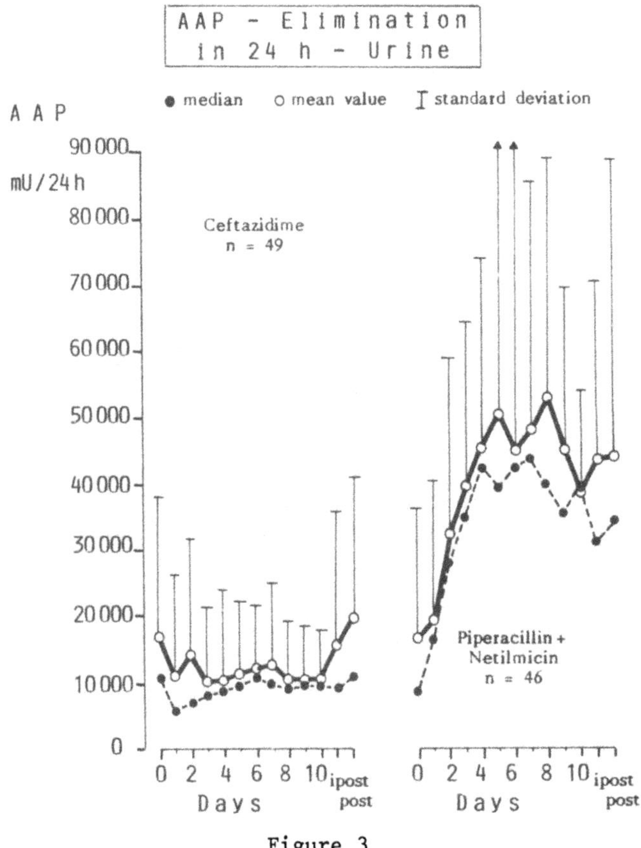

Figure 3

Additional treatment with furosemide

We investigated in both groups wether the combination of the studied drugs with furosemide revealed higher nephrotoxicity. Furosemide was given 40-80mg per day. In the CAZ group 8 patients who received additionally furosemide did not show marked increase of AAP elimination. In the PIP+NET group we found a tendency towards lower amounts of AAP in 24h urine. We assume that this effect is probably related to a higher wash out effect of the aminoglycosides. Any additive effects could not be demonstrated (figure 5).

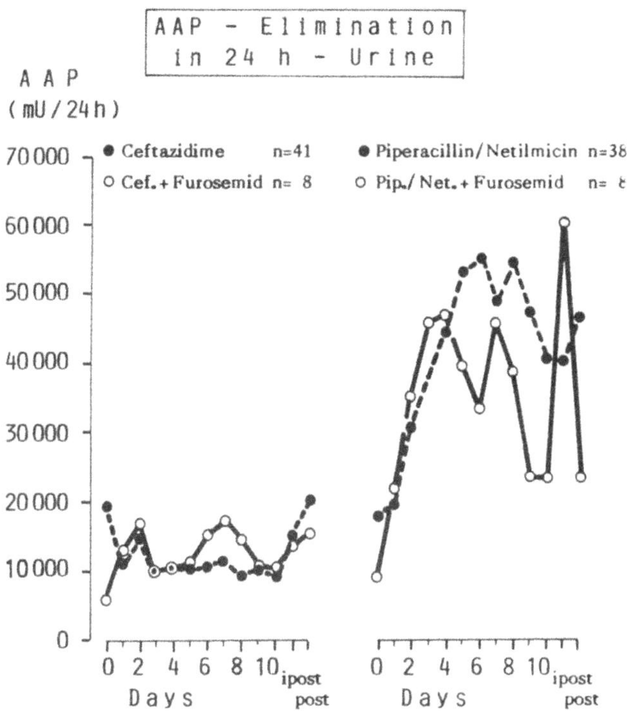

Figure 4. Creatinine in serum.

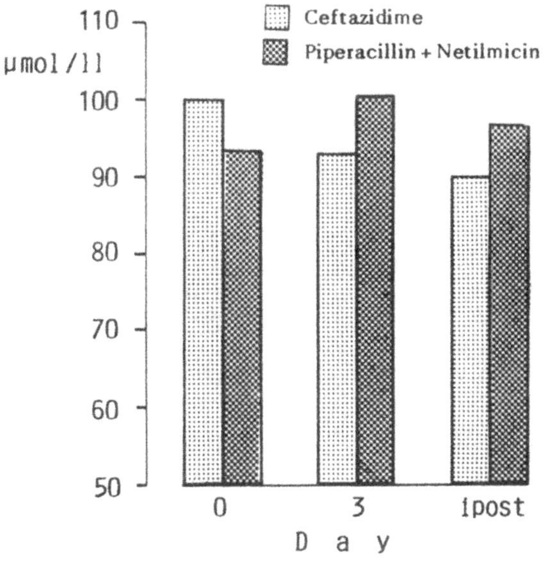

Figure 5

CONCLUSION

In a prospective open, randomized comparative multicenter study we evaluated the potential nephrotoxicity of ceftazidime (CAZ) as a single drug versus the combination of piperacillin (PIP) with netilmicin (NET). A total of 95 patients have been under investigation. The basic datas of 49 patients in the CAZ group and the 46 in the PIP+NET group were equally distributed. This was also true for the severity of main infection. Incidentally poor general status of health was more commonly seen in the PIP+NET group. The AAP activity in 24h urine before treatment in both groups was 3-5 times higher. This reflects the general morphological involvement of the kidney in the disease. Subsequently the treatment with CAZ resulted in no changes of the AAP elimination whereas in the PIP+NET group a significant increase could be demonstrated. In each group 8 patients received furosemide additionally. In the CAZ group AAP elimination was nearly uninfluenced. In the PIP+NET group a slight decrease could be seen. We assume that this decrease is obviously related to the higher wash out effect of the aminoglycosides. Any additive effect of the simultaneous application of furosemide with this antibiotics could not be seen.

LITERATURE

1. L.F. Prescott, Assessment of nephrotoxicity, Br.J.clin.Pharmacol. 13: 303-311 (1982).
2. R.G. Price, Urinary Enzymes, Nephrotoxicity and Renal Disease, Toxicology 23: 99-134 (1982).
3. U. Burchardt, G. Schinkothe, K. Meinel, D. Anton, I. Krebbel and L. Neef, Aminoglycosidnephropathie, Z. Gesmt Inn. Med. 37: 388-392 (1982).
4. A.W. Mondorf, W. Schoeppe, Is the Potential Nephrotoxicity of Drugs Predictable?, Contributions to Nephrology 42: 39-99 (1984).
5. A.W. Mondorf, J. Breier, J. Hendus, J.E. Scherberich, G. Mackenrodt, P.M. Shah, W. Stille, W. Schoeppe, Effect of amonoglycosides on proximal tubular membranes of the human kidney, Eur. J. Clin. Pharmacol. 13: 133-142 (1978).
6. F.W. Falkenberg, U. Mondorf, D. Pierard, C. Gauhl, A.W. Mondorf, U. Mai, G. Kantwerk, U. Meier, A. Rindhage, M. Rohracker, Identification of Fragments of Proximal and Distal Tubular Cells in the Urine of Patients und Cytostatic Treatment by Immunoelectronmicroscopy with Monoclonal Antibodies, American Journal of Kidney Diseases, Vol IX, No 2: 129-137 (1987).
7. P.S. Mitrou, A.W. Mondorf, U. Otto, K. Völker, B. Simon, cis-Platinum nephrotoxicity: effect o excretion of tubular membrane enzyme alanine aminopeptidase, 11th Int. Congr. Chemother., vo. 2: 1709-1711 (1979).
8. P.G. Davey, A.M. Geddes, D.M. Cowley, Study of alanine aminopeptidase excretion as a test of gentamicin nephrotoxicity, J. Antimicrob. Chemother. 11: 455-465 (1983).
9. A.W. Mondorf, Urinary enzymatic marker of renal damage, in Whelton, Neu, The aminoglycosides, Dekker, New York: 283-301 (1982).
10. G. Heinert, A.W. Mondorf, Quantiative enzymatic and immunologic histophotometry of diseased human kidney tissues using TV-camera and computer-assisted image processing systems, Proc. 1st Int. Symp. Med. Imaging and Image Interpretation: 232-238 (1982).
11. M. Nakamura, T. Itoh, K. Miyata, T. Uchisaka, T. Tanabe, M. Aono, K. Kimura, Protection by Glycerol of Urinary -L-Alanine Aminopeptidase Activity from Freezing and Thawing Inactivation, Toxicology Letters 21: 321-324 (1984).

MECHANISM OF THE MITOCHONDRIAL RESPIRATORY TOXICITY OF CEPHALOSPORIN ANTIBIOTICS

Bruce M. Tune

Department of Pediatrics
Stanford University
Stanford, California, USA

INTRODUCTION

The beta-lactam antibiotics exert their antimicrobial action by acylating and inactivating several functionally important bacterial membrane-bound proteins (Waxman and Strominger, 1983). This action is highly specific, and the beta-lactams have, in general, very favorable toxic-therapeutic ratios. However, several cephalosporins (Tune, 1986), and the new thienamycin antibiotic imipenem (Birnbaum et al., 1985), can cause acute renal failure when given under high-risk conditions. This toxicity is seen as an acute proximal tubular necrosis (Silverblatt et al., 1970), occurs in proportion to the concentrative uptake of the antibiotics by the tubular cell (Tune, 1975), and is prevented by inhibitors of this secretory transport (Tune and Fravert, 1980a).

There is circumstantial evidence that the toxic cephalosporins exert their nephrotoxic action by acylating tubular cell proteins (Browning and Tune, 1983). They reach concentrations in the tubular cell two to four orders of magnitude higher than in any other cell type, and they both acylate cellular proteins and are nephrotoxic in approximate proportion to their cellular concentrations (Tune, 1986) and beta-lactam reactivity (Yamana et al., 1976; Indelicato et al., 1977).

Cephalosporin-induced tubular necrosis follows an ultrastructural pattern (Silverblatt et al., 1970) closely resembling that of acute ischemic injury (Venkatachalam et al., 1978), and the cephalosporins may directly inhibit renal cortical mitochondrial respiration after in vitro or in vivo exposure. This mitochondrial toxicity affects respiration with succinate more than with glutamate plus malate as substrates (Tune and Fravert, 1980b). Because glutamate and malate contribute electrons to the respiratory chain proximal to succinate, the predominant involvement of succinate-driven respiration suggests a toxic injury outside the mitochondrial matrix.

Table 1. PATTERNS OF CEPHALOGLYCIN TOXICITY TO RENAL CORTICAL MITOCHONDRIA

Exposure	V_{max}[a]	K_m[b]
Control	262 ± 18	4.0 ± 0.3
In vitro[c]	229 ± 13	13.3 ± 3.1
	NS	P < 0.005
In vivo[c]	108 ± 9	2.0 ± 0.2
	P < 0.001	P < 0.001

a. V_{max} of oxygen consumption (µatom Eq/min per g prot) with succinate as substrate, calculated from double reciprocal plots of substrate concentration vs rate (ADP present).
b. K_m as 10^{-3} M.
c. Cephaloglycin 1000 µg/ml in vitro, 200 mg/kg in vivo.

There are certain important differences (Table 1) between the mitochondrial toxicity of the cephalosporins seen after in vitro or in vivo exposure (Bendirdjian et al., 1982). In vitro toxicity occurs with both nontoxic and nephrotoxic cephalosporins, is immediate in onset, and is reversed by increases in respiratory substrate concentration. In vivo toxicity is specific to the nephrotoxic cephalosporins, is delayed in onset, and is not overcome by substrate excess.

A hypothesis developed to explain these features of respiratory toxicity proposes that all of the cephalosporins can fit the carriers for mitochondrial anionic substrate uptake (Tune, 1986). In the intact kidney, where natural substrates are abundant, this fit causes limited or transient respiratory inhibition with the nontoxic cephalosporins. In vivo toxicity, which is seen after later isolation and washing of the mitochondria, develops with the comparatively sequestered and reactive cephalosporins that acylate these carriers, causing irreversible injury to substrate uptake.

METHODS AND RESULTS

To test this hypothesis we studied the uptake of 14-C-succinate and 3-H-adenosine diphosphate (ADP) by renal cortical mitochondria from New Zealand white rabbits using the method of sieve filtration (Palmieri and Klingenberg, 1979). Uptake was studied after in vivo and in vitro exposure to cephaloglycin (Cgl), which is highly nephrotoxic, and cephalexin (Clx), which is nontoxic (Tune et al., 1988). For studies of in vivo toxicity, animals were killed one hour after intravenous administration of vehicle or 300 mg/kg body weight of cephaloglycin or cephalexin. For studies of in vitro toxicity, mitochondria from vehicle-treated animals were studied before and immediately after the addition of concentrations of the antibiotics (1000 μg/ml of Cgl and 2000 μg/ml of Clx) that produce comparable respiratory inhibition.

Mitochondria were prepared by established methods (Tune et al., 1979) at 4° C in a pH 7.4 solution of (mM) 260 sucrose, 5 Tris-HCl, and 0.2 EDTA. Studies of mitochondrial substrate uptake and respiration were done in a 20°C, pH 7.4 medium: 220 sucrose, 20 Tris-HCl, 10 sodium phosphate, and 5 potassium chloride -- plus the substrates, inhibitors and tracers indicated in individual protocols.

In studies of uptake, mitochondria were incubated at 20°C in 2 ml aliquots of aerated respiration medium for 0.25 to 5 minutes. For studies of succinate uptake (from a 1.2×10^{-6} M medium concentration), no ADP was added and 5 μg/ml of antimycin A was used to block succinate metabolism. For studies of ADP uptake (from a 4.4×10^{-10} M concentration), the nucleotide was added to the medium without succinate.

The incubations were terminated by pouring the suspensions through 0.65 μ Millipore filters on a vacuum manifold. The filters were washed twice with 5 ml of iced respiration medium containing antimycin A, then transferred to liquid scintillation cocktail and counted. Mitochondrial succinate and ADP content were calculated from the counts per filter and counts in identically quenched standards of known specific activity.

Intramitochondrial water was determined from the difference between the 3-H-water (or total aqueous) and 14-C-sucrose (or extramitochondrial) spaces. Succinate and ADP uptake were thereby calculated per gram protein and per liter water. Mitochondrial water was not significantly altered by either in vivo or in vitro cephalosporin intoxication. Measurements of substrate uptake were therefore not affected by whether calculations were made per unit protein or water. Because of limitations of space, only the results per volume water will be given here.

In vivo and in vitro cephalosporin toxicity to respiration were measured in separate aliquots of mitochondria, using a platinum electrode assembly, in a respiration medium containing 1 mg/ml mitochondrial protein, 10 mM succinate, and 0.125 mM ADP. Rotenone (5 μg/ml) was added to block respiration through NADH dehydrogenase -- proximal to succinate entry into the respiratory chain.

Figure 1 illustrates the effects of in vivo cephaloglycin exposure on mitochondrial substrate transport. Succinate uptake was reduced approximately 70% at all three sampling times (§ $P < 0.005$). ADP uptake was reduced approximately 10% at one and five minutes (* $P < 0.05$).

Figure 2 shows the toxicity of in vitro cephaloglycin to succinate and ADP uptake. Succinate uptake was reduced to a similar degree to that seen with in vivo toxicity, but there was no significant effect on ADP uptake.

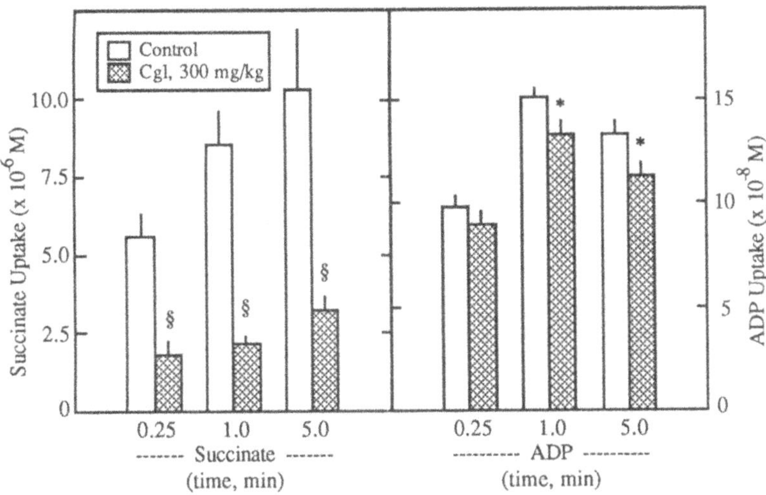

Figure 1. EFFECTS OF IN VIVO CEPHALOGLYCIN ON RENAL CORTICAL MITOCHONDRIAL SUBSTRATE UPTAKE

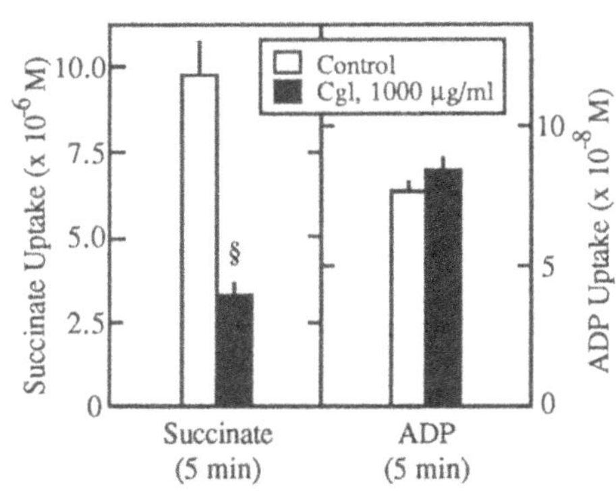

Figure 2. EFFECTS OF IN VITRO CEPHALOGLYCIN ON RENAL CORTICAL MITOCHONDRIAL SUBSTRATE UPTAKE

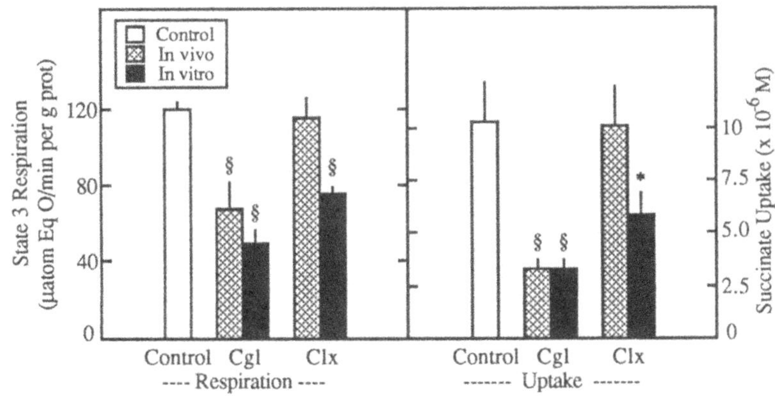

Figure 3. TOXICITY OF CEPHALOSPORINS TO MITOCHONDRIAL RESPIRATION AND SUBSTRATE UPTAKE

Table 2. SUCCINATE EFFLUX FROM CEPHALOGLYCIN-INTOXICATED MITOCHONDRIA

Treatment	Slope of washout	t-1/2[a]
Control	- 0.075 ± 0.017	4.0 min
Cephaloglycin	- 0.074 ± 0.012	4.1 min
	NS	

a. Half-life of mitochondrial washout.

Figure 3 shows the effects on respiration with and the uptake of succinate caused by in vivo and in vitro exposure to both cephalexin and cephaloglycin. In every instance, respiration and uptake were reduced in parallel patterns -- by both routes of exposure to cephaloglycin, but only by in vitro cephalexin.

These studies have measured the net uptake of succinate. To determine whether reduced uptake was due to decreased entry or increased efflux, we measured the washout of succinate in mitochondria exposed in vivo to cephaloglycin. Mitochondria were incubated five minutes with succinate and antimycin. The samples were trapped on Millipore filters, washed for three different times, ranging from 3 to 9 minutes, with 20°C medium containing antimycin, and then counted. The slopes of the logs of concentration against time, calculated by linear regression analysis in paired control and cephaloglycin-exposed samples, indicated no increased efflux resulting from cephaloglycin (Table 2). We conclude that the decreased net uptake of succinate seen with cephaloglycin intoxication is the result of reduced substrate entry.

As a test of the specificity of the pattern of cephaloglycin-induced mitochondrial injury, we examined the effects of three other insults to respiration (Figure 4) ($n = 8$-12 each). Potassium cyanide (1 mM), an inhibitor of cytochrome c oxidase (Slater, 1967), oligomycin (2 µm/g mitochondrial protein), an inhibitor of phosphorylating respiration (Slater, 1967), and unilateral ischemia (25 minutes, followed by 5 minutes of reflow) all reduced ADP-dependent respiration significantly. However, the respiratory chain inhibitors had no significant effect on the 5-minute uptake of succinate. While ischemic injury reduced net succinate transport (Figure 4) about as much as did cephaloglycin (Figure 1), it increased succinate efflux three-fold, from - 0.037 ± 0.006 to - 0.113 ± 0.021 (t-1/2's of 8.1 and 2.7 minutes, respectively) ($P < 0.005$). [The slower control effluxes in the ischemia studies, compared to those in Table 2, may have been a result of functional maturation of the mitochondria (Holtzman and Moore, 1975). Much larger rabbits (2.2-3.0 kg vs 1.6-2.0 kg, or 12-16 weeks vs 8-10 weeks of postnatal age) were used for the studies of arterial occlusion, to provide sufficient mitochondria for paired ischemic and contralateral control samples.]

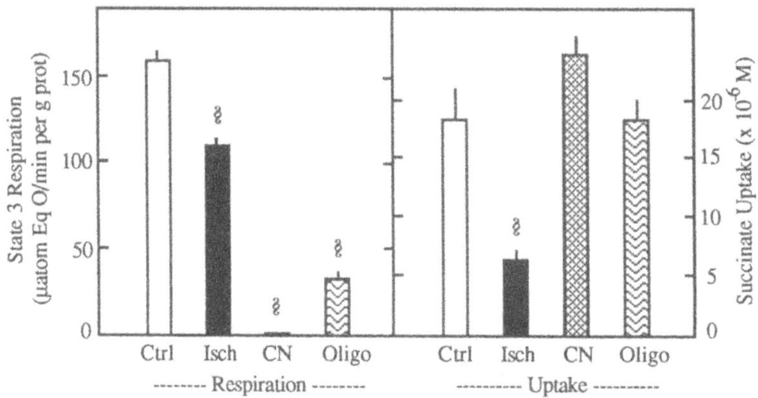

Figure 4. EFFECTS OF ISCHEMIA AND RESPIRATORY TOXINS ON MITOCHONDRIAL SUBSTRATE UPTAKE

Table 3. EFFECTS OF FRAGMENTATION ON CEPHALOGLYCIN-INTOXICATED MITOCHONDRIAL RESPIRATION

Protocol	Control	In vivo	In vitro
Intact Rate (I)	116 ± 5	61 ± 3	50 ± 8
Freeze-Thaw			
F-T Rate	115 ± 6	83 ± 5	91 ± 13
F-T/I Ratio	*1.00 ± 0.05*	*1.40 ± 0.11*	*1.89 ± 0.29*
		P < 0.005[a]	P < 0.02[a]
CCCP			
CCCP Rate	147 ± 10	70 ± 4	
CCCP/I Ratio	*1.26 ± 0.06*	*1.16 ± 0.03*	

a. P-values from t-tests comparing intoxicated to control F-T/I ratios.

In further studies, designed to allow easier access of substrate to intramitochondrial respiratory enzymes, control and cephaloglycin-intoxicated mitochondria were frozen and thawed in liquid nitrogen 3 times prior to measurement of respiration with succinate. Because fragmentation causes uncoupling of respiration, a comparison was also made between fragmented and chemically uncoupled intact mitochondria exposed to 10^{-7} M carbonyl cyanide chlorophenylhydrazone (CCCP) (Hanstein, 1976).

Table 3 shows the effects of these manipulations on respiratory rates. The ratios of freeze-thawed-to-intact and CCCP-to-intact rates are also presented. Fragmentation increased respiratory rates by 40 percent with in vivo cephaloglycin toxicity and 89 percent with in vitro cephaloglycin, which was significantly greater than control in each case. CCCP produced a slight increase of respiration that was no greater in intoxicated mitochondria than in controls. It is not clear whether the failure of fragmentation to normalize respiration completely occurred because the transporter normally functions as a receptor, facilitating substrate access to the respiratory chain, or resulted from a toxic effect of cephaloglycin on the respiratory chain itself.

SUMMARY/CONCLUSIONS

In summary, cephaloglycin, a nephrotoxic cephalosporin, produces a specific pattern of mitochondrial toxicity, decreasing both respiration with and the net uptake of succinate in renal cortical mitochondria after either in vivo or in vitro exposure, with no effect on succinate efflux. There is little or no reduction of ADP uptake by the same toxic exposures. Cephalexin, which is not toxic in vivo, inhibits respiration and uptake only with in vitro exposure. Fragmentation of mitochondria, which allows access of succinate to intramitochondrial enzymes without the need for carrier-mediated uptake, partially corrects the respiratory toxicity of cephaloglycin. We conclude that cephalosporin toxicity to succinate transport parallels the pattern of injury to mitochondrial respiration and may be pathogenic in this respiratory toxicity. These observations are consistent with the hypothesis that a) both nephrotoxic and nontoxic cephalosporins can fit the carriers for mitochondrial anionic substrate transport, and b) in situ nephrotoxicity develops as inhibition of transport becomes irreversible through acylation of these carriers.

ACKNOWLEDGMENTS: The data in Figures 1 to 3 and Tables 2 and 3, modified from Tune et al., 1988 © American Society for Pharmacology and Experimental Therapeutics, are reproduced with permission. This work was supported by grants from the National Institutes of Health (DK 33814) and the American Heart Association (85-0979) with funds contributed by the Northern California Heart Association.

REFERENCES

Bendirdjian, J.-P., Prime, D.J., Browning, M.C., and Tune, B.M.: The mitochondrial respiratory toxicity of cephalosporins - Molecular properties and pathogenic significance. In: Nephrotoxicity, ototoxicity of drugs. J.-P. Fillastre (Ed.), Editions INSERM, Universite de Rouen, France, 1982, pp. 303-319.

Birnbaum, J., Kahan, F.M., Kropp, H., and MacDonald, J.S.: Carbapenems. A new class of beta-lactam antibiotics. Discovery and improvement of Imipenem/Cilastatin. Amer. J. Med., 78 (suppl 6A): 3-21, 1985.

Browning, M.C., and Tune, B.M.: Reactivity and binding of beta-lactam antibiotics in rabbit renal cortex. J. Pharmacol. Exper. Therap., 226:640-644, 1983.

Hanstein, W.G.: Uncoupling of oxidative phosphorylation. Biochim. Biophys. Acta, 456:129-148, 1976.

Holtzman, D., and Moore, C.L.: Respiration in immature rat brain mitochondria. J. Neurochem., 24:1011-1015, 1975.

Indelicato, J.M., Dinner, A., Peters, L.R., and Wilham, W.L.: Hydrolysis of 3-chloro-3-cephems. Intramolecular nucleophilic attack in cefaclor. J. Med. Chem., 20:961-963, 1977.

Palmieri, F., and Klingenberg, M.: Direct methods for measuring metabolite transport and distribution in mitochondria. Meth. Enzymol., 56:279-301, 1979.

Silverblatt, F., Turck, M., and Bulger, R.: Nephrotoxicity due to cephaloridine: A light- and electron-microscopic study in rabbits. J. Infect. Dis., 122:33-44, 1970.

Slater, E.C.: Application of inhibitors and uncouplers for a study of oxidative phosphorylation. Meth. Enzymol., 10:48-57, 1967.

Tune, B.M.: The nephrotoxicity of cephalosporin antibiotics -- Structure-activity relationships. Comments on Toxicology, 1:145-170, 1986.

Tune, B.M.: Relationship between the transport and toxicity of cephalosporins in the kidney. J. Infect. Dis., 132:189-194, 1975.

Tune, B.M., and Fravert, D.: Mechanisms of cephalosporin nephrotoxicity. A comparison of cephaloridine and cephaloglycin. Kidney Int., 18:591-600, 1980a.

Tune, B.M., and Fravert, D.: Cephalosporin nephrotoxicity. Transport, cytotoxicity and mitochondrial toxicity of cephaloglycin. J. Pharmacol. Exper. Therap., 215:186-190, 1980b.

Tune, B.M., Sibley, R.K., and Hsu, C.-Y.: The mitochondrial respiratory toxicity of cephalosporin antibiotics. An inhibitory effect on substrate uptake. J. Pharmacol. Exper. Therap., in press.

Tune, B.M., Wu, K.-Y., Fravert, D., and Holtzman, D.: Effect of cephaloridine on respiration by renal cortical mitochondria. J. Pharmacol. Exper. Therap., 210:98-100, 1979.

Venkatachalam, M.A., Bernard, D.B., Donohoe, J.F., and Levinsky, N.G.: Ischemic damage and repair in the rat proximal tubule: Differences among the S_1, S_2, and S_3 segments. Kidney Int., 14:31-49, 1978.

Waxman, D.J., and Strominger, J.L.: Penicillin binding proteins and the mechanism of action of beta-lactam antibiotics. Ann. Rev. Biochem., 52:825-869, 1983.

Yamana, T., and Tsuji, A.: Comparative stability of cephalosporins in aqueous solution: Kinetics and mechanisms of degradation. J. Pharmaceut. Sci., 65:1563-1574, 1976.

DRUGS-INDUCED RENAL DISEASES: PERSONAL CONTRIBUTION

E. Lusvarghi, M. Leonelli, L. Furci, and A. Baraldi

Nephrology and Dialysis Unit
University of Modena, Italy

INTRODUCTION

Renal disease induced by drugs (1-12) have increased in geometrical progression over the last 20 years.
The incidence of acute drug-induced renal disease has risen from 5 to 25% in this period; the drugs most commonly involved continue to be antibiotics, followed by $NSAID_S$ radiocontrast agents and analgesic mixtures (1,2,6,7,13,15).
Predisposing factors towards acute renal failure (ARF), generally responsible for intrarenal plasma flow, have been identified in previous diuretic therapy, sodium depletion, congestive heart failure, underlying chronic renal failure, hypotension, diabetes, hepatocellular insufficiency and old age (that hinders reconstruction of damaged tubular cells) (15).
Chronic nephropathies mainly arise from incorrect or excessive use of analgesic mixtures and/or $NSAID_S$. Analgesic nephropathy (AN) shows striking geographical differences, according to local use and consumption, and the greater predisposition found in certain populations (9-11).
Thus the incidence of AN may vary from 1.7% in hemodialysed patients from the Philadelphia area to 30% in transplanted patients in Queensland, Australia.
This retrospective study was performed in order to focus attention on the incidence of drug-induced nephropathy, its clinical importance and the need to carry out effective prevention.

MATERIALS AND METHODS

In the period 1978-1987 we observed 133 cases of drug-induced nephropathy, of which 59 with acute renal failure and 74 with chronic course. This study gives a clinical evaluation of 39 patients with ARF, 73 with AN and 1 with nephrotic syndrome from gold salts.
Renal biopsy was performed in 12 cases: histologic study was indicated when the acute picture persisted beyond 2 weeks and in the chronic

Tab. I - **DRUG-ASSOCIATED ACUTE RENAL FAILURE (I)**

Number of cases = 39
mean age 61.39 ± 15.3
m=29 f=10 (mf=2.91:1)
ARF occurrence = home 22; hospital 17

predisposing factors	
dehydration	56.4%
underlying CRF	20.5%
hypotension	12.0%
diabetes	12.8%
hepatocell.insuff.	7.6%

ATN = 30		AIN = 5		PN = 2		GV = 2
aminoglycoside	19	cefuroxime	1	NSAID	2	cephalosporins
NSAID	7	rifampicin	1			penicillins
cotrimoxazole	2	nefopam	1			aminoglycosides
other drugs	8	propyphenazone	1			cotrimoxazole
		sulindac	1			NSAID

ATN = Acute Tubular Necrosis; AIN = Acute Interstitial Nephrites; PN = Papillary Necrosis; GV = Granulomatous Vasculitis.

nephropathies when the etiology was uncertain.
Statistical evaluation of data was performed with the chi square test, taking values of $p < 0.05$ as significant.

RESULTS

Table I shows the series of patients with ARF: mean age 61.39 ± 15.3 (limits 25-86), with a male/female ratio 1.9:1. In 22 cases the drug was taken at home, in 17 in hospital.
22/39 patients presented dehydration: in 20/22 the dehydration appeared in hospital. 8/39 presented underlying nephropathy, 5 hypertension, 3 hepatocellular insufficiency and 5 type I or II diabetes.
The drugs most frequently employed were the aminoglycosides and $NDAID_S$.
9/39 patients (22.8%) had taken one or more drugs.

Tab. II - **DRUG-INDUCED ACUTE RENAL FAILURE (II)**

signs and symptoms (n = 39)

oliguric	46.1%	leucocyturia	74.3%
non oliguric	53.9%	proteinuria	64.1%
duration oligoanuric period > 10 days	43.5%	anemia	43.5%
edema	15.3%	DIC	7.6%
hypertension	17.9%	peptic ulcera	5.1%.
macrohematuria	17.9%	fever, arthralgias, skin rash, pruritus	12.8%
microhematuria	53.9%		

clinical outcome

		ATN	AIN	PN	GV
full renal recovery	17 (43.5%)	14/30	3/5	-	-
recovery of previous renal function	5 (12.8%)	4/30	-	1/2	-
permanent renal damage	9 (23.0%)	4/30	2/5	1/2	2/2
chronic hemodialysis	1 (2.5%)	1/30	-	-	-
death	7 (17.9%)	7/30	-	-	-

Table II illustrates clinical course and outcome: ARF was oliguric in 18/39 patients (46.1%) and non-oliguric in 21 (53.9%). Non-oliguric ARF was common in the patients treated with aminoglycosides (58.8%). The anuric period exceeded 10 days in 17 patients (43.5%).

Hypertension appeared in 17.9% of patients, 43.5% presented anemia with hematocrit less than 30%, 3/39 patients developed DIC and 2 peptic ulcera(5.1%). Macroscopic hematuria appeared in 17.9%, microhematuria in 58.9%, non-nephrotic proteinuria in 64.1% and leucocyturia in 74.3%.

During the ARF period 69.2% patients underwent one or more hemodialysis treatment. Renal biopsy was performed in 8 cases: the histological finding was acute interstitial nephritis in 3 cases, acute tubular necrosis in 3 cases and granulomatous vasculitis in 2 cases.

In a follow-up of 1-9 years the outcome was: complete recovery in 17/39 patients (43.5%), recovery of previous renal function in 5 (12.88%), permanent renal damage in 9 (23.0%), death in 7 (17.9%).

One patient was put on regular dialysis treatment. The 7 patients who died and the 7/9 with permanent renal damage were over 60 years of age.

The two patients with granulomatous vasculitis underwent immunosuppressive therapy and partly regained renal function.

Table III shows the factors influencing mortality: significant were the anuria time ($p < 0.05$), creatininemia above 500 micromol/l ($p < 0.005$) and previous use of antibiotics ($p < 0.05$).

TAB. III - **DRUG ASSOCIATED ACUTE RENAL FAILURE** (III)

factor influencing the mortality rate

factors	X_2	p
age > 60 years	2.90	ns
oligoanuria	0.11	ns
duration of oligoanuria period > 10 days	4.55	< 0.05
maximum serum creatinine > 500 micromol/l	8.53	< 0.005
antibiotic administration	4.00	< 0.05
hepatocell. insuff.	0.36	ns
previous CRF	0.82	ns
hyperuricemia	0.12	ns

Tabel IV gives the cases of chronic drug-induced nephropathy. A nephrotic syndrome appeared in a woman who had long been taking gold salts for rheumatoid arthritis: renal biopsy revealed membranous glomerulonephritis; on sospension of the drug complete remission was obtained in 4 months.

73/74 (98.6%) of patients presented a chronic interstitial nephritis (CIN) from analgesic or $NSAID_s$ abuse. Diagnostic criteria were: (1) quantity of drug taken (more than 5 tablets per week); (2) time of abuse (at least 10 years continuous use); (3) bio-functional findings (hypostenuria, enzymuria, tubular acidification defect, urine sediment abnormality; (4) radiologic and ecographic findings and biopsy in cases of uncertain etiology (4 cases).

TAB. IV - **DRUG ASSOCIATED CHRONIC NEPHROPATHY** (I)

GN MEMBRANOUS n. 1 (gold salts)

ANALGESIC NEPHROPATHY (AN) - epidemiol. incidence in province of Modena (586.000 inhabitants)

Subjects examined for nephropathy	3952
Subjects with CRF	1562 (39%)
Subjects with AN	73 (1.84%)
mean age 54.9 (33-78)	
females 57 - males 16 (3.5:1)	
incidence in all patients in CRF	4.6%
incidence in all patients in RDT	14.9%

kind of analgesic abused: distribution in 73 patients

Saridon	39	Lonarid	1
Saridon plus other	18	Optalidon	3
Cibalgina	2	Various mixture	9
Knapp	1		
		Total	73

The patients mean age was 54.9 ± 16 (limits 33-78), with a female/male ratio of 3.5:1. The incidence of patients with CRF presenting in our clinic was 4.6%; that of all patients in hemodialysis 14.9%. The types of analgesic most commonly used were mixtures of phenacetin-propyphenazone-caffeine and paracetamol-propyphenazone-caffeine.

Table V illustrates the predominant symptoms and clinical course. The signs and symptoms most frequently observed were: anemia, hypertension, psychiatric disorders, proteinuria, leucocyturia, and early isostenuria.

TAB. V - **DRUG ASSOCIATED CHRONIC NEPHROPATHY** (II)

signs and symptoms (n = 73)			
anemia	55.3%	renal colic	6.9%
hypertension	33.1%	dementia	5.5%
dyspeptic syndrome	19.4%	splenomegaly	1.3%
psychiatric disorders	16.6%	proteinuria	36.1%
insomnia	13.8%	leucocyturia	36.1%
urinary infection	12.4%	hypostenuria	34.7%
polyneuritis	8.3%	erythrocyturia	18.0%
macrohematuria	6.9%		

clinical course

without RF	with RF		RDT
7	38		28 (+4)
	abuse stopped	abuse continued	
	22	16	

RF = Renal Failure; RDT = Regular Dialysis Treatment

Clinical course was as follows: 28/73 patients were put on periodic hemodialysis; 16/73 currently present progressive renal failure, 22/73 have CRF stationary following suspension of drug and 7/73 show only slightly impaired tubular function; 4/73 developed neoplasia of the urothelium; 4 patients died.
Lastly, a study performed in collaboration with Savi of Parma on a sample of 10 families of patients abusing analgesic mixtures failed to identify any association between a aplotype of the HLA system and analgesic nephropathy (16).

DISCUSSION AND CONCLUSIONS

The incidence of the drug-induced ARF studied by us amonts to 20% of all ARF observed over the last 10 years and agrees with literature data (1,2,7,12). Despite the high mortality rate (40-50%) of ARF in general, drug-induced ARF shows a lower mortality (below 20%) and more frequent, more rapid recovery of previous renal function (1,2,6,7,13,15).
Among our patients mortality was 17.9%, full and partial recovery were 56.3%. In agreement with the literature, the most commonly involved drugs were the aminoglycosides and antibiotics in general. User of these latter is significantly related to the mortality rate, as already pointed out by Kleinknecht (15). It should also be remembered that 43.5% of our patients took the drugs in hospital and 89% of these patients presented dehydration.
A study recently performed by our unit on 20.000 families in the province of Modena showed that 15% of the population habitually use analgesic mixtures and $NSAID_S$ and 1.3% (4615 people) abuses these.
The experience and knowledge acquired over the four decades since drugs began to be scientifically employed make it impossible to neglect the toxic effects of drugs: it is time to establish norms of primary and secondary prevention from the various categories of drug.
Obviously the nephrologist cannot forbid the use of nephrotoxic drugs, but it is his duty to enjoin upon his colleagues a live of pratice that will assist in preventing or reducing acute and chronic nephropaties.
For example:

1) describing the nephrotoxic syndromes of the drug in question;
2) evaluating renal function with Cockroft's formula (18), before the drug is administered;
3) identifying patients at risk and avoiding use of nephrotoxic drugs or reducing the doses;
4) keeping the patient hydrated;
5) informing government authorities and setting up campaigns against abuse of analgesic mixtures and $NSAID_S$.

REFERENCES

1. J. Wellington, J.R. Manaligod, L.T. Gerardo, The renal biopsy in drug-induced nephropaties, Seminars in Nephrology 5: 264 (1985).
2. K. Cooper, W.M. Bennet, Nephrotoxicity of common drugs used in clinical practice, Arch. Intern. Med. 147: 1213 (1987).
3. M.D. Clive, J.S. Stoff, Renal Syndromes associated with nonsteroidal antinflammatory drugs, N. Engl. J. Med. 310: 563 (1984).

4. J. Carmichael, S.W. Shankel, Effects of non steroidal anti-inflammatory drugs on prostaglandins and renal function, Am.. J. Med. 78: 992 (1985).
5. K. Solez, L.C. Racusen, S. Olsen, The pathology of drug nephrotoxicity, J. Clin. Pharmacol. 23: 484 (1983).
6. M.E. De Bose, Prevention of aminoglycoside nephrotoxicity, Proc. EDTA 22: 959 (1985).
7. Societè de Nephrologie. D. Kleinknecht (coordinator), P. Landais, B. Goldfarb (methodologists): Drug-associated acute renal failure. A prospective multicentre report Proc. EDTA 22: 1002 (1985).
8. D. Kleinknecht, Ph. Vanhille, L. A. Kanfer, V. Lamaire, J. Ph. Mery, J. Laederich, P. Callard, Le nephrites interstitielles aigues immuno-allergiques d'origine medicamenteuse: aspects actuels, in: "Actualité nephrologiques de l'Hospital Necker", Flammarion ed., Paris (1982).
9. U.C. Dubach, Analgesic Nephropathy. Proc. EDTA 22: 977 (1985).
10. S.F. Maher, Analgesic nephropathy. Observations, interpretations and perspective on the incidence in America. Am. J. Med. 76: 345 (1984).
11. V.M. Jr. Buchalew, H.M. Schey, Analgesic nephropathy: a significant cause of morbility in the United States, Am. J. Kidn. Dis. 7: 164 (1986).
12. M.E. De Broe, G.A. Porter, Drug-induced nephrotoxicity: an internation symposium. Am. J. Kidn. Dis. 8: 283 (1986).
13. H.L. Corwin, R.S. Teplick, M.J. Schreiber, L.S.T. Fang, J.V. Bonventre, C.H. Coggins, Prediction of autcome in acute renal failure. Am. J. Nephrol. 7: 8 (1987).
14. N. Làmeire, E. Matthys, R. Vanholder, K. De Keyser, W. Pauwels, H. Nachtergaele, L. Lambrecht, S. Ringoir, Causes and prognosis of acute renal failure in elderly patients, Nephr. Dial. Transplant. 2:316(1987).
15. D. Kleinknecht, P. Landais, B. Goldfarb, Aspetti fisiopatologici e clinici della necrosi tubulare acuta da farmaci nell'uomo, in: "Attualità nefrologiche e dialitiche", Wichtig ed., Milano (1985).
16. M. Savi, E. Rossi, A. Lo Russo, E. Lusvarghi, D. Bonucchi, M. Minari, T.M. Neri, Lack of association between analgesic nephropathy and HLA. Preliminary results of a family study. Abstract Ninth Intern. Histocompatibility Workshop and Conference, München-Wien 9W 043 (1984).
17. E. Lusvarghi, D. Bonucchi, L. Vandelli, M. Minari, G. Malmusi, M. Savi, Analgesic abuse: epidemiologic evidence in the District of Modena, in: "Prevention in nephrology", G. Buccianti ed., Masson Italia, Milano (1987).
18. D.W. Cockroft, M.N. Gault, Prediction of creatinine clearance from serum creatinine, Nephron, 16: 31 (1976).

THE EFFECT OF PARATHYROID HORMONE ON CISPLATIN NEPHROTOXICITY

Giovambattista Capasso, Dario R. Giordano, Natale G. De Santo, and Shaul G. Massry

Chair of Pediatric Nephrology, Department of Pediatrics, Ist Faculty of Medicine, University of Naples, Italy

INTRODUCTION

The clinical use of cisplatin as an antineoplastic agent is limited by its nephrotoxicity that, in many cases, includes acute tubular necrosis and renal wasting of various electrolytes (1-4). Several studies have been performed to account for the various disorders of renal function induced by cisplatin. The decrease in GFR, for example, has been found to be related to a reduction in renal blood flow and to a lowered effective filtration pressure (5). The reported concentrating defect and the observed impaired sodium reabsorption have been associated to a defect in papillary hypertonicity found in cisplatin treated rats (6), while the potassium wasting effect is in part due to a negative potential difference induced by cisplatin in late distal segments (6). Finally the pathogenesis of cisplatin induced hypomagnesemia has been attributed to pathological changes confined to the straight portion (S_3 segment) of superficial nephrons (7). On the other hand many therapeutic strategies have been tested to reduce its nephrotoxic action: the fall in GFR, for example, can be modified by hydration, mannitol diuresis (8) and by the administration of atrial natriuretic peptide (9); moreover compounds that provide SH groups have been reported to reduce the cisplatin associated renal injury (10).

Since PTH has been implicated in some of the biochemical changes peculiar of the injured cells, in the present paper we have examined if parathyroidectomy and/or administration of exogenous PTH could affect cisplatin nephrotoxicity.

METHODS AND RESULTS

All studies were performed on male Wistar rats (Morini, Reggio Emilia, Italy). Animals received standard rat chow and had free access to water. In order to evaluate the effects of PTH on CP nephrotoxicity three experimental protocol were designed. In study I CP was injected in parathyroidectomized (PTX) rats and their renal function was compared to sham PTX rats.In study II the renal effect of exogenous PTH administration was tested on CP treated rats.In study III verapamil,a well known calcium channel blocker,was used before and after CP administration.

In the study I the rats were parathyroidectomized by electrocautery during ether anesthesia.The success of the procedure was assessed,three days later,by a decrease in plasma calcium levels of at least 2 mg/dl below pooled preoperative values.Thereafter these rats had free access to water containing 50 gr/liter of calcium gluconate. This procedure is adeguate to normalize plasma calcium levels in PTX.Another group of rats underwent sham-PTX surgical procedure. Nine days after the surgery both groups of animals were injected intraperitoneally with cisplatin (Platinex,Bristol) using 10 mg/kg BW of CP and studied 72 hours later. The results of this set of experiments are reported in Table I.

Table I Effect of parathyroidectomy on BUN and serum creatinine of cisplatin treated rats.

	Sham-PTX	PTX
BUN (mg/dl)	115 $\pm$ 19	76 $\pm$ 5 *
S_{cr} (mg/dl)	2.91 $\pm$ 0.56	1.99 $\pm$ 0.14 *

* $p<0.05$

The study II was designed to ascertain if the effect of parathyroidectomy on CP nephrotoxicity was related to the absence of PTH. To this end we injected 50 IU twice daily of bovine 1-84 PTH (Sigma,S.Louis,USA) for a total of 9 days,four days prior and five days after CP (6 mg/kg BW) administration.Rats were studied 5 days after CP and their renal function was compared to rats that underwent the same cisplatin treatment,but that were injected only with PTH diluent (Sham-PTH).The results of this set of experiments are reported in table II.

Table II Effect of PTH administration on cisplatin nephrotoxicity.

	Sham-PTH	PTH
BUN (mg/dl)	97 $\pm$ 20	153 $\pm$ 22 *
S_{cr} (mg/dl)	1.63 $\pm$ 0.19	2.23 $\pm$ 0.16 *

* $p<0.05$

In the third set of experiment we wanted to test if PTH effects on CP nephrotoxicity could be mediated by an increase in intracellular calcium concentration,related to an activation of voltage dependent calcium channels.We therefore injected verapamil to a group of rats that have received CP.Since it has been reported (11) that in the ischemic model of acute renal failure (ARF) verapamil has a beneficial effect only when it was given before the induction of ARF, the rats were treated with 4 mg/kg of verapamil nine days before and three days after CP administration (10 mg/kg BW).In this case the rats were studied 72 hours after the CP treatment and their renal function was compared with a sham-verapamil group.The results of these experiments are reported in table III.

Table III Effect of verapamil on cisplatin nephrotoxicicty

	Control	Verapamil
BUN (mg/dl)	84 ± 10	113 ± 9
S_{cr} (mg/dl)	1.34 ± 0.05	1.49 ± 0.012

DISCUSSION

Cisplatin (CP) is a recently developed antineoplastic agent that has a remarkable broad spectrum of clinical activity in the treatment of solid tumors (1). However the clinical use of the drug is largely hampered by its nephrotoxicity. In fact the degree of renal toxicity rather than the therapeutic response often determines the dosage of this therapeutic agent (2).

Very recently Bennet (12) using renal functional criteria and renal cortical slices transport as well as renal morphology,has shown that parathyroidectomy modifies experimental gentamicin nephrotoxicity.Moreover the same author has reported that parathyroid hormone given to a separate group of parathyroidectomized rats eliminated the protective effect of parathyroidectomy on renal structure and function.

Indeed using renal functional criteria such as BUN and S_{cr} we were able to demonstrate an important role of PTH in the drug nephrotoxicity.Although in parathyroidectomized rats it was not possible to prevent renal failure enterely,the absence of parathyroid hormone significantly reduced cisplatin nephrotoxicity both in the short and in the long term courses of cisplatin treated rats. Furthemore the exogenous administration of PTH,in the presence of unchanged blood calcium levels,clearly increased the susceptibility of the renal tissue to cisplatin injury. Taking together the data collected in these two set of experiments are consistent with the hypothesis that parathyroid hormone suppression is a mediator of beneficial effect on cisplatin nephrotoxicity.

Since PTH increase calcium influx across plasma membrane,thereby raising the cytosolic calcium concentration (22), and because intracellular calcium levels have been postulated as a major determinant of cell death (14),it is conceivable to suppose that the deleterious effect elicited by PTH on cisplatin nephrotoxicity could be mediated by an increase in intracellular calcium level. Indeed the hypothesis that alterations in cellular Calcium homeostasis could be identified as the primary pathogenetic mediator of cellular injury has received experimental supports in the last few years.It has been proposed that the increase of intracellular free calcium to toxic levels transforms cellular injury from a potentially reversible to an irreversible state (15).Although calcium may enter the cell in a variety of ways,the presence of voltage dependent fast and slow channels is an important and a very effective route of calcium transport through a cell membrane that is relatively calcium impermeable. In this respect the recent advent of agents that modulate calcium entry by acting on specific classes of calcium channels,has provided an important tool by which it is possible to elucidate the nature of the cellular processes involved in the control of cytosolic calcium,also in pathophysiological conditions. Verapamil is one of these substances.It selectively impedes calcium entrance into cells via voltage-dependent slow calcium channels.The rationale to use verapamil in our studies was also strenghtened by the results of Burke and coll. (11) who demonstrated that verapamil protect kidneys from acute ischemic renal failure induced by norepinephrine.However, in our experiments,when we treated the rats with verapamil before and after the injection of cisplatin,no beneficial effect on renal function was detected. Such negative results can be interpreted at least in three ways:first,it is enterely possible that the protective effects of verapamil could be present,but at earlier stage.In this regard the experiments of Offerman and coll. are rilevant (16).These investigators have shown that when verapamil was given to patients with testicular cancer that were treated with four cisplatin chemotherapy course,it was able to prevent the early changes in renal function during the first cisplatin treatment. However although verapamil was given for the whole study period it failed to reduce the fall in renal function later on.Second,the data could also indicate that calcium could have entered the injured cells,not through specific channels,but utilizing unspecific leaks formed in a plasma membrane that had become more permeable. This possibility is not unreasonable since serum creatinine and BUN were significantly elevated three days after cisplatin injection, i.e.there was an already established acute renal failure with a very likely derangement of the membrane structure.

A third possible interpretation of the verapamil results is that intracellular calcium is not the mediator of cellular injury,at least in cisplatin nephrotoxicity.Indeed current evidences suggest that cytosolic free calcium does not increase during toxic injury (17). The present experiments cannot prove or disprove such hypothesis that deserves,in any case,a great deal of attention.

REFERENCES

1. Einhorn LH,Williams SD : The role of cisplatinum in solid tumor therapy. New Engl J Med 300:289-291,1978.
2. Madias NE,Harrington JT : Platinum nephrotoxicity. Am J Med 65:307-314,1978.
3. Chopra S,Kaufman J,Jones TW,Hong WK,Gehr MK,Hamburger RJ,Flammenbaum W,Trump BF :Cis-diamminedichloroplatinum induced acute renal failure in the rat. Kidney Int 21:54-64,1982.
4. Gordon JA,Peterson LN,Anderson RJ : Water fluid metabolism after cisplatin in the rat. Am J Physiol 243:F36-F43,1982.
5. Winston JA,Safirstein R : Reduced renal blood flow in cisplatin induced acute renal failure in the rat. Am J Physiol 249:F490-F496,1985.
6. Allen GG,Barrat LJ : Effect of cisplatin on the transepithelial potential difference of rat distal tubule. Kidney Int 27:842-847,1985.
7. Mavichak V,Wong NLM,Quamme GA,Magil AB,Sutton RAL,Dirks JH : Studies on the pathogenesis of cis-platin induced hypomagnesemia in rats. Kidney Int 28:914-921,1985.
8. Ozols RF,Corden BJ,Jacob J,Wesley MN,Ostchega Y,Young RC : High-dose cisplatin in hypertonic saline. Ann Intern Med 100:19-24,1984.
9. Capasso G,Anastasio P,Giordano DR,Albarano L,De Santo NG : Beneficial effects of atrial natriuretic factor on cisplatin induced acute renal failure in the rat. Am J Nephrol 7:228-234,1987.
10. Borch R,Pleasants ME : Inhibition od cis-platinum nephrotoxicity by diethyl-dithiocarbamate rescue in a rat model. Proc Natl Acad Sci USA 76:6611-6614,1979.
11. Burke TJ,Arnold PE,Gordon JA,Bulger RE,Dobyan DC,Schrier RW : Protective effect of intrarenal calcium membrane blockers before and after renal ischemia. Functional,morphological and mitochondrial studies. J Clin Invest 74:1830-1841,1984.
12. Bennet WM,Pulliam JP,Porter GA,Houghton DC : Modification of experimental gentamicin nephrotoxicity by selective parathyroidectomy. Am J Physiol:F832-F835, 1985.
13. Nagata N,Rasmussen H : Parathyroid hormone,3',5'-AMP, Ca^{2+} and renal gluconeogenesis. Proc Natl Acad Sci USA 65:368-374,1970.
14. Schanne FAX,Kane AB,Young EE,Farber JL : Calcium dependence of toxic cell death: a final common pathway. Science 206:700-702,1979.
15. Farber JL : The role of calcium in cell death. Life Sci 29:1289-1295,1981.
16. Offerman JJG,Meijer S,Sleijfer DTh,Mulder NH,Donker AJM,Schraffordt Koops H,Van Der Hern GK : The influence of verapamil on renal function in patients treated with cisplatin. Clinical Nephrology 24:249-255,1985.
17. Cheung JY,Bonventre JV,Malis CD,Leaf A : Calcium and ischemic injury. N Engl J Med 314:1670-1676,1986.

EFFECT OF ANTIHYPERTENSIVE AGENTS ON RENAL FUNCTION AND ON SODIUM-VOLUME STATUS

Vito M. Campese

University of Southern California
Department of Medicine
2025 Zonal Avenue
Los Angeles, California 90033

The relationship between the state of sodium-volume balance and the genesis and maintenance of hypertension is very complex. One established notion is that any sustained rise of blood pressure is associated with an adaptation of the renal sodium excretion mechanisms, as mainfested by a rightward shift of the renal function curve (1). Thus, the kidney exerts a pivotal role in the genesis and/or maintenance of any forms of hypertension independent of its etiology. This implies that the ability of an antihypertensive agent to sustain a decrease in blood pressure depends in large part on its effects on renal function.

Some have postulated that the abnormality in the renal function curve preceeds the development of hypertension and it is related to a primary inhability of the kidney to excrete a sodium load (2-3); according to this hypothesis hypertension is needed to maintain a normal sodium-volume balance in response to an increased dietary sodium load.

This concept is based on several observations. First, isolated kidneys from "pre-hypertensive" DAHL'S salt-sensitive rats excrete less sodium than kidneys from resistant rats (3). Second, renal cross-transplant studies in different strains of genetically hypertensive rats have shown that hypertension is transferred with the "hypertensive kidneys" (4-6). Third, normotensive siblings of hypertensive patients display a delayed excretion of an acute salt load (7). Finally, weanling SHR excrete less sodium than WKY rats (8). Among the renal intrinsic factors that may cause a shift to he right of the renal function curve are: increased vascular resistance, changes in glomerular basement membrane filtration coefficient, changes in renal tubular reabsorption and reduced kidney mass (9).

In patients with essential hypertension the shift of the renal function curve is more likely linked to changes in renal tubular function and/or increased vascular resistance. Increased proximal renal tubular reabsorption, measured by the renal lithium clearance, was found in patients with essential hypertension (10). Na+-K+ ATPase activity was greater in renal tubules of 5 week old SHR than in WKY (11).

Changes in renal vascular resistance have also been clearly documented in human subjects with essential hypertension. Hollenberg, et al (12-13) have shown significant abnormalities of renal blood blow (RBF) measured by the xenon wash-out technique in patients with essential hypertension of different age. In a group of young hypertensives under the age of 35 years, they found a bimodal distribution of renal blood flow. In a subgroup, representing about two thirds of young hypertensive patients, they observed an average reduction in RBF of 20%. Due to the striking variability of RBF in hypertensive but not in normotensive and to the reversibility of this abnormality after the administration of phentolamine they attributed this reduction to increased activity of the sympathetic nervous system (SNS). In a smaller subset of patients, renal blood flow was increased (11). Other investigators have also observed increased RBF in younger patients with essential hypertension (13). No convincing explanation for this renal functional abnormality has been put forward.

In older patients with advanced nephrosclerosis, renal blood flow was decreased and it was not significantly affected by intrarenal administration of vasodilators such acetylcholine, dopamine, or phentolamine (14). This suggests that the renal vascular abnormalities in advanced nephrosclerosis are largely fixed and related to organic changes.

Several lines of evidence, on the other hand, suggest that the deranged renal function curve may be a consequence of hypertension and of its underlying pathophysiologic mechanisms, rather than the cause. In this case, the right ward shift of the natriuresis curve would represent a physiologic adaption of the kidneys to maintain a normal sodium- volume balance in the face of increased blood pressure. Without this adaptation, a pronounced natriuresis and diuresis would ensue leading to volume depletion. Among the known factors that could be responsible for the rise in blood pressure and for the adaptation of the renal function curve are the renin-angiotensin-aldosterone and the sympathetic nervous system. Several observations support the concept that the increased activity of the sympathetic nervous system may be responsible for these renal functional abnormalities in hypertension. First, there is convincing evidence that this system may be involved in the pathogenesis of hypertension both in human subjects (15-17) and in rats with congenital hypertension (18-22). Second, as previously stated, the abnormalities in renal vascular resistance in young subjects with hypertension appear to be related to increased activity of the SNS (11). Third, enhanced activity of the SNS may inhibit renal sodium excretion by changes in renal blood flow, by activation of the renin-angiotensin system or by direct effects on renal tubules (23-26). Forth, SHR display enhanced renal nerve activity in response to stress and/or to increased dietary sodium intake (18). Finally, renal devervation or pharmacologic inhibition of the SNS can prevent the development of hypertension, and, presumably, the renal functional abnormalities in SHR (27).

The recent work of Kimura et al (28) provides the strongest evidence yet, that extrinsic factors can be responsible for the deranged renal function curve in hypertension. These investigators have recently observed abnormal renal function curves in patients with primary aldosteronism and with renovascular hypertension, which normalized after surgical correction of these diseases.

Finally, it needs to be pointed out that essential hypertension is not an homogeneous disease, but it includes subsets of patients with different pathophysiologic mechanisms. Thus, different intrinsic or extrinsic factors may alter the renal function curve in different patients. For example, the slope of the renal function curve is different in salt-sensitive than in salt-resistant patients with essential hypertension. Moreover, salt-sensitive patient display an abnormal relationship between sodium intake and plasma norepinephrine; while plasma levels of norepinephrine are suppressed during high sodium intake in normal subjects and in salt-resistant patients, they tend to rise in salt-sensitive subjects. These observations, raise the possibility that high dietary sodium intake may enhance the SNS activity and possibly the renal nerve activity in salt-sensitive patients (29). On one hand this would lead to a rise in blood pressure and to pressure-diuresis; on the other hand, the increased renal sympathetic activity would result in sodium retention. The net result is a rise in blood pressure without any significant change in sodium-volume balance.

EFFECT OF ANTI HYPERTENSIVE AGENTS ON RENAL FUNCTION

The complexity of the relationship between blood pressure and the volume-sodium state in hypertension needs to be taken into account when evaluating the effects of antihypertensive agents on renal function and on electrolyte balance. Moreover, antihypertensive agents can directly or indirectly affect renal function through a variety of frequently opposing mechanisms (Table I). Since the ability of an antihypertensive agent to cause a sustained decrease in blood pressure depends in large part on its effect on renal function, it is essential to study the renal effects of every antihypertensive agent. The purpose of this paper is to review the effects on renal function and on the sodium volume state of the most commonly used anti-hypertensive agents.

TABLE 1 POTENTIAL EFFECTS OF ANTIHYPERTENSIVE AGENTS ON RENAL FUNCTION

Alterations of systemic or intrarenal hemodynamics
Alterations of the renin-angiotensin-aldosterone system
Changes of the renal sympathetic activity
Direct effect on intrarenal adrenoceptors
Direct renal tubular effects
Alterations of vasopressine
Changes of sodium-volume state

Thiazide Diuretics

The thiazide diuretics initially lower blood pressure by reducing plasma and extracellular fluid volume and cardiac output. With long-term use, plasma volume returns to pretreatment levels while, at the same time, peripheral resistance and renal vascular resistance decrease (30,31). The decrease in vascular resistance is probably related to decreased vascular reactivity to stimuli (32). RBF, GFR and filtration fraction were also unchanged whereas PRA and urine kallikrein increased significantly after prolonged therapy with thiazides (31).

Recent multicenter trials have raised concern regarding the use of thiazide diuretics as first line choise in the management of essential hypertension, due to the fact that these trial have failed to show any reduction in ischemic heart disease or in sudden death, in spite of lowered blood pressure (33-36). This unfavorable outcome has been attributed to the undesirable side effects of diuretics which include hypokalemia, hyperglycemia, hyperuricemia and increased plasma triglycerides and total cholesterol (37). On the other hand, indapamide, a methylindole diuretic, appears to favorable affect the lipid profile (38).

Vasodilators

Non specific vasodilators include hydralazine, minoxidil, diazoxide and sodium nitroprusside.

They all cause renal vasodilation and no significant effects on glomerular filtration rate (39). Despite the favorable effect on renal vascular resistance these agents cause significant sodium retention which may offset the favorable effect on peripheral vascular resistance and mitigate the hypotensive action. Minoxidil, the most potent oral vasodilator commercially available, may cause marked sodium and fluid retention which may lead to peripheral edema and, in the most severe cases, to congestive heart failure and pericardial effusion (40).

Calcium Channel Blocking Agents

Acute administration of nifedipine causes a substantial increase in renal blood flow, no change in GFR and a brisk diuresis and natriuresis (41). In patients with the lowest RBF and GFR there was little response, probably reflecting advanced renal vascular changes. Acute administration of other calcium channel blocking agents cause similar acute renal hemodynamic changes (42-46). Chronic administration of these agents appears to have little or no effects on RBF and GFR (45,46,47). Leonetti, et al observed a rise in RBF but no changes in GFR in hypertensive patients given felodipine acutely (48). The increase in RBF and the decrease in renal vascular resistance was still present after 7 days of treatment with 10 mg twice daily of this agent. They also observed a marked natriuresis during the first and second day, but not thereafter. The sodium and potassium balance remained negative for the full duration of the study. Higher doses of felodipine can decrease GFR and cause sodium retention. Most calcium channel antagonists have little effect on potassium balance. The mechanisms for the renal hemodynamic effects of these agents are complex; however, the observed changes may be at least partly related to inhibition of the intrarenal effects of norepinephrine and angiotensin II (45,49-52). However, DiBona (53) has demonstrated that felodipine has diuretic and natriuretic properties which are due to its direct effect on renal tubular water and sodium reabsorption both in dogs and rats.

These agents appear to interfere with both proximal and distal sodium reabsorption. A proximal site of action has been suggested in experiments with nicardipine in the dogs (54). Huang (55) has shown that verapamil decreased tubular reabsorption of sodium in the proximal and/or distal tubules in the non-clipped kidney of Goldblatt hypertensive rats. Micropuncture studies have shown that felodipine interferes with sodium reabsorption in the distal renal tubule of the rat (53).

It is possible that not all calcium channel blocking agents have the same effects on renal hemodynamic. Blakshear, et al (49) have compared the effects of diltiazem and nifedipine on renal function in response to decreased blood pressure in the anesthetized dog. Diltiazem has less effects on renal perfusion and GFR than nifedipine and it activates the sympathetic and renin-angiotensin-aldosterone systems to a lesser degree than nifedipine.

Zanchetti and Leonetti (43,56) have observed that doses of nifedipine and verapamil which cause a comparable fall in blood pressure have different effects on renal function. Nifedipine increased water and sodium excretion by 100%, whereas verapamil had minimal and insignificant effects.

Beta Adrenergic Blocking Agents

Beta-adrenergic receptor blocking drugs produce variable effects on renal function. This variability cannot be accounted for by the presence or absence of cardioselectivity, nor by the effect on cardiac output, or on renin secretion.

Propranolol

Intravenous administration of propranolol reduced renal blood flow and glomerular filtration rate both in man (57), and in dogs (58). Chronic (at least 1 month) oral administration of this drug also resulted in significant decrease in glomerular filtration rate (59-60) and in renal blood flow (60-62).

Creatinine clearance in patients taking propranolol, did not reflect the magnitude of reduction in glomerular filtration rate; the fractional excretion of creatinine was inversely related to inulin-clearance suggesting increased tubular secretion with propranolol (60). The change in renal blood flow during treatment with propranolol correlated inversely with pretreatment renal blood flow, suggesting that the decrease in renal perfusion is more likely to occur in patients with higher baseline renal blood flow that in hypertensive patients with already impaired renal blood flow (61). The reduction in renal function is probably not of clinical importance in subjects with essential hypertension and normal renal function, although it may lead to reduced capacity to handle a sodium load (62) and to occasional sodium retention. The decrease in renal function, however, can occasionally become clinically significant in patients with already impaired renal function prior to administration of the drug (63). Conflicting results are available on the effect of propranolol on the sodium-volume state. Gordon (64) observed that propranolol administered for 1 month in small doses (10 mg 3 times daily) caused significant expansion of plasma volume; with higher doses, the changes in plasma volume were inconsistent. Other investigators have shown no change in plasma volume when added to diuretics (66). Wilkinson et al (67) found no changes in body weight, exchangeable sodium, and exchangeable potassium when propranolol was administered for 1 month in doses of 120 to 480 mg/day.

Atenolol

As opposed to propranolol, atenolol, a Beta 1-cardioselective adrenoceptor blocking drug, does not appear to alter significantly the renal function. In one study, atenolol did not affect glomerular filtration rate measured by 51Cr-EDTA, or effective renal blood flow measured by 125I-hyppurate clearance, in 10 hypertensive subjects treated with atenolol in doses of 50-200 mg daily for 8 weeks (68). Wilkinson et al (67) found also no changes in creatinine clearance in patients given atenolol in doses of 25-100 mg 3 times daily for 2 months. In one study, long-term administration of atenolol in elderly (65 years) hypertensive patients resulted in a 25 percent increase in effective renal blood flow (69).

No changes in exchangable sodium, exchangeable potassium, total body potassium and body weight occurred in patients treated with atenolol for 2 months (67). In a study of 13 patients with creatinine clearance ranging betwen 15 and 80 ml/min we were also unable to demonstrate any significant effect of atenolol on creatinine, inulin and para-amino-hippurate clearance, nor on exchangeable sodium or on plasma volume (see Table II).

TABLE 2 EFFECT OF ATENOLOL ON RENAL HEMODYNAMICS AND SODIUM-VOLUME STATUS

	PLACEBO	ATENOLOL
Inuline Clearance	84±12.6	83±11.5
PAH	637±136	553±89
Exchangeable Na mEq/kg	38.5±1.4	37.7±3.1
Plasma Volume	36.3±3.1	43.1±2.7

Nadolol

Nadolol administered intravenously to hypertensive patients and to healthy volunteers while ingesting 10 mEq/day of sodium induced a significant, dose-related increase in renal blood flow (70). Based on the time-course and the parallel decrease in plasma renin activity these investigators postulated that the renal vasodilation reflects the reversal of angiotensin influence on the renal arterial vasculature.

Renal perfusion was found to be preserved during chronic administration of nadolol (71). O'Connor et al (77) have found an inverse correlation between the long-term change (five to seven weeks) in renal blood flow after nadolol and pretreatment blood flow. This suggests that patients with pretreatment higher blood flow are more likely to manifest a decrease in renal blood flow during administration of nadolol. O'Callaghan et al (69) observed that nadolol reduced the effective renal blood flow by an average of 20 percent in 10 elderly patients with hypertension.

Timolol

There is little information on the effect of timolol, a non-selective beta-adrenergic blocking drug, on renal function. In one study, serum urea increased from 28±2.7 mg/dl to 34±2.4 mg/dl ($p<0.05$), and serum creatinine increased from 0.73±0.07 mg/dl to 0.98±0.08 mg/dl, in 24 patients treated with the drug for 4 weeks (73). Mean body weight increased from 73±3.8 to 75±3.3 kg.

Labetalol

This antihypertensive agent combines beta and alpha adrenergic blocking properties. Several studies have shown no significant effect of this agent on glomerular filtration rate and renal blood flow in patients with various degrees of renal function (74). Wallin (74) has also shown that this agent does not alter free water clearance and maximum urine osmolality. Larsen and Pedersen (75) have shown that labetalol does alter the change in GFR and RPF that occurs during exercise.

Converting Enzyme Inhibitors

In normotensive subjects, these agents increase RBF but have no effect on GFR, irrespective of the state of sodium balance. Under conditions of salt loading and salt depletion, biphasic saluretic response occurs which parallels the urinary excretion of the drug; this suggests a direct interference with tubular sodium reabsorption (39,76). In patients with essential hypertension these agents induce an increase in RBF twice that observed in normal subjects, despite a greater fall in arterial pressure (77), without any significant change in GFR (39). Reams and Bauer (78) have shown that inulin clearance was unchanged during enalapril treatment in patients with initial clearance less that 80 ml/min.

Navis, et al (79) studied the effect of enalapril on renal sodium excretion in hypertensive patients on 200 or 50 mmol sodium diet. On 50 mmol of dietary sodium intake, the GFR and the filtered load of sodium were lower and tubular reabsorption of sodium was higher than 200 mmol. Enalapril corrected the decrease in GFR and in filtered load of sodium, but not the increased sodium reabsorption observed during the 50 mmol sodium intake. Prolonged administration of enalapril for 12 weeks caused negative sodium balance (80). Others have shown that enalapril given for 72 hrs to patients with mild to moderate hypertension caused an increase in effective renal blood flow and fractional sodium excretion without any change in GFR, a decrease in filtration fraction and in exchangeable sodium (81).

When used in the treatment of congestive heart failure these agents may cause sodium and water diuresis, and may correct the hyponatremia (82). These effects have been attributed to the hemodynamic improvement which follows the administration of these drugs. However, it has been postulated that these agents may have unique direct effect on renal tubular function. Suki and Rose, (83) for example, have shown the captopril and enalaprilat, inhibit the hydro-osmotic effect of vasopressine on the isolated cortical collecting tubule of rabbit microperfused in vitro. This effect appears to be dependent upon activation of prostaglandin synthesis since it can be abolished by prior administration of indomethacin.

Alpha 1 Adrenergic Blocking Agents

Renal perfusion, as well as glomerular filtration rate, are generally well preserved during chronic treatment of hypertension with this drug (84-85).

Koshy, et al (86) found a small but significant increase in plasma volume in patients whose blood pressure failed to respond to prazosin; however, in patients whose blood pressure decreased after administration of the drug, there was no change in inulin or PAH clearance nor in plasma volume. Thus, it appears that this agent may decrease renal vascular resistance. Ibsen et al (87) found a significant increase in plasma volume and extracellular fluid volume when prazosin was given to hypertensive patients already receiving propranolol. A mild increase in body weight has also been shown after 3 weeks of administration of prazosin (3 mg/day), (88). Prazosin may improve renal function in patients with chronic congestive heart failure (89).

Centrally Acting Anti-Adrenergic Agents

Methyldopa

Numerous studies have examined the effects of methyldopa on renal function. Earlier studies, failed to demonstrate any significant change in renal blood flow or in glomerular filtration rate during treatment with methyldopa (90). In one study, methyldopa given in doses of 1 to 1.75 g/day for 7-10 days produced an increase in renal blood flow and in urine volume both in the supine and tilted position, in patients with decreased glomerular filtration rate (20).

More recently Grabie et al (91) have shown that acute administration of methyldopa reduced GFR and sodium excretion without altering renal blood flow in hypertensive subjects with normal GFR. These changes occurred before any demonstrable effect on blood pressure, suggesting a direct effect of the drug on renal circulation. Chronic administration of methyldopa for 1 week resulted in similar changes in renal hemodynamics and in sodium retention. The antinatriuresis was interpreted to be the result of decreased filtration of sodium and, possibly, of enhanced proximal tubular sodium reabsorption. In a similar study, Cruz et al (92) have also observed a reduction in inulin clearance and in filtration fraction without any changes in renal blood flow, free-water clearance and maximal concentrating ability in 6 hypertensive subjects with normal renal function treated with methyldopa, 250-750 mg 3 times daily for 10 days.

Guanabenz

Animal experiments have shown that guanabenz has a diuretic effect. When administered in high doses (1 mg/kg/i.v) in hypertensive rats, guanabenz lowered blood pressure, increased urine flow while decreasing urine osmolality (93). Micropuncture studies in rat indicated that guanabenz inhibits water reabsorption primarily in the collecting duct. The excretion of sodium, potassium and total solutes was also increased (93).

In the anesthetized dog, guanabenz increased water and sodium excretion and glomerular filtration rate (GFR). The increase in water excretion appears to be the result of both decreased anti-diuretic hormone (ADH) secretion and inhibition of its hydrosmotic effect on the renal collecting duct. In the anesthetized dog, guanabenz increased GFR without changing renal blood flow. The increase in sodium excretion could partially be the result of increased GFR and partially of a direct inhibition of renal tubular sodium reabsorption (94). The diuretic effect of guanabenz depends upon stimulation of alpha-2 receptors, since it is blocked by yohimbine, an alpha-2 receptor antagonist. On the contrary, neither the increase in GFR nor the increase in sodium excretion by guanabenz are prevented by alpha-1 adrenergic blockage (94). The renal effects of guanabenz are not altered by meclofenamate (93) or by indomethacin (94).

More conflicting are the data from human experiments. Acutely, after a single oral dose of 16 mg, guanabenz reduced GFR, fractional excretion of sodium and clearance of free water. In hypertensive patients, preconditioned with prior saline loading, guanabenz caused an increase in sodium excretion, in fractional sodium excretion, and in free water clearance without any change in GFR (95). Chronic administration of the drug (for 1 week to months) resulted in reduction or no changes in GFR without any significant change in renal blood flow, body weight plasma volume, sodium balance or free water clearance (96).

Clonidine

Clonidine is an antihypertensive agent whose hypotensive action has been attributed primarily to its effect on the central sympathetic nervous system. The antihypertensive effect was associated with a decrease in cardiac output, in total peripheral vascular resistance and in renal vascular resistance (97), without any significant alteration in renal blood flow or glomerular filtration rate both after acute (97), or chronic administration (98-99). In some studies, a moderate but significant decrease in creatinine clearance was observed after chronic administration of the drug (100-101).

The effect of clonidine on sodium and water balance is less clear. In rats and in dogs, acute administration of clonidine resulted in diuresis, increased urinary excretion of sodium, chloride, and potassium, and in increased free water clearance (102). These effects have been attributed to decreased ADH release and to increased intrarenal synthesis of prostaglandins, which antagonize the response to ADH. Clonidine also reduced water intake in rats by a central action which was prevented by alpha adrenergic receptor blocking agents such as tolazoline, phentolamine etc., (102).

In contrast to the findings in animal studies, the observations in man are more controversial. Acute administration of clonidine in man produced sodium and water retention (97, 103). Chronic administration of the drug has been shown to produce a small degree of water and salt retention in some studies (102) but not in others (99). In a study performed while patients were in metabolic balance, we have shown that administration of clonidine for 6 weeks in patients with essential hypertension and normal renal function resulted in a decrease in exchangeable sodium, plasma volume, and body weight (100). On the contrary, in patients with mild to moderate renal failure (GFR <80 ml/min/1.73 m_2), clonidine resulted in mild, even though not significant, rise in plasma volume and exchangeable sodium (101). Thus, the effect of this drug on the state of sodium balance may depend upon the experimental conditions and upon the degree of renal function prior to the administration of the drug.

The mechanism(s) of the natriuretic effect of clonidine and guanabenz are complex. The natriuretic action could be in part related to the action of these agents on the SNS. The influence of the SNS on the renal regulation of sodium excretion is well established (104). Acute exposure to air jet stress leads to an increase in renal sympathetic nerve activity and to antinatriuresis; this is more pronounced in SHR than WKY (18). The antinatriuretic response to air stress in conscious SHR is abolished by surgical renal denervation and it is prevented by intracerebroventricular administration of alpha 2-adrenoceptor agonists, such as clonidine (105).

Suki et al (106) have shown that clonidine in a concentration of 10^{-4}M inhibits the reabsorption of sodium in the isolated proximal convoluted tubules of rabbits microperfused in vitro. Clonidine also inhibits ADH action in the collecting tubule (107).

REFERENCES

1. Guyton AC, Coleman TG, Cowley AW Jr, Scheel KW, Manning RD Jr, Norman RA Jr: Arterial pressure regulation overriding dominance or the kidneys in long-term regulation and in hypertension. Am J Med 52:584-594, 1972.
2. Blaustein MP, Hamlyn JM: Role of a natriuretic factor in essential hypertension: A hypothesis. Ann Int Med 98:785-792, 1983.
3. Tobian L, Johnson MA, Lange J, Magraw S: Effect of varying perfusion pressures on the output of sodium and renin and the vascular resistance in kidney of rats with "post-salt" hypertension and Kyoto spontaneous hypertension. Circ Res (Suppl I): 36, 37:161-170, 1975.
4. Dahl LK, Heine M: Primary role of renal homografts in setting blood pressure levels in rats. Circ Res 36:692-696, 1975.
5. Kawabe K, Watanabe TX, Shiono K, Sokabe H: Influence of blood pressure of renal isografts between spontaneously hypertensive and normotensive rats, utilizing the F hybrids. Jap Heart J 19:886-893, 1978.
6. Bianchi G, Fox U, DiFrancesco GF, Giovannetti AM, Pagetti D: Blood pressure changes produced by kidney

crosstransplantation between spontaneously hypertensive rats (SHR) and normotensive rats (NR). Clin Sci Mol Med 47:435-448, 1974.
7. Grim CE, Luft FC, Miller JL, Brown PL, Gannon MA, Weinberger MH: Effects of sodium loading and depletion in normotensive first-degree relatives of essential hypertension. J Lab Clin Med 94:764-771, 1979.
8. Beierwalters WH, Arendshorst W, Klemmer PJ: Electrolytes and water balance in young spontaneously hypertensive rats. Hypertension 4:908-915, 1982.
9. Guyton AC: Renal function curve. A key to understanding the pathogenesis of hypertension. Hypertension 10:1-6, 1987.
10. Weber AB: Red-cell lithium-sodium counter transport and renal lithium clearance in hypertension. N Engl J Med 314:198-201, 1986.
11. Cangiano JL, Rodriguez-Sargent C, Opava-Stitzer S, Martinez-Maldonado M: Renal Na_{+}-K_{+}-ATPase in weanling and adult spontaneously hypertensive rats. Proc Soc Exp Biol Med 177:240-246, 1984.
12. Hollenberg NK, Borucki LJ, Adams DF: The renal vasculature in early essential hypertension: Evidence for a pathogenetic role. Medicine 57:167-178, 1978.
13. Bianchi G, Cusi D, Guidi E: Renal hemodynamics in human subjects and in animals with genetic hypertension during the prehypertensive stage. Am J Nephrol 3:73-79, 1983.
14. Hollenberg NK, Adams DF, Solomon H, Chenitz WR, Burger BM, Abrams HL, Merrill JP: Renal vascular tone in essential and secondary hypertension: Hemodynamic and angiographic response to vasodilators. Medicine 54:29-44, 1975.
15. Louis WJ, Doyle AE, Anavekar S: Plasma norepinephrine levels in essential hypertension. New Engl J Med 288:599-601, 1973.
16. Dequattro V, Campese VM, Miura Y, Meier D: Increase plasma catecholamines in high renin hypertension. Am J Cardiol 38:801-804, 1976.
17. Goldstein DJ: Plasma norepinephrine in essential hypertension: A study of the studies. Hypertension 3:48-52, 1981.
18. Lundin S, Thoren P: Renal function and sympathetic activity during mental stress in normotensive and spontaneously hypertensive rats. Acta Physiol Scand 115:115-124, 1982.
19. McCarty R, Kopin IJ: Alterations in plasma catecholamines and behavior during acute stress in spontaneously hypertensive and Wistar-Kyoto normotensive rats. Life SCi 22:997-1006, 1978.
20. Grobecker H, Saavedna JN, Roized HF, Weise V, Kopin IJ, Axelrod J: Peripheral and central catecholamines neurons in genetic and experimental hypertension in rats. Clin Sci Mol Med 51:377S-380S, 1976.
21. DeChamplain J, Krakoff LR, Axelrod J: Interrelationships of sodium intake, hypertension, and norepinephrine storage in the rat. Circ Res 24 (Suppl I): 75-92, 1969.
22. Anderson DE: Interactions of stress, salt and blood pressure. Ann Rev Physiol 46:143-153, 1984.
23. DiBona GF: The functions of the renal nerves. Rev. Physiol Biochem Pharmacol 94:75-181, 1982.

24. Bello-Reuss E: Effect of catecholamines on fluid reabosption by the isolated proximal convoluted tubule. Am J Physiol 238:F347-F352, 1980.
25. Schrier RW: Effects of adrenergic nervous system and catecholamines on systemic and renal hemodynamics, sodium and water excretion and renin secretion. Kidney Int 6:291-306, 1974.
26. Weinberger MD, Luft FC, Henry DP: The role of the sympathetic nervous system in the modulation of sodium excretion. Clin Exp Hypert A4:719-735, 1982.
27. Winternitz SR, Katholi RE, Oparil S: Role of the renal sympathetic nerves in the development and maintenance of hypertension in the spontaneously hypertensive rat. J Clin Invest 66:971-978, 1980.
28. Kimura G, Saito F, Kojima S, et al: Renal function curve in patients with secondary forms of hypertension. Hypertension 10:11-15, 1987.
29. Campese VM, Romoff MS, Levitan D, Saglikes Y, Friedler RM, Massry SG: Abnormal relationship between sodium intake and sympathetic nervous activity in salt-sensitive patients with essential hypertension. Kidney Int 21:371-378, 1982.
30. Conway J, Lauwers P: Hemodynamics and hypotensive effects of long-term therapy with chlorothiazide. Circulation 21:21-27, 1960.
31. O'Connor DT, Preston RA, Stone RA: Renal vascular resistance falls during long-term thiazide treatment of essential hypertension. Clin Res 27:17A, 1979.
32. Aleksandrow D, Wysznacka W, Gajewski J: Influence of chlorothiazide upon arterial responsiveness to norepinephrine in hypertensive subjects. N Engl J Med 261:1052-1055, 1959.
33. Veterans Administration Cooperative Study Group on antihypertensive agents: Effect of therapy on morbidity in hypertension. JAMA 202:1028-1034, 1967.
34. Australian National blood pressure study management committee: The Australian therapeutic trial in mild hypertension. Lancet 1:1261-1267, 1980.
35. Multiple Risk Factor Intervention Trial Researh Group: Multiple Risk Factor Intervention Trial: Risk factors changes and mortality results. JAMA 248:2465-2477, 1982.
36. Medical Research Council Working Party: MRC trial of treatment of mild hypertension. Principal results. Br Med J 291:97-104, 1985.
37. Kaplan NM: Clinical hypertension. Williams & Wilkins, Baltimore, 1986.
38. Meyer-Sebellek W, Gotzen R, Heitz J, Arntz HR, Schulte KL: Serum lipoprotein levels during long-term treatment of hypertension with indapamide. Hypertension 7 (Suppl II) II170-II174, 1985.
39. Hollenberg NK: Vasodilators, antihypertensive therapy, and the kidney. Circulation 75 (Suppl V), V-39-V-42, 1987.
40. Campese VM: Minoxidil: A review of its pharmacoligical properties and therapeutic use. Drugs 22:257-278, 1981.
41. Klutsch VK, Schmidt P, Grobwendt J: Der Einflub von bay a 1040 auf die nierenfunktion des hypertonikers. Arzneimittelforschung 22:377-380, 1972.
42. Kinoshita M, Kukusawa R, Shimono Y, Motomura M, Tomonaga G, Hoshino T: Effects of diltiazem hydrochloride on

renal hemodynamics and urinary electrolyte excretion. JPN Circ J 42:553-560, 1978.
43. Zanchetti A, Leonetti G: Natriuretic effect of calcium antagonists. J. Cardiovasc Pharmacol 7: (Suppl 4) 33-37, 1985.
44. Schmitz A: Acute renal effects of oral felodipine in normal man. Eur J Clin Pharmacol 32:17-22, 1987.
45. Bauer JH, Sunderrajan S, Reams G: Effects of calcium entry blockers on renin-angiotensin-aldosterone system, renal function and hemodynamics, salt and water excretion and body fluid composition. Am J Cardiol 56:62H-67H, 1985.
46. Chaignon M, Bellet M, Lucsko M, Rapoud C, Guedon J: Acute and chronic effect of a new calcium inhibitor, nicardipine, on renal hemodynamics in hypertension. J Cardiovasc Pharmacol 8:892-897, 1986.
47. Austin MB, Robson RA, Bailey RR: Effect of nifedipine on renal function of normal subjects and hypertensive patients with renal functional impairment. New Zeland Med J 96:829-831, 1983.
48. Leonetti G, Grandi KR, Terzoli L, Fruscio M, Rupoli L, Cuspidi C, Sampieri L, Zanchetti A: Effects of single and repeated doses of the calcium antagonist felodipine on blood pressure, renal function, electrolytes and water balance, and renin-angiotensin aldosterone system in hypertensive patients. J Cardiovasc Pharmacol 8:1243-1248, 1986.
49. Blackshear JL, Orlandi C, Williams GH, Hollenberg NK: The renal response to diltiazem and nifedipine: Comparison with nitroprusside. J Cardiovasc Pharmacol 8:37-43, 1986.
50. Steele TH, Challoner-Hue L: Renal interactions between norepinephrine and calcium antagonists. Kidney Int. 26:719-724, 1980.
51. Bell PD, Navar LG: Cytoplasmic calcium in the mediation of macula densa tubuloglomerular feedback responses. Science 215:670-673, 1982.
52. Blanc E, Sraer J, Sraer JD, Baud L, Arddillod R: Ca_{2+} and Mg_{2+} dependence of angiotensin II binding to isolated rat renal glomeruli. Biochem Pharmacol 27:517, 1978.
53. DiBona GF: Effects of felodipine on renal function in animals. Drugs 29 (Suppl 2):168-175, 1985.
54. Abe Y, Komori T, Miura K, et al: Effects of the calcium antagonist nicardipine on renal function and renin release in dogs. J Cardiovasc Pharmacol 5: 254-259, 1983.
55. Huang WC: Effects of verapamil alone and with captopril on blood pressure and bilateral renal function in Goldblatt hypertensive rats. Clin Sci 70:453-460, 1986.
56. Leonetti G, Cuspidi C, Sampieri L, Terzoli L, Zanchetti A: Comparison of cardiovascular renal, and humoral effects of acute administration of two calcium channel blockers in normotensive and hypertensive subjects. J Cardiovasc Pharmacol 4:319-324, 1982.
57. Sullivan JM, Adams DF, Hollenberg NK: -adrenergic blockade in essential hypertension: Reduced renin release despite renal vasoconstriction. Circ Res 39:532-536, 1976.
58. Nies AS, McNeil JS, Schrier RW: Mechanism of increased sodium reabsorption during propranolol administration. Circulation 44:596-604, 1971.

59. Ibsen H, Sederberg-Olsen P: Changes in glomerular filtration rate during long-term treatment with propranolol in patients with arterial hypertension. Clinical Science 44:129-134, 1972.
60. Bauer JH, Brooks CS: The long-term effect of propranolol therapy on renal function. Am J Med 66:405-410, 1979.
61. Pedersen EB: Effect of sodium loading and exercise on renal haemodynamics and urinary sodium excretion in young patients with essential hypertension before and during propranolol treatment. ACTA Med Scand 201:365-373, 1977.
62. O'Connor DT, Preston RA: Urinary kallikrein activity, renal hemodynamics, and electrolyte handling during chronic beta blockade with propranolol in hypertension. Hypertension 4:742-749, 1982.
63. Warren DJ, Swanson CP, Wright N: Deterioration in renal function after beta blockade in patients with chronic renal failure and hypertension. Brit. Med J 2:193-194, 1974.
64. Gordon RD: Effects of beta-adrenoreceptor blocking drugs on plasma volume, renin and aldosterone as components of their antihypertensive action. Drugs 11 (Suppl):156-163, 1976.
65. Tarazi RC, Frolich ED, Dustan HR: Plasma volume changes with long-term beta-adrenergic blockade. Am Heart J 82:770-766, 1971.
66. Bravo EL, Tarazi RC, Dustan HP: Beta-adrenergic blockade in diuretic-treated patients with essential hypertension. New Engl J Med 292:66-70, 1975.
67. Wilkinson R, Stevens IM, Pickering M, Robson V, Hawkins T, Kerr DNS, Harry JD: Renal function exchangeable sodium, potassium and plasma renin in essential hypertensive treated with atenolol and propranolol. In: Cruickshank JM, McAinsh J, Caldwell ADS, Eds. Atenolol and Renal Function. R Soc Med Int Congr Symp Ser #19, Academic Press, London, pp. 45-49, 1980.
68. Waal-Manning HJ, Bolli P: Atenolol (vs) placebo in mild hypertension. Renal, metabolic and stress antipressor effects. Brit J Phamacol 9:553-560, 1980.
69. O'Callaghan WG, Laher MS, McGarry K, O'Brien ET, O'Malley K: Antihypertensive and renal haemodynamic effects of atenolol and nadolol in elderly hypertensive patients. Brit J Clin Pharmacol 14:135P-136P, 1982.
70. Hollenberg NK, Adams DF, McKinstry DN, Williams GH, Borucki LJ, Sullivan JM: Beta-adrenoceptor blocking agents and the kidney: Effect of nadolol and propranolol on the renal circulation. Brit J Clin Pharmacol 7: (Suppl 2):219s-222s, 1979.
71. Textor SC, Fouad FM, Bravo EL, Tarazi RC, Vidt DG, Gifford RW, Jr: Redistribution of cardiac output to the kidneys during oral nadolol administration. New Engl J Med 307:601-605, 1982.
72. O'Connor DT, Barg AP, Duchin KL: Preserved renal perfusion during treatment of essential hypertension with beta blocker nadolol. J Clin Pharmacol 22:187-195, 1982.
73. Lubbe WF: Antihypertensive therapy with timolol and alpha methyldopa. A double-blind trial in patients with moderately severe hypertension. South African Med J 50:279-285, 1976.
74. Wallin JD: Antihypertensive and their impact on renal function. Am J Med 80 (Suppl 419):103-106, 1983.

75. Pedersen EB, Larsen JS: Effect of propranolol and labetalol on renal hemodynamics at rest and during exercise in essential hypertension. Postgrad Med J 56:27-32, 1980.
76. Lant AF, McNabb RW, Noormohamed FH: Kinetic and metabolic aspects of enalapril action. J Hypertension (Suppl 2):S37-S42, 1984.
77. Williams GH, Hollenberg NK: Accentuated vascular and endocrine response to SQ 20881 in hypertension. N Engl J Med 297:184-188, 1977.
78. Reams GP, Bauer JH: Long-term effects of enalapril monotherapy and enalapril/hydrochlorothiazide combination therapy on blood pressure, renal function, and body fluid composition. J Clin Hypertension 2:55-63, 1986.
79. Navis G, DeJong PE, Donker AJ, Van Der Hem GK, DeZeeuw D: Moderate sodium restriction in hypertensive subjects: Renal effects of ACE-inhibition. Kidney Int 31:815-819, 1987.
80. Navis GJ, DeZeeuw D, DeJong PE: Enalapril and the kidney: Renal vasodilation and natriuresis due to the inhibition of angiotensin II formation. J Cardiovasc Pharmacol 8:(Suppl 1) S30-S34, 1986.
81. Sanchez RA, Marco E, Gilbert HB, Raffaele P, Brito M, Gimenez M, Moleao LI: Natriuretic effect and changes in renal hemodynamics induced by enalapril in essential hypertension. Drugs 30 (Suppl 1):49-58, 1985.
82. Packer M, Medina N, Yushak M: Correction of dilutional hyponatremia in severe chronic heart failure by converting-enzyme inhibition. Ann Int Med 100:782-789, 1984.
83. Suki WN, Rouse D: Renal tubular actions of antihypertensive agents. Kidney Int (In Press).
84. Preston RA, O'Connor DT, Stone RA: Prazosin and renal hemodynamics: Arteriolar vasodilatation during therapy of essential hypertension in man. Journal of Cardiovascular Pharmacology 1:277-286, 1979.
85. McNair A, Rasmussen S, Nielsen PE, Rasmussen K: The antihypertensive effect of prazosin on mild to moderate hypertension, changes in plasma volume, extracellular volume and glomerular filtration rate. ACTA Med Scand 207:413-416, 1980.
86. Koshy MC, Mickley D, Bourgoignie J, Blaufox MD: Physiologic evaluation of a new antihypertensive agent: Prazosin HCl. Circulation. 55:533-537, 1977.
87. Ibsen H, Rasmussen K, Aerenlund Jensen H, Leth A: Changes in plasma volume and extracellular fluid volume after addition of prazosin to propranolol treatment in patients with hypertension. Scand J Clin Lab Invest 38:425-429, 1978.
88. Barbieri C, Ferrari C, Caldara R, Rampini P, Crossignani RM, Bergonzi M: Effects of chronic prazosin treatment on the renin-angiotensin-aldosterone system in man. J Clin Pharmacol 21:418-423, 1981.
89. Myers JB, Morgan TD, Walker JN: Effect of prazosin on renal function in chronic congestive cardiac failure. Med J Australia 2:290-291, 1981.
90. Mohammed S, Hanenson IB, Magenheim HG, Gaffney TE: Effects of alpha-methyldopa on renal function in hypertensive patients. Amer Heart J 76:21-27, 1968.
91. Grabie M, Nussbaum P, Goldfarb S, Walker BR, Goldberg M, Agus ZS: Effects of methyldopa on renal hemodynamics and

tubular function. Clin Pharmacol Ther. 27:522-527, 1980.
92. Cruz F, O'Neill WM Jr, Clifton G, Wallin JD: Effect of labetalol and methyldopa on renal function. Clin Pharmacol Ther 30:57-63, 1981.
93. Kauker ML: Inhibition of water reabsorption in the collecting tubule by guanabenz, an antihypertensive drug. Kidney Int 21:279A, 1982.
94. Strandhoy J, Morris M, Buckalew VM: Renal effects of the antihypertensive, guanabenz, in the dog. J Pharmacol Exp Ther. 221:347-352, 1982.
95. Gehr M, MacCarthy EP, Goldberg M: Guanabenz; a centrally acting, natriuretic antihypertensive drug. Kidney Int 29:1203-1208, 1986.
96. Bosanac P, Dubb J, Walker B, Goldberg M, Agus ZS: Renal effects of guanabenz: A new antihypertensive. J Clin Pharmacol 16:631-636, 1976.
97. Onesti G, Schwartz AB, Kim KE, Paz-Martines V, Swartz C: Antihypertensive effect of clonidine. Circ Res (Suppl II) 28-29: II 53-II 69, 1971.
98. Bock KD, Merguet P, Heimsoth VH: Effect of clonidine on regional blood flow an its use in the treatment of hypertension. In: 26th Hahnemann Symposium: Hypertension Mechanisms and Management Eds. G. Onesti KE, Kim JH, Moyer, New York, Grune & Stratton, pp. 395-403, 1973.
99. Thananopavarn C, Golub MS, Eggena P, Barrett JD, Sambhi MP: Clonidine, a centrally acting sympathetic inhibitor, as monotherapy for mild to moderate hypertension. Am J Cardiol 49:153-158, 1982.
100. Campese VM, Romoff M, Telfer N, Weidmann P, Massry SG: Role of sympathetic nerve inhibition and body sodium-volume in the antihypertensive action of clonidine in essential hypertension. Kidney Int. 18:351-357, 1980.
101. Campese VM, Levitan D, Romoff MS, Saglikes Y, Sajo I, Massry SG: Effect of sympathetic nerve inhibition on the state of sodium-volume balance in hypertensive patients with normal or impaired renal function. Clin Sci 63:301s-303s, 1982.
102. Schmitt H: The pharmacology of clonidine and related products. In: Antihypertensive agents. Eds. F. Gross, Berlin, Heidelberg, New York, Springer-Verlag, pp. 299-396, 1977.
103. Davidov M, Kakaviatos N, Finnerty FA: The antihypertensive effects of an imidazoline compound. Clin Pharmacol Ther. 8:810-816, 1967.
104. DiBona GF: Neurogenic regulation of renal tubular sodium reabsorption. Am Physiol 233:F73-F81, 1977.
105. Koepke JP, DiBona GF: Central adrenergic receptor control of renal function in conscious hypertensive rats. Hypertension 8:133-141, 1986.
106. Rouse D, Suki WN: Alpha -Adrenergic inhibition of fluid absorption in the rabbit proximal convoluted renal tubule Kidney Int (In Press).
107. Krothapalli RK, Suki WN: Functional characterization of the alpha adrenergic receptor modulating the hydroosmotic effect of vasopressine on the rabbit cortical collecting tubule. J Clin Invest 73:740-749, 1984.

MISCELLANEOUS TOPICS

CHARACTERIZATION OF BILATERAL RENAL RESPONSE TO ATRIAL NATRIURETIC PEPTIDE IN 2-KIDNEY, 1 CLIP HYPERTENSIVE RATS

Wann-Chu Huang and Jian-Nan Wu

Department of Physiology and Biophysics
National Defense Medical Center, Taipei
Taiwan, Republic of China

INTRODUCTION

The atrial natriuretic peptide (ANP) released from the cardiocytes of mammalian atria has been implicated in the regulation of blood pressure and body fluid balance[1,2]. Previous studies have shown that this peptide can produce vasodepressor effect through a direct arterial vasodilation or reduced cardiac output and attenuation of endogenous vasoconstrictors[2-5]. Also, it can induce a striking natriuretic and diuretic effect by changing the renal hemodynamics and tubular function[1,2,6,7]. The hypotensive and renal effects of ANP may be prominent in conditions with elevated activity of the renin-angiotensin system[7-9].

It is recognized that the renal effect of an antihypertensive agent is an important issue of concern in the management of hypertension, particularly in the case of a deranged kidney function. We have previously demonstrated that the 2-kidney, 1 clip Goldblatt hypertensive rat is an angiotensin-dependent hypertensive model, and both kidneys are characterized with different perfusing pressure and renin and angiotensin contents[10-12]. Furthermore, the excretory function of the stenotic kidney is highly dependent on the perfusing pressure. When the arterial blood pressure is reduced toward normal range by angiotensin converting enzyme inhibitors or calcium channel blockers, the excretory function of the stenotic kidney is consistently depressed whereas the nonclipped kidney always exhibits an enhanced excretory function[10,11,13,14]. Some studies, on the other hand, showed that both kidneys had different capabilities of autoregulation of renal blood flow in response to reductions in arterial pressure[15,16]. In order to investigate if ANP produces differential renal responses between kidneys in this hypertensive model, we thus performed the present study to characterize the effect of ANP on the blood pressure and the excretory function of both the stenotic kidney and the nonstenotic kidney.

MATERIALS AND METHODS

Two-kidney, one clip Goldblatt hypertensive rats (n=16) were prepared by unilaterally constricting the renal artery of Sprague-Dawley rats with 0.25 mm silver clip 4 weeks prior to study. The contralateral kidney remained intact. The sham-operated rats (n=9) served as controls. All rats were fed a commercial chow and were allowed tap water ad libitum.

At the time of the acute experiments, both hypertensive and control rats which by then weighed between 250-350 g were anesthetized with Inactin (100 ug/kg, i.p.) and were prepared for bilateral renal clearance experiments as described previously[10,13]. Inutest (polyfructosan, Laevosan-Gesellschaft, Linz, Austria) clearance was used as glomerular filtration rate (GFR). The femoral arterial pressure was monitored using a Statham P23DC transducer (Gould-Statham Instruments, Inc., Hato Ray, Puerto Rico, USA) and recorded on a P7D Grass polygraph (Grass Instrument Co., Quincy, Mass, USA).

Experiments were performed on one control group of 9 rats and two hypertensive groups each consisted of 8 rats. In control rats and the first group of hypertensive rats, ANP (atriopeptin II, 2.5-10 ug/kg) with randomized order was administered intravenously after two control clearance periods. The second dose of ANP was administered when the arterial pressure and urine flow had recovered. Two clearance collections were taken during each injection of ANP. In the second group of hypertensive rats, the unclipping procedure was carried out before ANP administration. After two initial control periods, the clip on the left kidney was removed carefully. Five minutes were allowed to elapse before proceeding with four subsequent 30-min clearance collections. ANP was then administered and the blood pressure and bilateral renal clearance were followed as aforementioned.

Plasma and urine polyfructosan concentrations were measured with an anthrone colorimetric method as described previously[14]. Plasma sodium and potassium concentrations were determined with a flame photometer (model 943, Instrumentation Laboratory, Mass., USA). Plasma and urine osmolalities were measured with an osmometer (model 3DII, Advanced Instrument, Inc., Mass., USA). GFR, electrolyte excretion rate and free water and osmolar clearances were calculated according to standard clearance formulas. The data were analyzed using both paired and unpaired analysis where applicable. The results are expressed as mean ± SEM.

RESULTS

The effects of ANP administration on the mean arterial blood pressure of both hypertensive and control rats are illustrated in Fig 1. In both

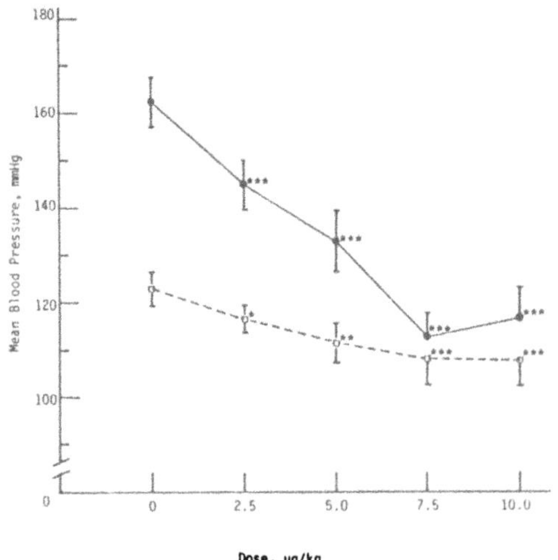

Fig.1 Effect of ANP on the mean blood pressure in hypertensive(●) and normal(○) rats. *$p<0.05$; **$p<0.01$; ***$p<0.001$ as compared to control level.

groups of rats, administration of ANP produced a dose-dependent hypotensive effect. However, the magnitude of decrease in blood pressure was greater in the hypertensive group than that in the control group.

The nonclipped kidney weighed 1.29±0.05 g which was significantly greater than that of the clipped kidney (1.03±0.04 g) but did not differ from that of the corresponding kidney of normal rats (1.13±0.04 g). The effects of ANP administration on GFR, urine flow and free water reabsorption in both the clipped kidney and the nonclipped kidney of hypertensive rats are shown in Fig 2. ANP administration caused significant increases in GFR, urine flow, free water reabsorption rate and osmolar clearance in the nonclipped kidney. There was, however, no significant change in these renal indices in the clipped kidney.

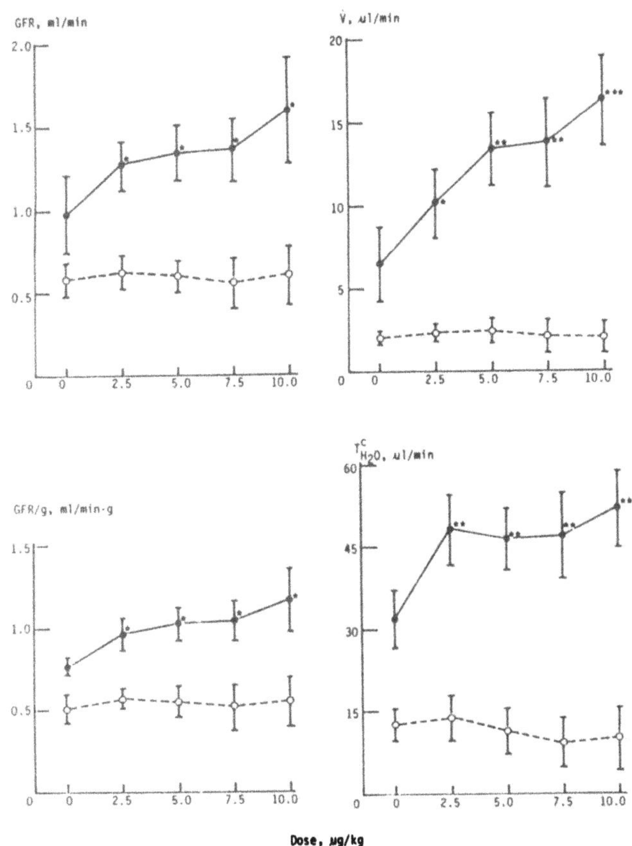

Fig. 2 Effects of ANP on glomerular filtration rate (GFR), urine flow (V) and free water reabsorption rate ($T^{C}_{H_2O}$) in hypertensive rats. ●—● the nonclipped kidney; O---O the clipped kidney; GFR/g=GFR per gram of kidney weight. Statistical notations see Fig. 1.

Fig 3 depicts the effects of ANP on the absolute and the fractional excretion rates of sodium and potassium in hypertensive rats. In the nonclipped kidney, ANP administration increased the absolute and the fractional amounts of sodium excretion. The natriuretic response was dose-related. Small dose (2.5 ug/kg) of ANP caused a kaliuresis but larger dose did not significantly change potassium excretion. In the clipped kidney, there was no significant alteration in sodium and potassium excretion rates following ANP injections.

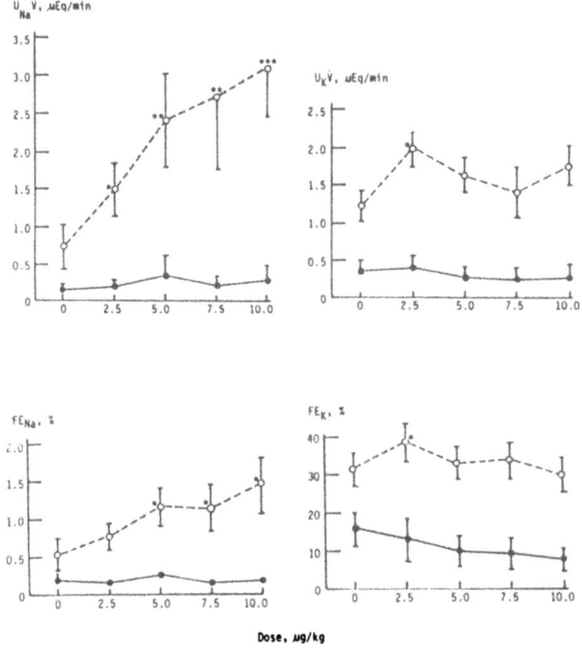

Fig. 3 Effects of ANP on the excretions of absolute sodium ($U_{Na}V$), fractional sodium (FE_{Na}), absolute potassium (U_KV) and fractional potassium (FE_K) in hypertensive rats. 0——0 the nonclipped kidney; ●--● the clipped kidney. Statistical notations see Fig. 1.

The bilateral renal responses to ANP administration in control rats are illustrated in Fig 4 and Fig 5. Significant increases in GFR and excretory function in response to ANP administration were observed in both kidneys of control rats. The increased renal function was dose-dependent. There was no significant difference in functional response to ANP between the left kidney and the right kidney.

Table 1 shows the effect of unclipping and subsequent administration of ANP on the blood pressure and bilateral renal function in a separate group of hypertensive rats. Removal of the clip reduced the arterial blood pressure and increased the function of the newly unclipped kidney. In contrast, the excretory function of the contralateral kidney was gradually declined. Subsequent administration of ANP further decreased the blood pressure but did not significantly alter the function of both kidneys.

DISCUSSION

The most interesting finding in the present study is that ANP induced

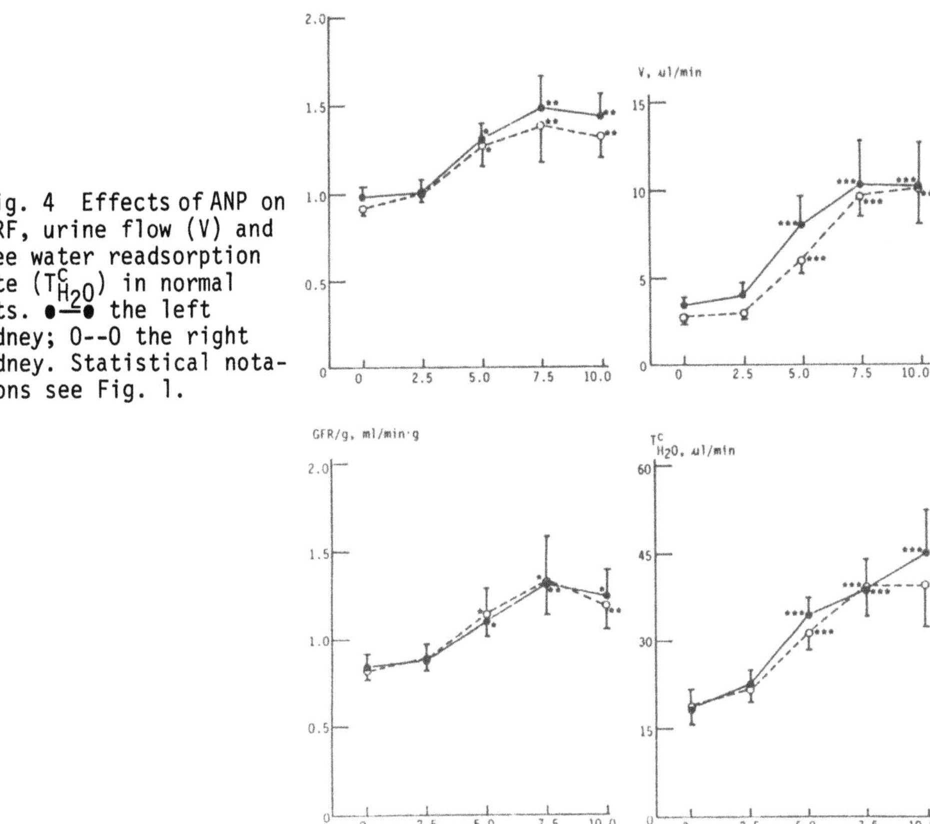

Fig. 4 Effects of ANP on GRF, urine flow (V) and free water readsorption rate ($T^{C}_{H_2O}$) in normal rats. ●—● the left kidney; O--O the right kidney. Statistical notations see Fig. 1.

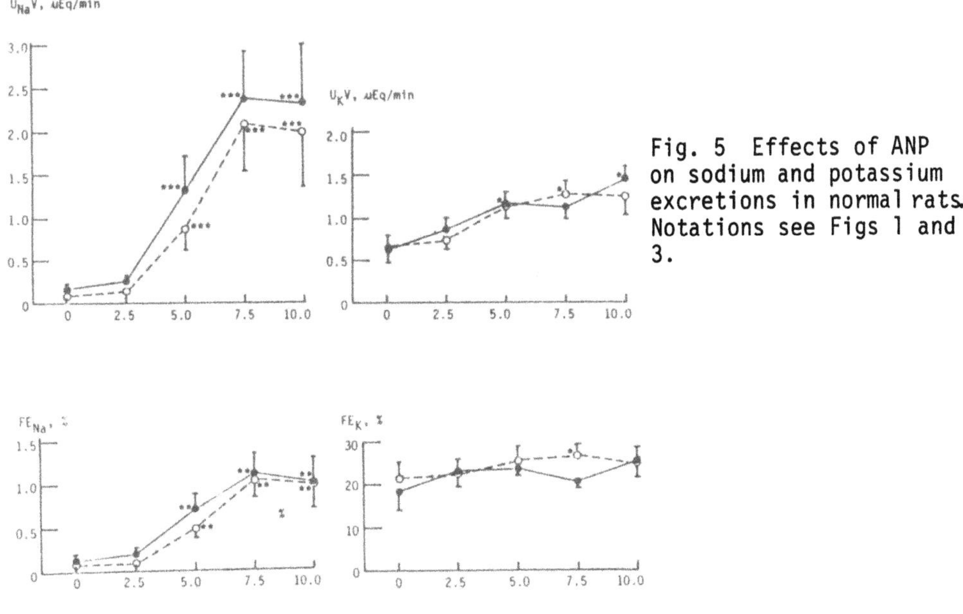

Fig. 5 Effects of ANP on sodium and potassium excretions in normal rats. Notations see Figs 1 and 3.

Table 1. Effects of unclipping and subsequent administration of ANP on blood pressure and bilateral renal function of hypertensive rats.

	Control	Unclipping		ANP injection (ug/kg)		
		1 hr	2 hr	2.5	5	10
BP, mmHg	167±4	148±6***	136±7***	120±6+	120±9+	111±8+
V, ul/min						
nonclipped	7.0±1.1	4.4±0.6*	3.7±0.4*	3.5±0.5	3.6±0.5	4.8±0.8
clipped	1.6±0.3	11.8±2.5**	9.2±2.5**	6.7±1.1	6.9±0.8	6.7±1.2
GFR, ml/min						
nonclipped	1.2±0.1	1.2±0.1	1.0±0.1	1.0±0.1	1.1±0.1	1.2±0.1
clipped	0.6±0.1	1.1±0.1*	1.1±0.1*	1.1±0.1	1.1±0.1	1.1±0.1
$U_{Na}V$, uEq/min						
nonclipped	1.18±0.37	0.52±0.12*	0.46±0.11*	0.44±0.11	0.60±0.17	0.93±0.28
clipped	0.09±0.04	2.07±0.79*	1.84±0.91*	1.22±0.41	1.16±0.23	0.90±0.18
U_KV, uEq/min						
nonclipped	1.67±0.34	1.27±0.26*	0.89±0.16*	0.83±0.13	0.74±0.13	0.85±0.16
clipped	0.35±0.07	1.37±0.21*	1.14±0.16*	1.02±0.14	0.93±0.07	0.85±0.10

Abbreviations: BP=blood pressure; V=urine flow; GFR=glomerular filtration rate; $U_{Na}V$=absolute sodium excretion rate; U_KV=absolute potassium excretion rate. *$p<0.05$; **$p<0.01$; ***$p<0.001$ (vs control); + $p<0.05$ (vs 2 hr after unclipping).

a distinct renal responses in the 2-kidney, 1 clip Goldblatt hypertensive rats. Graded doses of ANP significantly increased GFR and caused striking natriuresis and diuresis in the nonclipped kidney. Moreover, the enhanced renal function occurred despite pronounced reductions in the blood pressure. In contrast, GFR and the excretory function of the clipped kidney did not change significantly. No such distinct renal responses to ANP were noted between the kidneys of control rats. The reason for such differential renal responses in hypertensive rats is unclear; however, it may be related to the difference in the preexisting pressure perfusing the clipped kidney and the nonclipped kidney. It has been shown that the postclip perfusion pressure to the clipped kidney is within normal range despite elevations in the systemic arterial pressure[17] and that the autoregulatory capability of the stenotic kidney is impaired in this hypertensive model[16]. As shown in Fig 1, ANP administration caused a marked reductions in the arterial blood pressure. If no effective adjustment in renal vascular resistance occurred during ANP administration, the profound fall of systemic blood pressure is expected to counteract the direct action of ANP on the clipped kidney and renders this kidney to fail to exhibit a normal response. Nevertheless, it is worthy to note that ANP enhances renal function of the nonclipped side without compromizing the function of the clipped kidney. This is in contrast to those seen in the earlier studies using angiotensin converting enzyme inhibitor or calcium channel blocker[11,13,14]. The latter two agents increase the nonclipped kidney function whereas simultaneously deteriorate the clipped kidney function.

ANP administration produced a profound reductions in the arterial blood pressure and the hypotensive response was greater in hypertensive rats than in normal rats. Previous studies suggested that the vasodepressor effect could be due to direct vasodilation or decrease in cardiac output[2-4]. Also, it has been shown that ANP can blunt the action of endogenous vasoconstrictors[5]. Thus, in the angiotensin-dependent 2-kidney, 1 clip hypertensive model, attenuation of angiotensin-induced vasoconstriction by ANP may partly account for the greater hypotensive response. In addition, the marked natriuresis and diuresis may also contribute to vasodepressor effect of ANP.

Removal of the renal arterial clip induced a rapid fall of arterial blood pressure enhanced the function of the ipsilateral kidney and depressed the function of the contralateral kidney. These observations are consistent with those of other and our previous studies[13,18]. Some studies suggested that the mechanism responsible for the vasodepressor response is not related to the urinary loss of sodium and water or the alterations in the status of the renin-angiotensin system, the prostaglandin system or the kallikrein-kinin system[19,20]. Other studies support the concept that renal mudullary vasodepressor factor(s) may be released and responsible for the reduction in blood pressure following unclipping[21-23]. The enhanced function of the newly unclipped kidney is expected because of relief of arterial stenosis whereas the mechanism for the decreased function of the contralateral kidney remains unknown. It could be due to a precipitus decreases in blood pressure in response to unclipping since the nonclipped kidney needs a higher perfusing pressure for maintaining a normal function as elucidated previously[10,15,16]. Nevertheless, it isinteresting that subsequent administration of ANP failed to enhance the renal excretory function as that seen in rats without unclipping. Whether unclipping process induces a mechanism counteracting against or overriding the primary action of ANP merits further investigation.

REFERENCES

1. A.J. de Bold, H.B. Borenstein, A.T. Veress, and H. Sonnenberg, A rapid and potent natriuretic response to intravenous injection of atrial myocardial extracts in rats, Life Sci., 28:84 (1981).
2. B.J. Ballermann and B.M. Brenner, Role of atrial peptides in body fluid homeostasis, Circ. Res., 58:619 (1986).
3. R. Garcia, G. Thibault, M. Cantin and J. Genest, Effect of a purified atrial natriuretic factor on rat and rabbit vascular strips and vascular beds, Am. J. Physiol., 247:R34 (1984).
4. C.L. Huang, J. Lewicki, L.K. Johnson and M.G. Cogan, Renal mechanism of action of rat atrial natriuretic factor, J. Clin. Invest., 75:769 (1985).
5. H.D. Kleinert, T. Maack, S.A. Atlas, A. Januszewicz, J.E. Sealey and J. H. Laragh, Atrial natriuretic factor inhibits angiotensin-, norepinephrine and potassium-induced vascular contractility, Hypertension, 6(suppl I): I143 (1984).
6. H. Sonnenberg, W.A. Cupples, A.J. de Bold and A.T. Veress, Intrarenal localization of the natriuretic effect of cardiac atrial extract, Can. J. Physiol. Pharmacol., 60:1149 (1982).
7. L.N. Peterson, C. de Rouffignac, H. Sonnenberg and D.Z. Levine, Thick ascending limb response to dDAVP and atrial natriuretic factor in vivo, Am. J. Physiol., 252:F374 (1987).
8. M. Volpe, G. Odell, H.D. Kleinert, et al., Effect of atrial natriuretic factor on blood pressure, renin and aldosterone in Goldblatt hypertension, Hypertension, 7(suppl I):I43 (1985).
9. B.S. Edwards, T.R. Schwab, R.S. Zimmerman, D.M. Heublein, N.S. Jiang and J.C. Burnett, Jr., Cardiovascular, renal and endocrine response to atrial natriuretic peptide in angiotensin II mediated hypertension, Circ. Res., 59:663 (1986).

10. W.C. Huang, D.W. Ploth, P.D. Bell, J. Work and L.G. Navar, Bilateral renal function responses to converting enzyme inhibitor (SQ20881) in two-kidney, one clip Goldblatt hypertensive rats, Hypertension, 3:285 (1981).
11. W.C. Huang, D.W. Ploth and L.G. Navar, Angiotensin-mediated alterations in nephron function in Goldblatt hypertensive rats, Am. J. Physiol., 243:F553 (1982).
12. L.G. Navar, W.C. Huang, K.D. Mitchell, C.A. Jackson and D.W. Ploth, Renal mechanisms of hypertension, in "Proceedings of the first congress of the Asian and Oceanian Physiological Societies", C. Pholpramool and R. Sudsuang, ed., The Physiological Society, Thailand, pp. 253 (1987).
13. W.C. Huang and L.G. Navar, Effects of unclipping and converting enzyme inhibition on bilateral renal function in Goldblatt hypertensive rats, Kidney Int., 23:816 (1983).
14. W.C. Huang, Effects of verapamil alone and with captopril on blood pressure and bilateral renal function in Goldblatt hypertensive rats, Clin. Sci., 70:453 (1986).
15. D.W. Ploth, N.R. Richard, W.C. Huang and L.G. Navar, Impaired renal blood flow and cortical pressure autoregulation in contralateral kidneys of Goldblatt hypertensive rats, Hypertension, 3:67 (1981).
16. B.M. Iversen, K.J. Heyeraas, I. Sekse, K.-J. Andersen and J. Ofstad, Autoregulation of renal blood flow in two-kidney, one-clip hypertensive rats, Am. J. Physiol., 251:F245 (1986).
17. W.R. Murphy, T.G. Coleman, T.L. Smith, and K.A. Stanek, Effects of graded renal arterial constriction on blood pressure, renal artery pressure, and plasma renin activity in Goldblatt hypertension, Hypertension, 6:68 (1984).
18. H. Thurston, R.F. Bing, E.S. Marks and J.D. Swales, Response of chronic renovascular hypertension to surgical correction or prolonged blockade of the renin-angiotensin system by two inhibitors in the rat, Clin. Sci., 58:15 (1980).
19. G.I. Russell, R.F. Bing, J.D. Swales and H. Thurston, Indomethacin or aprotinin infusion: Effect on reversal of chronic two-kidney, one-clip hypertension in the conscious rat, Clin. Sci., 62:361 (1982).
20. R. Dietz, G.J. Mast, A. Schomig, J.B. Luth and W. Rascher, Reversal of renal hypertension: Effects on renin, salt and water balance. Klin. Wochenschr., 56(suppl 1):23 (1978).
21. E.E. Muirhead, Antihypertensive functions of the kidney, Hypertension, 2:444 (1980).
22. R.F. Bing, G.I. Russell, J.D. Swales, H. Thurston and A. Fletcher, Chemical renal medullectomy: Effect upon reversal of two-kidney, one-clip hypertension in the rat, Clin. Sci., 61:335s (1981).
23. G. Gothberg, S. Lundin and B. Folkow, Acute vasodepressor effect in normotensive rats following extracorporal perfusion of the declipped kidney of two-kidney, one-clip hypertensive rats, Hypertension, 4 (suppl II):II-101 (1982).

THE EFFECTS OF HYDROCORTISONE ON THE MESONEPHROS PROXIMAL TUBULE CELLS

Mirella Bertossi, Beatrice Nico, Luisa Roncali, Daniela Virgintino, Lucia Mancini, Domenico Ribatti and Pasquale Coratelli*

Institute of Histology and General Embryology and (*)Institute of Nephrology
University of Bari-Polyclinics
Bari, Italy

INTRODUCTION

The mesonephros is the first excretory organ to function during the chick embryo development; its nephrons differentiate between the 3rd and 6th incubation days (i.d.), and are active before their differentiation is over, since filtration by glomeruli and concentration by proximal tubules have been proved to be effective on the 5th i.d. (Chambers and Kempton, 1933; Romanoff, 1960; Friebovà-Zemanovà, 1981; Friebovà-Zemanovà and Gonkarevskaya, 1982; Narbaitz and Kapal, 1986). The mesonephros reaches the zenith of its activity on the 11th i.d., then it begins to degenerate being supplanted by metanephros or permanent kidney (Lillie, 1952; Salzgeber and Weber, 1966; Narbaitz and Kacew, 1978).

The present ultrastructural study was carried out in order to analyze the effects of hydrocortisone on the reabsorption of proteins by the proximal tubule cells utilizing horseradish peroxidase (HRP) as marker of epithelial permeability. The chick embryo mesonephros can be considered a suitable model for this study since its nephrons both differentiate following the same steps described for avian and mammalian metanephric nephrons (Larsson, 1975; Narbaitz and Kacew, 1978; Friis, 1980; Narbaitz and Kapal, 1986) and show morphofunctional properties very similar to those of adult kidney (Chambers and Kempton, 1933; Gibley and Chang, 1967; Maunsbach, 1973).

MATERIAL AND METHODS

Twelve chick embryos incubated under routine conditions were utilized.
I) Four normally developed embryos (controls) were killed by decapitation at the 10th i.d., and their mesonephros, removed by dissection, were fixed in a sodium cacodylate-buffered mixture of 2% glutaraldehyde and 2% paraformaldehyde, postfixed in sodium cacodylate-buffered 1% OsO_4.
II) Four normally developed embryos were sacrificed at the 10th i.d., ten minutes after an intravascular injection of horseradish peroxidase (0.3 mg HRP Sigma Type II/gram body weight in 0.1 ml of saline solution).
III) Four embryos received 10 μg of hydrocortisone (Flebocortid,Richter) dissolved in 50 μl of saline solution onto the chorioallantoic membrane, at

the 5th and at the 6th i.d., and were killed, at the 10th i.d., ten minutes after an intravascular injection of HRP.
The mesonephroi of the II and III group embryos were fixed in a sodium cacodylate buffered mixture of 2% glutaraldehyde and 2% paraformaldehyde, cut by vibrotome, and the slices were processed according to the Graham and Karnovsky method (1967) to evidentiate the HRP reaction product.

All the specimens were embedded in Epon 812, and cut with an LKB V ultramicrotome; the ultrathin sections were stained with lead citrate, and observed under a 9A Zeiss electron microscope.

RESULTS

I. In the mesonephros of control embryos (Fig. 1), the proximal tubule cells (PTCs), welded by iuxtaluminal tight junctions, show a well developed brush border, a relevant amount of tubular invaginations of the apical plasmalemma, both small and large cytoplasmic vacuoles, mitochondria and lysosomes. These features correspond to those of the proximal tubule in mammalian adult kidney, whose cells are characterized by remarkable endocytic and digestive activities.

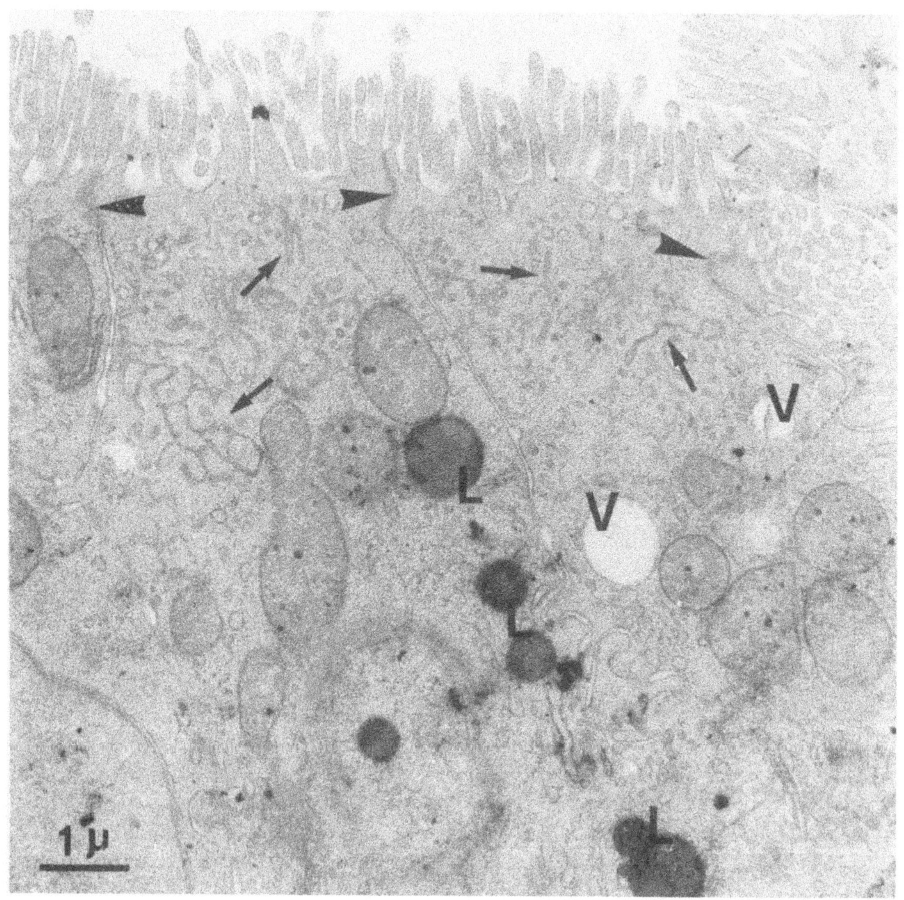

Fig. 1. Apical region of proximal tubule cells in a control embryo mesonephros (I); tight junctions (▲), tubular invaginations (↑), lysosomes (L), and large apical vacuoles (V) are seen.

II. The steps of the protein reabsorption and degradation processes can be clearly documented in the PTCs of the embryos intravascularly injected with HRP; the marker, which passes the glomerular filtration barrier, reaches the luminal surface of the proximal tubule. Here the tracer is endocytosed at the level of the tubular cell apical invaginations, which give rise to small apical vacuoles merging, in turn, to form large apical vacuoles; the latter, finally, fuse with primary lysosomes, whose enzymes degradate the marker molecules (Fig. 2). HRP is also detectable at the basal front of the PTCs, coming from the peritubular capillary network (Fig. 2) since their endothelial cells allow the extravasation of the marker. HRP penetrates the interendothelial clefts, is never endocytosed at the basal and lateral surfaces of the tubular cells, and is prevented from passing into the tubular lumen by the tight junctions of the PTCs.

III. In hydrocortisone treated embryos, the PTCs are on the whole thinner than in the controls and somewhat detached owing to the presence of intercellular spaces crowded by microvillous expansions (Fig. 3). Microdetachments of the joined plasmalemmas are, at times, recognizable at the level of the tight junctions apically welding the epithelial cells (Fig. 4).

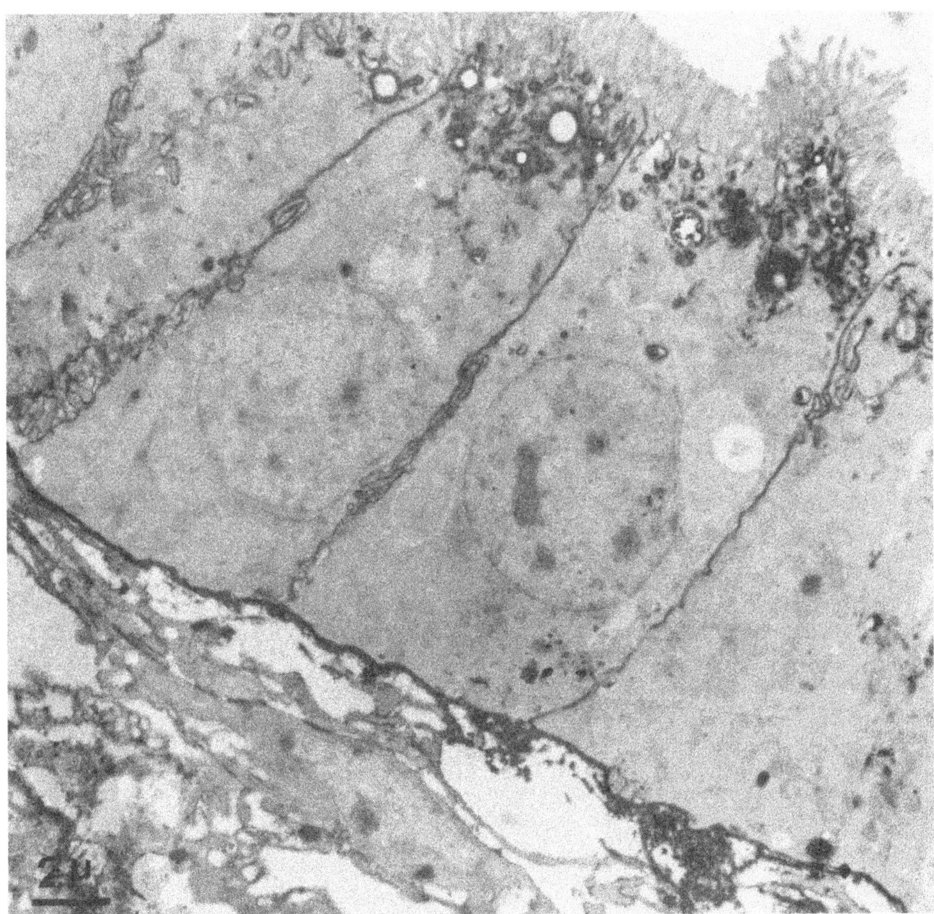

Fig. 2. Tubular epithelium in the mesonephros of a normal embryo intravascularly injected with HRP (II). The marker is detectable in the apical tubular invaginations, in small and large vacuoles, and along basal and lateral surfaces of the epithelial cells.

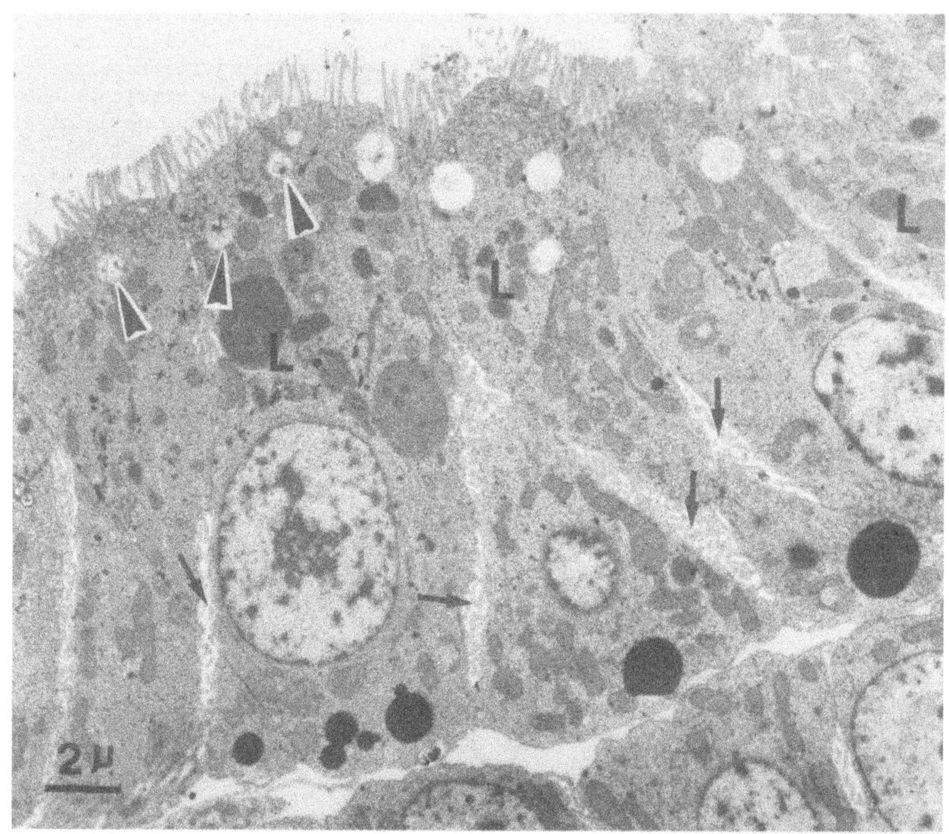

Fig. 3. Proximal tubule cells of a hydrocortisone treated and HRP injected embryo (III). Somewhat wide intercellular spaces (↑) separate the cells, in which medium-sized and partially HRP-labeled vacuoles (▲) as well as primary lysosomes (L) are distributed in the apical cytoplasm; large and completely HRP-filled vacuoles are detectable in the basal cytoplasm.

Atypical cells are seen scattered among apparently normal PTCs. They are rounded in their apical front, poor in microvilli, containing few mitochondria and a relevant amount of free ribosomes (Fig. 5).

As concerns morphological evidence of endocytic and digestive properties in PTCs under hydrocortisone treatment, it can be observed that apical endocytic vacuoles containing the marker are less numerous than under the normal developmental situation (Fig. 2, 3); lysosomes are gathered around the HRP-marked vacuoles with which they seldom seem to fuse (Fig. 6 a); vacuoles of various sizes and shapes, which contain a various amount of HRP mixed with lysosome matrix, are scattered throughout the cell cytoplasm (Fig. 6 b), and round-shaped vacuoles, completely filled with electrondense material, are frequently seen in the basal portion of the PTCs (Fig. 3, 6 b).

DISCUSSION

Our observations confirm great similarity in the PTC ultrastructural features of chick mesonephros and other vertebrate metanephros (Gibley and Chang, 1967; Narbaitz and Kapal, 1986), and demonstrate that protein endocytosis and degradation take place in the same way described for adult mammalian kidney (Straus, 1964; Graham and Karnovsky, 1966; Maunsbach, 1973).

As to the main aim of our research, it seems that hydrocortisone treatment causes an impairment of protein endocytosis and of lysosomal activities, the fusion processes between apical endocytic vacuoles and primary lysosomes being reduced, and the enzymatic digestion of the tracer within secondary lysosomes incomplete. Moreover the ultrastructural features observed in some PTCs of hydrocortisone treated embryos (t.i., few microvilli and mitochondria, and a quantity of free ribosomes) suggest that hydrocortisone,

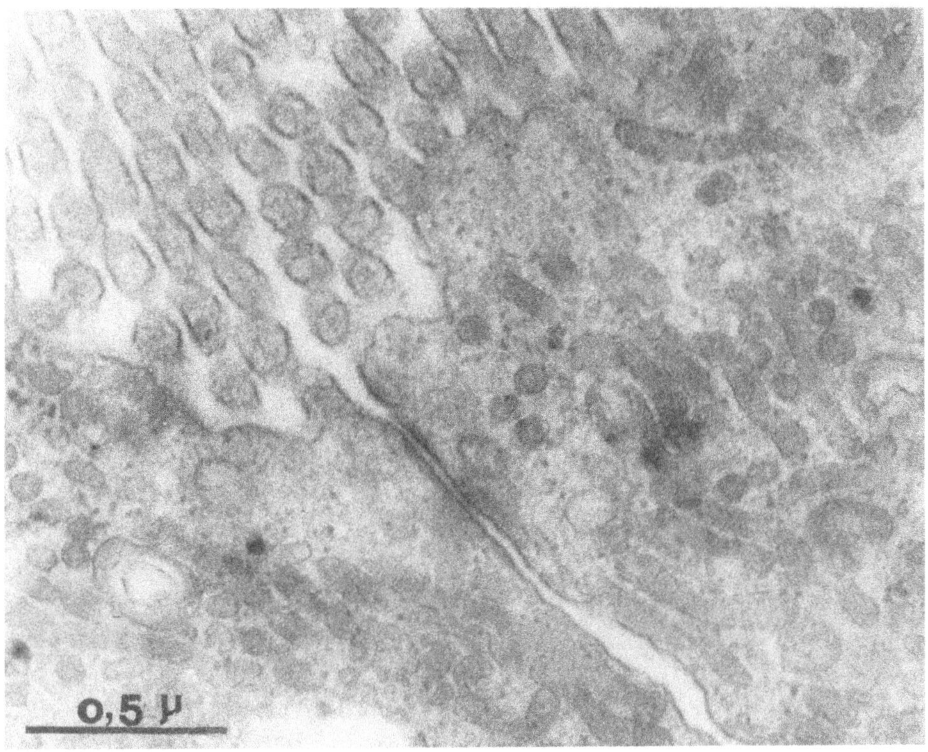

Fig. 4. An altered tight junction in the proximal tubule of a hydrocortisone treated and HRP injected embryo (III).

twice administered at the 5th and 6th i.d. when some nephrons are still developing (Friebovà-Zemanovà, 1981), causes the failure of maturation processes in those cells which, at that time, have not yet started to differentiate. Both the effects observed in this experimental condition may actually have a common cause, as the hydrocortisone, affecting the process of protein synthesis, may produce disturbances in the lysosomal activities of fully-differentiated PTCs and blockage in the differentiation of the immature ones.

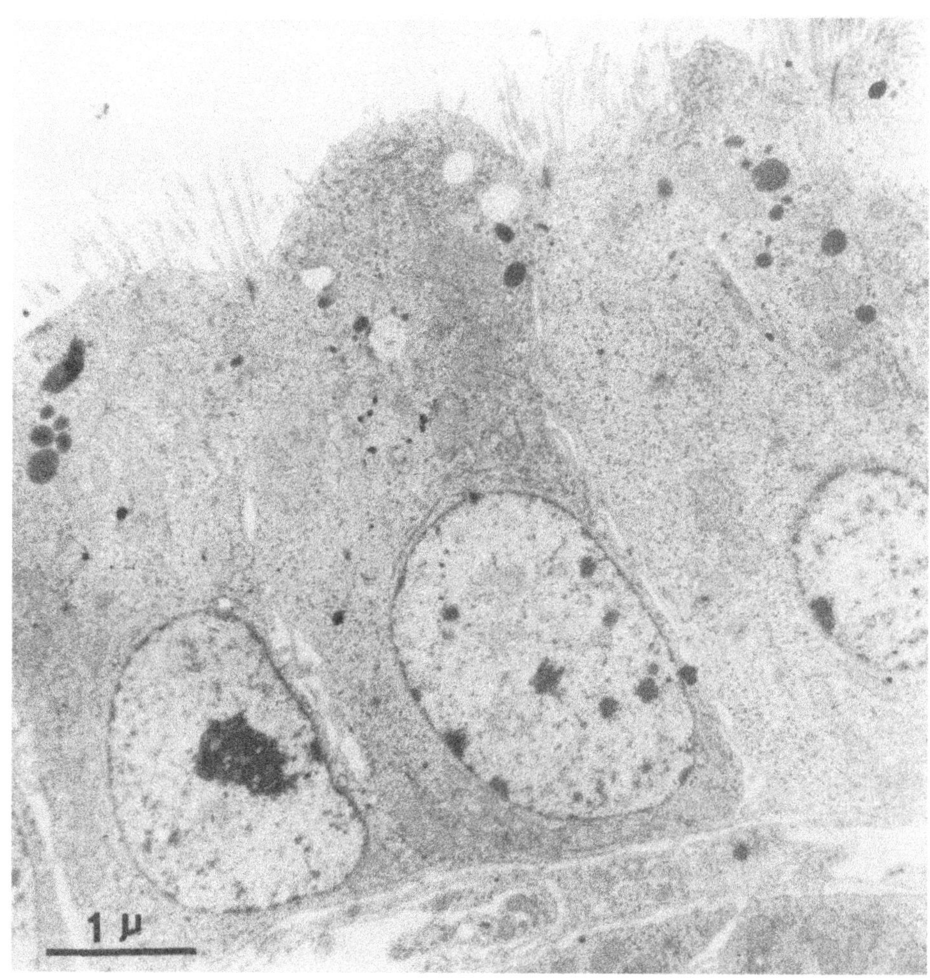

Fig. 5. Hydrocortisone treated and HRP injected embryo mesonephros (III). Part of a proximal tubule bordered by "undifferentiated" cells, poor in microvilli and rich in polysomes.

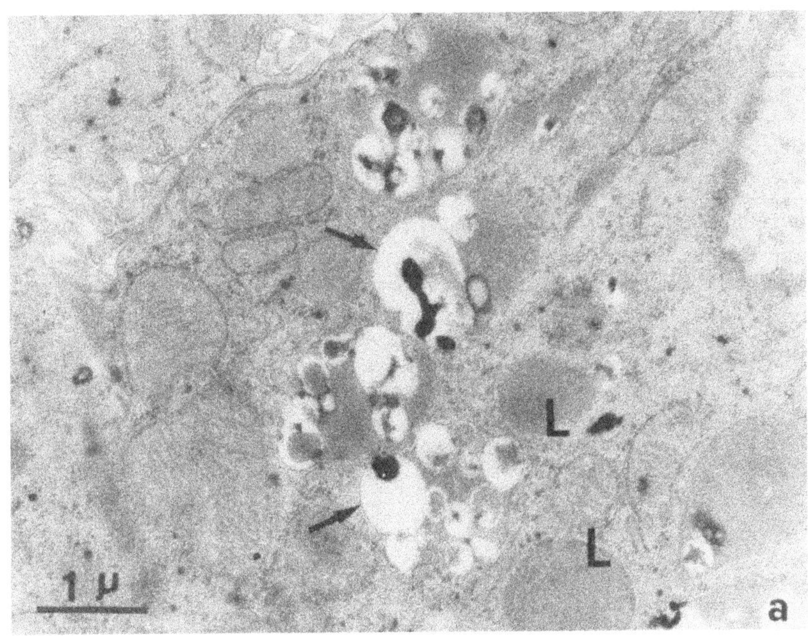

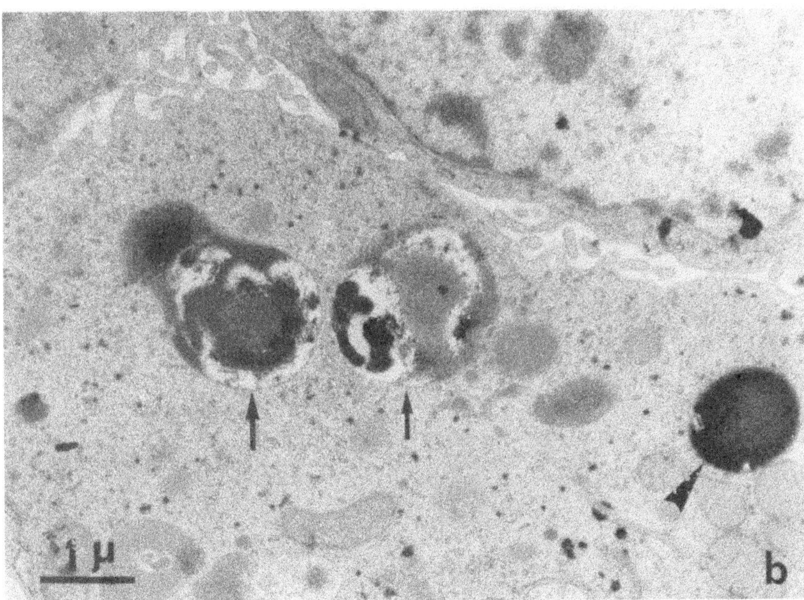

Fig. 6. Hydrocortisone treated and HRP injected embryo PTCs (III). Note in (a): primary lysosomes (L), and small and large vacuoles partially filled with HRP (↑), and in (b): secondary lysosomes containing HRP reaction product mixed with their matrix (↑) as well as one vacuole completely filled by homogeneous electrondense material (▲).

REFERENCES

Chambers, R., and Kempton, R.T., 1933, Indications of function of the chick mesonephros in tissue culture with phenol red, J.cell comp.Physiol., 3:131.

Friebovà-Zemanovà, Z., 1981, Formation of the chick mesonephros. 4. Course and architecture of the developing nephrons, Anat.Embryol., 161:341.

Friebovà-Zemanovà, Z., and Goncharevskaya, O. A., 1982, Formation of the chick mesonephros. 5. Spatial distribution of the nephron populations, Anat.Embryol., 165:125.

Friis, C., 1980, Postnatal development of the pig kidney: ultrastructure of the glomerulus and the proximal tubule, J.Anat., 130:513.

Gibley, C.W., and Chang, J.P., 1967, Fine structure of the functional mesonephros in the eight-day chick embryo, J.Morphol., 123:441.

Graham, R.C., and Karnovsky, M.J., 1966, The early stages of absorption of injected horseradish peroxidase in the proximal tubules of mouse kidney. Ultrastructural cytochemistry by a new technique, J.Histochem.Cytochem., 14:291.

Larsson, L., 1975, The ultrastructure of the developing proximal tubule in the rat kidney, J.Ultrastruct.Res., 51:119.

Lillie, F.R., 1952, "Development of the chick", Holt, Rinehart & Winston, New York.

Maunsbach, A.B., 1973, Ultrastructure of the proximal tubule, in: "Handbook of physiology", Geiger, ed., American Physiological Society, Washington.

Narbaitz, R., and Kacev, S., 1978, Ultrastructural and biochemical observations on the metanephros of normal and cultured chick embryos, Anat.Embryol., 155:95.

Narbaitz, R., and Kapal, V.K., 1986, Scanning electron microscopical observations on the differentiating mesonephros of the chick embryo, Acta Anat., 125:183.

Romanoff, A.L., 1960, "The Avian embryo. Structural and fuctional development", Mac Millan, New York.

Salzgeber, B., and Weber, R., 1966, La régression du mésonéphros chez l'embryon de poulet. Etude des activités de la phosphatase acide et de cathepsines. Analyse biochimique, histochimique et observations au microscope électronique, J.Embryol.exp.Morphol., 15:397.

Straus, W., 1964, Cytochemical observations on the relationship between lysosomes and phagosomes in kidney and liver by combined staining for acid phosphatase and intravenously injected horseradish peroxidase, J.Cell Biol., 20:497.

OXALATE DEPOSITS IN THE KIDNEY OF 5/6 NEPHRECTOMISED RATS SUPPLEMENTED BY LARGE DOSES OF VITAMIN C

Keiji Ono*, Hiroko Ono*, Yohko Hisasue*, Kazuhiko Kikawa** and Yukinori Oh***

*Ono Geka Clinic, **Fukuoka Tokushukai Hospital and ***Fukuoka Red Cross Hospital, Fukuoka, Japan

INTRODUCTION

The secondary oxalosis of renal failure has been recognised for more than 20 years (Bennett and Rosenblum, 1961), but details of its prevalence and clinical features have been addressed only recently(Salyer and Keren, 1973; Boer et al., 1984; Pru et al., 1985). Oxalate is a non-metabolisable end product of glycine and ascorbic acid metabolism(Elder and Wyngaarden, 1960) and virtually all of it is excreted by the kidneys. Renal insufficiency can produce oxalate loads that exceed renal excretory capacity. Protein binding of oxalate is minimal and most of it should be removed by hemodialysis. However, hemodialysis does not remove oxalate as fast as it is formed, leaving patients at risk from the complications which result from systemic oxalosis (Landwehr et al., 1987).

In addition to removing toxic substances from the blood hemodialysis also leads to the loss of essential nutrients such as vitamins and amino acids. Patients with renal failure who are treated in this way lose considerable amounts of ascorbic acid and are usually given a large dose of vitamin C as supplementation(Sullivan et al.,1972). However, as ascorbate is the main precursor of endogenous oxalate (Thompson and Weiman, 1984), hyperoxalemia in regular hemodialysis patients is aggravated by routine vitamin C supplementation (Ono, 1986). The present study was undertaken to see if this observation could be confirmed in experimental animals.

MATERIALS AND METHODS

Outbred male Wistar rats(7 weeks of age, weight 180 to 190 mg) were anesthetised with intraperitoneal pentobarbital sodium (3 mg/100 gm body weight). The abdomen was opened through a midline incision and the left kidney was separated from the adrenal gland and peritoneal fat. One third of the upper and lower poles of the left kidney were cauterised, leaving the pelvis and the hilum intact. The current intensity and duration of contact was adjusted to avoid tissue carbonisation. In this way two-thirds of the left kidney was excised during the first stage of the procedure, hemorrhage, a common post-operative complication, was not seen in this study. One week after cauterisation, the hilum of the contralateral intact kidney was ligated under ether anesthesia, leaving the animals with only one-sixth of their original renal mass. Post-operatively the animals received 4 ml of an isotonic saline solution containing 1 mg/ml of cephalothin sodium intraperitoneally.

Following surgery fifty rats were divided into two groups: 30 were allowed free access to drinking water containing 8 mg/ml of vitamin C and the remaining 20 given tap water without vitamin C. All animals were fed a standard diet with 24% protein. Serum creatinine, Hct, and body weight were measured monthly for 12 months using a micromethod and tail blood. Endogenous creatinine clearance was measured after 1, 3, 6, 8 & 11 months and plasma levels of oxalate, vitamin C urinary oxalate analysed in the 3rd and 8th post operative months. Plasma oxalic acid levels were determined by capillary gas chromatography as described by Wolthers and Hayer (1982). When animals developed renal failure severe enough to threaten survival, as suggested by weakness, involuntary movements, coarse hair, diarrhea and an oribital bloody discharge, they were sacrificed by abdominal aortic puncture under intraperitoneal anesthesia. In another six healthy rats, plasma levels of oxalate and vitamin C, creatinine clearance and urinary oxalate output were measured as for the controls. The heparinised blood was centrifuged immediately to separate the plasma and stored at -20°C for subsequent biochemical analysis. At the time of death the kidney was removed and fixed in 10% formalin for histological studies. Sections of this organ were stained with hematoxylin-eosin, PAS and Cong-red for light microscopy. All values are reported as mean ± SEM. Statistical comparisons were made using the Student's t test.

RESULTS

Operated rats recovered fully from surgery within 5 to 7 days and there was no post operative mortality, all rats surviving longer than one month.In this experiment body weight served as a good indicator of uremia as the degree of uremia paralleled the weight curves of the rats. After the first post operative month, all rats gained weight rapidly until the 5th month when the weight gain slowed. All animals started to lose weight after eight months when the serum creatinine started to increase progressively. The mean weight of treated rats paralleled that of non-treated animals (Fig. 1). During the first post operative month the serum creatinine level rose to from 0.4 mg to about 1.2 mg in both groups and remained fairly stable at 1.2 to 1.5 mg/dl for 6 months. Thereafter, it

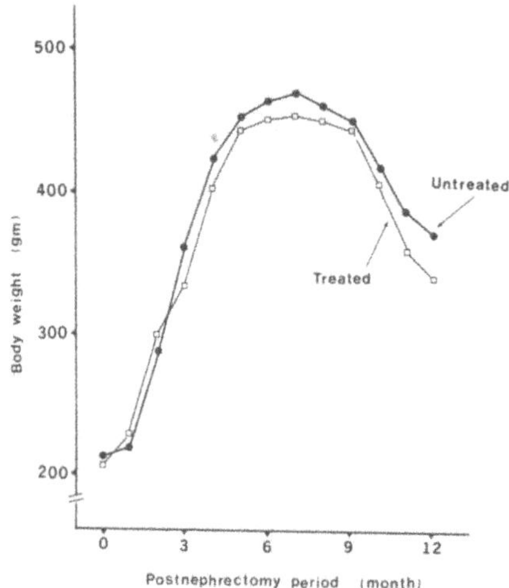

Fig. 1 Changes of body weight of 5/6 nephrectomised rats treated and untreated with vitamin C

rose progressively and rapidly as shown in Fig. 2. Serum creatinine levels in the vitamin C treated group were much higher than those of the non-treated rats upto the 11th and 12th post operative months. However, the number of non-treated rats at these stages were too small for statistical analysis.

Fig. 2 Changes in serum creatine of 5/6 nephrectomised rats treated and untreated with vitamin C. In parentheses: number of rats □ = treated grou, ● = non treated group. Mean ± SEM

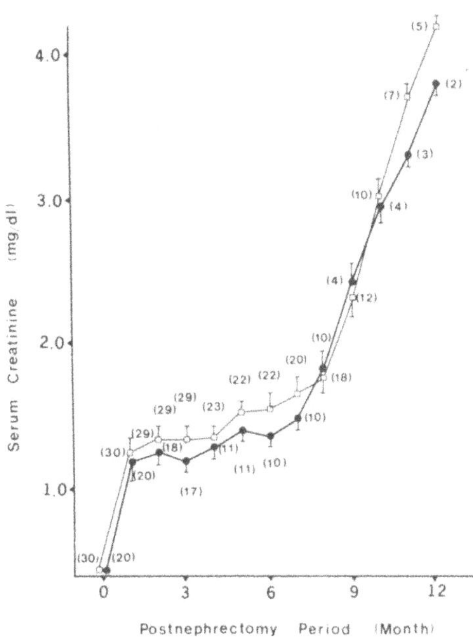

Plasma oxalate and vitamin C levels were increased because of decreasing renal function and their levels in treated rats were significantly higher than those of non-treated animals (Fig. 3,4).

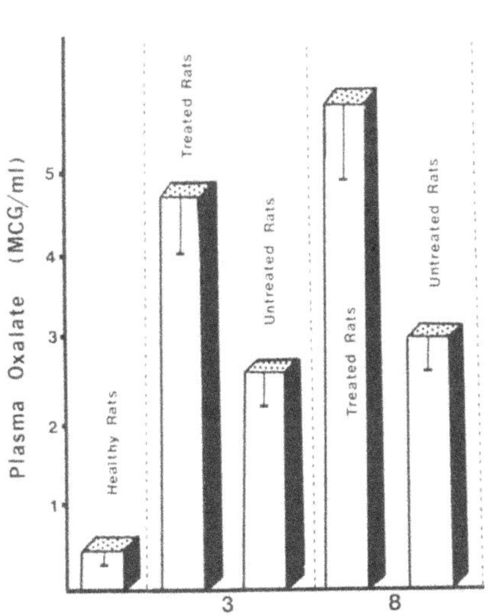

Fig. 3 Plasma oxalate levels of 5/6 nephrectomised rats treated and untreated with vitamin C. Mean ± SEM

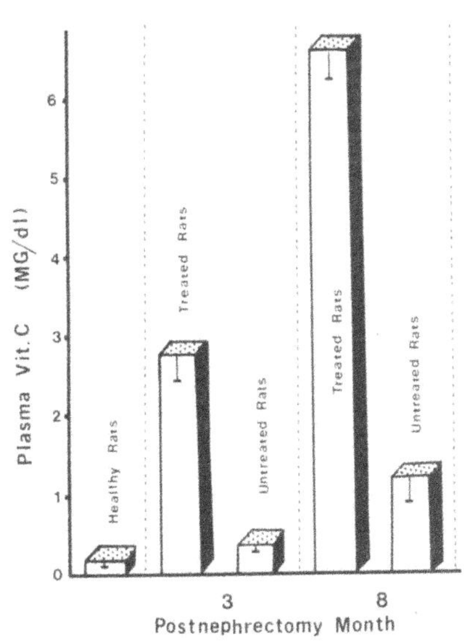

Fig. 4 Plasma vitamin C levels of 5/6 nephrectomised rats treated and untreated with vitamin C. Mean ± SEM

The histological findings of the renal remnant in both vitamin C treated and non-treated rats were practically the same except for one point. In the treated animals there was deposition of calcium oxalate crystals mainly in tubules of the remnant kidney of rats sacrificed after the 11th post operative months (Fig. 5a, 5b). However, glomerular and interstitial fibrosis and a marked inflammatory reaction and tubular dilatation were seen equally in both groups of rats (Fig. 5a, 5b).

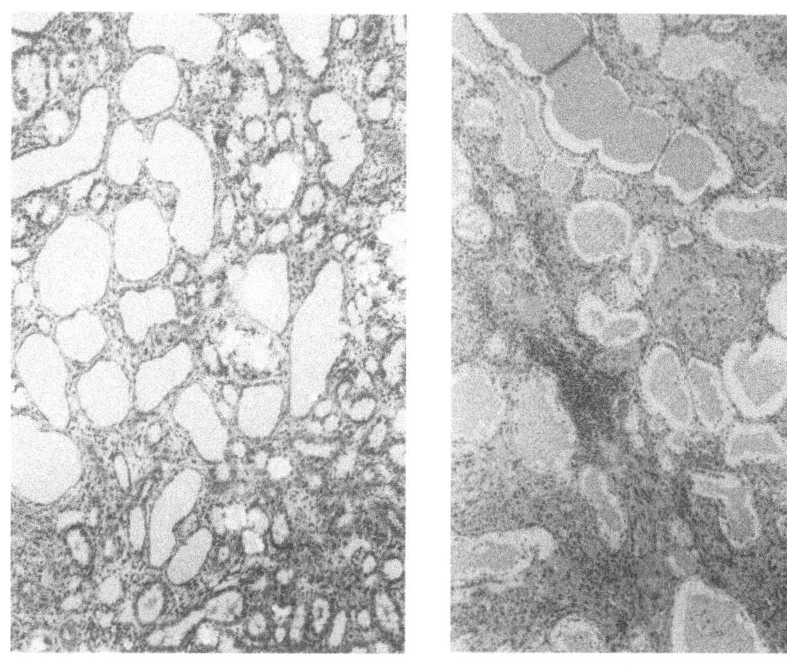

Fig. 5a Fig. 5b

Fig. 5a,5b. Photomicrograms of rat kidneys removed 11 months after 5/6 nephrectomy. Marked tubular dilatation and glomerular and interstitial fibrosis was seen in both treated (a) and untreated (b) specimens. However, intratubular calcium oxalate deposits were seen only in the vitamin C treated rats (a).
a: Hematoxylin-Eosin, in semipolarised light. X 100
b: Hematoxylin-Eosin, X 100

DISCUSSION

In the human, oxalic acid is a metabolic end product which can only be excreted by the kidney. It is not surprising, therefore, that in patients with renal insufficiency, oxalate accumulates in the body. The secondary oxalosis of renal failure is believed to be the result of a chronic elevation of the plasma concentration of oxalate. Autopsy studies of patients who have died of renal failure have suggested that the incidence and extent of calcium oxalate crystal deposition correlates closely with the duration of renal failure (Fayemi et al., 1979), although it is not known with certainty if there is a critical plasma concentration at which precipitation and tissue deposition occurs.

The conversion of ascorbic acid to oxalate was described many years ago (Lamden and Chrystowski, 1954) and it would seem a reasonable precaution to recommend screening for ascorbate induced hyperoxalemia in all hemodialysis patients taking vitamin C supplementation (Balcke et al.,

1980, 1982; Pru et al., 1985). Predialysis levels of vitamin C correlate well with the plasma oxalate levels (Pru et al., 1985) and there are several studies which suggest that the supplementation of large doses of vitamin C in regular dialysis patients contributes to the body oxalate burden (Balcke et al., 1980, 1982). However, we have recently found that even in pateints treated with a small dose of vitamin C (50 to 100mg/day) for 4 weeks, plasma oxalate levels are significantly higher than those of non-treated patients (Ono, 1986). These findings prompted us to perform an experimental sutdy designed to evaluate the effect of oral vitamin C supplementation on secondary oxalosis in rats in chronic renal failure induced by 5/6 nephrectomy. In the present study the most interesting finding was that oxalate depostis were seen only in vitamin C treated 5/6 nephrectomised rats. Although the functional deterioration and histological destruction of the remnant kidney was equal in both vitamin C treated and non-treated groups. Although the renal function of these rats progressively deteriorated, it was still much better than that of hemodialysis patients. In spite of this oxalate deposits were clearly seen in the remnant kidney in 5/6 nephrectomised rats which have been supplemented with massive doses of vitamin C (100 to 160 mg/24 hr/100 gm) orally. The effect of ascorbic acid administration on the plasma oxalic acid levels of 5/6 nephrectomised rats in our study was probably due to the augmented synthesis of oxalic acid from ascorbic acid and the decreased urinary output of oxalic acid due to renal failure. In this study we have shown, as far as we are aware, for the first time, in experimental animals that vitamin C supplementation caused or prompted the formation of oxalate crystals in kidneys with reduced function. Oxalate in the urine is a solution in a state of supersaturation, thus the kidney is the first organ to suffer crystalisation; the failing kidney may be likened to a selective sponge that accomodates most of the oxalate that is crystalised out.

In conclusion, these results confirm the clinical observation that vitamin C is definitely a precursor of oxalate in renal failure. Renal tubular oxalate deposition occurred if the 5/6 nephrectomised rats were supplemented with massive doses of vitamin C even though renal function was well above the levels of end stage renal failure which requires renal replacement therapy. Therefore vitamin C should be regarded as another potentially harmful vitamin in uremia, along with vitamin A (Ono 1984). We strongly believe that vitamin C supplementation should be restricted to the minimal dose necessary to correct ascorbic acid deficiency.

REFERENCES

1. Bennett,B., and Rosenblum,C., 1961, Identification of calcium oxalate crystal in the myocardium in patients with uremia, Lab. Invest.,10:947.
2. Salyer,W.R., Keren,D., 1973, Oxalosis as a complication of chronic renal failure, Kidney Int.,4:61.
3. Boer,P., Van Leersum,L., Hene,R.J., and Drohout Mees,E.J., 1984, Plasma oxalate concentration in chronic renal disease. Am.J.Kidney Diseas.,4:118
4. Pru,C., Eaton,J., Kjellstrand,C., 1985, Vitamin C intoxication and hyperoxalemia in chronic hemodialysis patients. Nephron 39:112.
5. Elder,T.D., Wyngaarden,J.B., 1960. The biosynthesis and turn of oxalate in normal and hyperoxaluric subjects. J.Clin.Invest.39:1337.
6. Landwehr, D.M., Brothis,J., Landwehr,G., Halbedl,S., and Costello, J., 1987, Increased oxalate appearance (OXA) in hemodialysis patients (Abstract), 20th Ann. Meeting Am. Soc. Nephrol.
7. Sullivan,J.E., Eisenstein,A.B., Mottola,C.M. and Mittal,A.K., 1972, The effect of dialysis on plasma and tissue levels of vitamin C.

Tans. Am. Soc. Artif. Organs 18:277.
8. Thompson,C.S., and Weiman,E.J., 1984, The significance of oxalate in renal failure. Am.J. Kidney Diseas.4:97.
9. Ono K., Secondary hyperoxalemia caused by vitamin C supplementation in regular hemodialysis patients. Clin.Nephrol. 26:239.
10. Wolthers, B.G., and Hayer,M., 1982, The determination of oxalic acid in plasma and urine by means of capillary gas chromatography. Clin. Chim. Acta 120;87.
11. Fayemi,A.O., Ali,M., and Braun,E.V., 1979, Oxalosis in hemodialysis patients. Arch. Pathol. Lab. Med. 103:58.
12. Lamden, M.P., and Chrystowski, G.A., 1954, Urinary oxalate excretion by man follwoing ascorbic acid ingestion. Proc. Soc. Exp. Biol. Med. 85:190.
13. Balcke, P., Schmidt,P., Zazgornik,J., Kopsa,H., and Deutsch,E., 1982, Secondary hyperoxalemia in chronic renal failure. Inter. J. Artif. Organs 5:141.
14. Balcke, P., Schmidt, P., Zazgornik, J., Kopsa,H., and Deutsch, E., 1980, Secondary oxalosis in chronic renal insufficiency. N. Engl. J. Med. 303:944.
15. Ono,K., 1984, Hypervitaminosis A toxicity in regular hemodialysis patients. Trans. Am. Sco. Artif. Intern. Organs 30:40.

EFFECTS OF CANRENONE ON Na^+,K^+ ATPase ACTIVITY, ARTERIAL PRESSURE AND PLASMA POTASSIUM CONCENTRATION IN UREMIC HEMODIALYZED PATIENTS

F. Quarello, R. Boero, C. Guarena, C. Rosati, G. Beltrame, P. Colombo, I.M. Berto, M. Aimino, M. Formica, and G. Piccoli

Institute of Nephrology, University of Torino. Dialysis Unit Nuova Astanteria Martini Hospital, Torino, Italy

INTRODUCTION

Canrenone is the main active metabolite[1] of the diuretic and antihypertensive drugs spironolactone and canrenoate-K, and competes with aldosterone for a common cytosolic receptor in distal and collecting tubules of the nephron.[2] In addition it has recently been demonstrated that canrenone *in vitro* may directly interfere with ouabain-sensitive Na^+,K^+ pump (Na^+,K^+ adenosine triphosphatase), acting as a partial agonist at the digitalis receptor site.[3,4] Moreover Garay et al.[4] showed that canrenone is able to restimulate *in vitro* the Na^+,K^+ pump of human red blood cells (RBC) blocked by high concentrations of ouabain.

Since the original reports by Welt and colleagues,[5,6] some authors have confirmed a derangement of Na^+,K^+ pump activity in erythrocytes (RBC) from patients with chronic renal failure,[7] and evidence has accumulated suggesting the presence in uremic plasma of a sodium pump inhibitor(s),[8-10] which has been related to a digoxin-like substance(s), whose secretion seems to be stimulated by fluid overload.[11,12]

The pathophysiological relevance of the Na^+,K^+ pump suppression in uremic patients is currently unknown. A defect in sodium transport could be implicated in the genesis of arterial hypertension, which is common in these patients, and often related to volume expansion.[13] In fact it has been described that, as a consequence of Na^+,K^+ inhibition in vascular smooth muscle cells, more sodium is accumulated inside the cells and is paralleled by calcium influx, enhancing both basal vascular tone and responsiveness to vasoconstrictor stimuli.[14] Moreover, the reduced Na^+,K^+ ATPase activity could also contribute to hyperkalemia, since a reduced intracellular translocation of potassium, which is mainly mediated by the Na^+,K^+ pump, has been shown in uremic patients.[15]

The aim of this study was then to evaluate the acute effects of canrenone on erythrocyte Na^+,K^+ pump, arterial pressure and plasma potassium in uremic hemodialyzed patients.

SUBJECTS AND METHODS

Seven uremic patients on hemodialysis, six males and one female, were investigated. Their age ranged from 49 to 76 years, mean 62 years;

dialytic age ranged from 20 to 83 months, mean 39 months. Residual renal function was absent in all patients. No patient was taking digitalis. Antihypertensive medications were withdrawn at least one week prior to the study. Chronic renal failure was due to glomerulonephritis (3), interstitial nephritis (3), nephroangiosclerosis (1). Patients were dialyzed 4 hours three times weekly using hollow fiber or plate (0.8-1.3 m^2) cuprophan disposable dialyzers. All patients were on bicarbonate hemodialysis (dialysate composition in mmol/l: Na 138, K 2, Ca 1.75, Mg 0.5, Cl 108.5, CH_3COO 5, HCO_3 31, Glucose 5.55).

Each patient received either placebo or canrenone (Phanurane®, Théraplix, France), 150 mg orally, in a cross-over randomized sequence, with the following protocol, performed at the mid-week dialysis: blood for erythrocyte electrolyte concentration and fluxes and for plasma potassium concentration was drawn before, three hours after drug administration and after hemodialysis, which was started immediately following the second sampling. At the same time arterial pressure was measured by a non invasive automated device (Nippon Colin BP 203); the values represent the mean of three consecutive measurements. Plasma potassium was evaluated by flame photometry. Informed consent was obtained from each subject included in the study.

Erythrocyte sodium concentration and fluxes

Blood was drawn from the arterio-venous fistula, collected into heparinized tubes, and immediately processed. Intraerythrocyte Na and K concentrations ($[Na_i]$ and $[K_i]$) were evaluated by hemolysing in deionized water a fixed volume of erythrocytes (100 µl), which had been washed three times with 110 mmol/l $MgCl_2$ solution at 4° C. The Na and K concentrations of the hemolysate were measured on a Perkin Elmer model 2380 atomic absorption spectrophotometer and expressed as mmol/l of packed red cells.

RBC Na efflux mediated by Na^+,K^+ pump was estimated in fresh cells according to Garay et al.,[4] as previously described.[9] The washed erythrocytes were resuspended in a cold magnesium-sucrose medium (mmol/l): 75 $MgCl_2$, 85 sucrose, 10 MOPS-Tris (pH 7.4 at 37° C) and 10 glucose, to a hematocrit of 20-25%. A portion of the cell suspension was added (final hematocrit 4-5%) to different cold solutions containing buffered magnesium-sucrose plus the following additions (mmol/l): (1) 2 KCl, (2) 0.1 ouabain. One set of tubes was kept in ice, in order to measure the baseline Na concentration (0 time), and another set was incubated at 37° for 30 min (medium 1) and 1 h (medium 2). After incubation tubes were transferred in an ice bath for 1' and then centrifuged at 1750 g for 5' at 4° C. The supernatant was carefully removed and the Na concentration was measured by atomic absorption spectrophotometry. Sodium efflux was taken as the difference between the Na content after incubation and the baseline Na content. The Na^+,K^+ pump activity was calculated by subtracting Na efflux in the presence from that in the absence of ouabain. The rate constant for ouabain-sensitive Na efflux was calculated dividing the Na efflux by the $[Na_i]$, and was expressed in h^{-1}. All measurements were performed in duplicate.

Statistical evaluation was carried out with the Wilcoxon matched pairs test. Data are expressed as means±SEM.

RESULTS

Main results are shown in tables 1 and 2.

Table 1. Intraerythrocyte Na and K concentration and Na^+,K^+ pump activity.

	Na^+,K^+ PUMP (rate constant h^{-1})	$[Na_i]$ (mmol/l RBC)	$[K_i]$ (mmol/l RBC)
BASELINE	0.205±0.018	9.3±0.9	105±2
PLACEBO	0.207±0.019	9.4±0.9	103±2
HEMODIALYSIS	0.232±0.021	10.0±0.9	106±2
BASELINE	0.208±0.020	9.2±0.9	100±1
CANRENONE	0.230±0.023*	9.2±0.9	104±1**
HEMODIALYSIS	0.267±0.025	9.6±1.0	103±1

* $p < 0.005$ vs baseline; ** $p < 0.01$ vs baseline

Table 2. Arterial pressure and plasma potassium concentration.

	ARTERIAL PRESSURE (mmHg)		PLASMA POTASSIUM (mmol/l)
	Systolic	Diastolic	
BASELINE	156±3	80±2	5.7±0.3
PLACEBO	160±3	80±2	5.7±0.3
HEMODIALYSIS	145±4	75±4	3.8±0.4
BASELINE	159±3	81±2	5.6±0.2
CANRENONE	160±3	78±2*	5.4±0.2**
HEMODIALYSIS	147±3	74±4	3.8±0.4

* $p < 0.05$ vs baseline; ** $p < 0.025$ vs baseline

DISCUSSION

A large body of evidence supports the hypothesis that volume expansion elicits in mammals the release of a circulating ouabain-like Na^+,K^+ pump inhibitor, which may play a role in the resultant increase in renal sodium excretion.[16] Even the Na^+,K^+ pump inhibition observed in uremia seems to be due, at least in part, to fluid overload; in fact it has been reported that hemodialysis[8,17,18] was able to acutely stimulate Na^+,K^+ pump activity in erythrocytes, and to reduce the plasma concentration of a digoxin-like factor(s);[19] moreover the amount of stimulation of the Na^+,K^+ pump was correlated to the degree of volume removal during hemodialysis. Thus it has been speculated that the trigger for the release of this Na^+,K^+ pump inhibitor is hypervolemia: predialysis fluid retention could stimulate the secretion of this substance, which is then lowered by volume removal during hemodialysis.

In a previous study we have observed a Na^+,K^+ pump inhibition after saline infusion in erythrocytes from normal subjects.[20] Moreover we demonstrated that the Na^+,K^+ pump inhibition was reproducible by incubating normal erythrocytes with their own plasma obtained after volume expansion[20]. This supports the hypothesis that Na^+,K^+ pump inhibition was due to a circulating factor(s). The administration of canrenone was able to prevent the RBC Na^+,K^+ pump inhibition induced by volume expansion.[21] Similar results were then found in a group of essential hypertensive patients investigated with a similar protocol; in these patients we observed also a significant reduction in arterial pressure after canrenone administration[22].

The present study confirms these results in uremic patients and suggests that administration of a single oral dose of 150 mg canrenone three hours before the beginning of hemodialysis may reverse the inhibition of erythrocyte Na^+,K^+ pump, which is present in these patients, probably due to volume expansion. Interestingly Na^+,K^+ pump activity after canrenone was similar to that observed after hemodialysis in the placebo study. Pharmacokinetic data indicate that canrenone is rapidly absorbed after oral administration, and its plasma concentration reaches a peak within two hours after the administration.[1]

Taken together, these observations suggest that the stimulating effect of canrenone on the suppressed Na^+,K^+ pump is due to a competition with an endogenous ouabain-like pump inhibitor. Our results fit well with the observation that canrenone *in vitro* behaves as a partial agonist of ouabain at the digitalis receptor site of Na^+,K^+ pump of human erythrocytes[3,4] and is able to restimulate a pump blocked by high concentrations of ouabain.[4]

Moreover our data are also in agreement with those obtained by Bianchi's group in Milan.[23] They administered chronically canrenoate-K, which is converted *in vivo* into canrenone, to essential hypertensive patients, in whom high concentrations of endogenous ouabain-like factors are hypothesized to play a pathogenetic role,[24] and observed after three months a significant increase in erythrocyte Na^+,K^+ pump activity, as compared to basal values.

Our results show that canrenone, in a therapeutical dose, may exert an acute antihypertensive effect; in fact, while following placebo blood pressure remained unchanged, after canrenone administration diastolic arterial pressure significantly fell ($p < 0.05$). One can speculate that the hypotensive effect of canrenone is mediated by the competition of the drug with an endogenous ouabain-like factor at the digitalis receptor site of the Na^+,K^+ pump at a vascular level, as inferred also by data from animals[25,26] and clinical studies in humans[23]. In fact it has been suggested that a reduction of Na^+,K^+ ATPase activity may play a role in the genesis of vasoconstriction in chronic uremia.[27,28]

However, it has been reported that canrenone may prevent the vasoconstriction, induced in smooth muscle cells with several agents, by means of other non specific membrane activities.[29] Moreover, paradoxically chronic treatment with canrenone in essential hypertensive patients potentiates the acute pressor effect of ouabain, through an unknown mechanism.[30] However the results of these studies do not rule out the possibility of an interaction between canrenone and endogenous ouabain-like factors at the level of Na^+,K^+ pump.

Interestingly plasma potassium concentration significantly fell after canrenone administration, despite the antialdosterone effect of the drug; this was paralleled by a concomitant significant increase of intra-erythrocyte potassium concentration. Since renal function was absent in all patients, these data suggest an increased intracellular potassium translocation, possibly mediated by restimulation of the Na^+,K^+ pump.

In conclusion, this study supports the hypothesis that canrenone protects the Na^+,K^+ pump against endogenous uremic inhibitors, and may favourably affect blood pressure and intra-extracellular redistribution of potassium. Obviously canrenone is contraindicated in renal failure, but may represent a useful tool for clinical studies on the pathophysiology of uremia.

REFERENCES

1. W. Sadée, M. Dagcioglu, and R. J. Schroder, Pharmacokinetics of spironolactone, canrenone and canrenoate-K in humans, Pharmacol. Exp. Ther. 185: 686-695 (1973).
2. D. Marver and J. P.Kokko, Renal target sites and the mechanism of action of aldosterone, Min. Electrolyte Metab. 9: 1-18 (1983).
3. P. Finotti and P. Palatini, Canrenone as a partial agonist at the digitalis receptor site of sodium potassium activated adenosine triphosphatase, J. Pharmacol. Exp. Ther. 217: 784-790 (1981).
4. R. P. Garay, J. Diez, C. Nazaret, G. Dagher, and J. P. Abitbol, The interaction of canrenone with the Na^+,K^+ pump in human red blood cells, Naunyn-Schmiedeberg's Arch. Pharmacol. 329: 311-315 (1985).
5. L. G. Welt, G. R. Sachs, J. J. Macmanus, An ion transport defect in erythrocytes from uremic patients, Trans. Assoc. Am. Phys. 77: 169-181 (1964).
6. L. G. Welt, E. K. M. Smith, M. J. Dunn, A. Szerwinski, H. Proctor, C. Cole, J. W. Balfe and H. J. Gitelman, Membrane transport defect: the sick cell, Trans. Assoc. Am. Phys. 30: 217-226 (1967).
7. A. P. Quintanilla, Alteration of Na,K pump in the uremic state. Int. J. Artif. Organs 10: 337-442 (1988).
8. H. Izumo, S. Izumo, M. DeLuise and J. Flier, Erythrocyte Na^+,K^+ pump in uremia. Acute correction of transport defect by hemodialysis, J. Clin. Invest. 74: 581-588 (1984).
9. F. Quarello, R. Boero, C. Guarena, C. Rosati, M.C. Deabate, T. Fidelio and G. Piccoli, Red blood cell Na^+,K^+ pump activity in patients on hemofiltration, Blood Purif. 2: 130-134 (1984).
10. C. H. Cole, J. W. Balfe and C. G. Welt, Induction of an ouabain sensitive ATPase defect by uremic plasma, Trans. Assoc. Am. Phys. 81: 213-221 (1968).
11. H. J. Kramer, J. Pennig, D. Klingmüller, J. Kipnowski, K. Glänzer and R. Düsing, Digoxin-like immunoreacting substance(s) in the serum of patients with chronic uremia, Nephron 40: 297-302 (1985).
13. J. H. Acosta, Hypertension in chronic renal failure, Kidney Int. 22: 702-712 (1982).
14. M. P. Blaustein, Sodium ions, calcium ions, blood pressure regulation and hypertension: a reassessment and a hypothesis, Am. J. Physiol. 232: C165-C173 (1977).
15. J. Fernandez, J. R. Oster and G. O. Perez, Impaired extrarenal disposal of an acute oral potassium load in patients with end stage renal disease on chronic hemodialysis, Min. Electrolyte Metab. 12: 125-129 (1986).
16. V. Buckalew and K. Gruber, Natiuretic hormone, in: "The Kidney in Liver disease", M. Epstein, ed., Elsevier Biomedical, New York (1983), p. 479-499.
17. J. M. Krzezinsky and G. Rorive, (letter), N. Engl. J. Med. 309: 987-988 (1983).
18. F. Quarello, R. Boero, C. Guarena, C. Rosati, G. Giraudo, F. Giacchino and G. Piccoli, Acute effects of hemodialysis on erythrocyte sodium fluxes in uremic patients, Nephron 41: 22-25 (1985).
19. G. Deray, M. G. Pernollet, M. A. Devynck, J. Zingraff, A. Touam, J. Rosenfeld and P. Meyer, Plasma digitalis-like activity in essential hypertension or end-stage renal disease, Hypertension 8: 632-638 (1986).
20. R. Boero, F. Quarello, C. Guarena, C. Rosati and G. Piccoli, Effects of an intravenous saline load on erythrocyte sodium transport in normal human subjects, Clin. Sci. 69: 709-712 (1985).
21. F. Quarello, R. Boero, C. Guarena, M. C. Deabate, M. C. Forneris, C.

Rosati, B. Rolando and G. Piccoli, Il canrenone previene l'inibizione della pompa Na^+,K^+ indotta dall'espansione del volume extracellulare, in: "Nefrologia Dialisi Trapianto", C. Giordano and N. DeSanto, eds., Wichtig, Milano (1986), p. 431-434.
22. R. Boero, C. Guarena, M. C. Deabate, B. Rolando, C. Rosati, F. Quarello and G. Piccoli, Erythrocyte Na^+,K^+ pump inhibition following saline infusion in essential hypertensive subjects: effects of canrenone administration, Int. J. Cardiology (in press).
23. G. Pati, E. Niutta, M. G. Tripodi, C. Barlassina, D. Cusi and G. Bianchi, Inibizione dell'azione delle sostanze endogene ad attività ouabaino-simile da parte del canrenoato di K nell'ipertensione arteriosa essenziale, in: "Atti XXVI Congresso Nazionale Società Italiana di Nefrologia", F. Mastrangelo, S. Rizzelli, V. De Blasi, L. Alfonso and D. Brancaccio, eds, Wichtig, Milano (1985), p. 247-250.
24. H. E. de Wardener and G. A. MacGregor, The natriuretic hormone and essential hypertension, Lancet 26: 1450-1454 (1982).
25. M. De Mendonca, M. L. Grichois, M. G. Pernollet, B. Thorman, P. Meyer, M. A. Devynck and R. Garay, Hypotensive action of canrenone in a model of hypertension where ouabain-like factors are present, J. Hypertension 3 (suppl. 3): 73-75 (1985).
26. M. L. Grichois, M. De Mendonca, I. Wauquier, M. G. Pernollet, B. Thorman, M. A. Devynck, P. Meyer and R. P. Garay, La canrénone: un antihypertenseur efficace dans le modèle expérimental d'hypertension où le transport actif du sodium est diminué, Arch. Mal. Coeur 6: 875-878 (1986).
27. J. Brod, J. Shaeffer, H. Hengtenberg and T. Kleinschmidt, Investigations on the Na+,K+ pump in erythrocytes of patients with renal hypertension, Clin. Sci. 66: 351-355 (1984).
28. R. Boero, C. Guarena, I. M. Berto, M. C. Deabate, C. Rosati, F. Quarello and G. Piccoli, Erythrocyte Na^+,K^+ pump activity and arterial hypertension in uremic dialyzed patients (submitted).
29. P. Salvati, F. Vaghi, M. Colombo and G. Bianchi, The interaction of canrenone with the Na,K pump in isolated rabbit renal arteries, in: "Abs. Xth Int. Congr. Nephrol.", London (1987), p. 300.
30. S. Laurent, P. Hannaert, X. Girard, M. Safar and R. P. Garay. Chronic treatment with canrenone in essential hypertensive patients potentiates the acute pressor effect of ouabain, J. Hypertension 5: S173-S175 (1987).

RENAL EXCRETION OF ARGININE-VASOPRESSIN IN MICROALBUMINURIC DIABETIC PATIENTS

Giovanni Maria Narelli, Mauro Cignarelli, Adriano Paternostro, Vittoria Romanazzi, Giuseppe Passavanti*, Rosaria Cospite, Giovanni De Pergola, Pasquale Coratelli*, and Riccardo Giorgino

Clinica Medica III, *Istituto di Nefrologia,
Università di Bari Policlinico, Bari, Italy

INTRODUCTION

Enhanced activity of haemodynamic hormones have been reported to be involved in the development of renal lesions of diabetic kidney[1,2]. Apart from other pressor factors even plasma arginine-vasopressin (AVP) have been found to be increased in uncontrolled diabetic patients very probably reflecting both a hypovolemic status and an increase in "effective" extracellular fluid osmolality; however, high circulating AVP levels have also been observed in certain well controlled diabetic patients thus suggesting that an alteration of mechanisms regulating AVP secretion exists in diabetes mellitus[3,4].

AVP administration induces glomerular haemodynamic changes[5] and a permeselective defect of glomerular basal membrane[6] similar to those occuring in the early stage of diabetic nephropathy.

Thus, we have studied the daily AVP renal output in 63 metabolically stable nonazotemic type 2 diabetics and the relationship with urinary albumin excretion (the best marker of early renal damage) was also investigated.

We chose non-insulin dependent diabetic patients (NIDDM) in order to eliminate the effect of insulin administration on the body sodium-fluid status and on AVP secretion[7] and the measurament of urinary AVP, since it gives a more accurate estimation of AVP secretion. AVP, indeed, is secreted episodically[8] and plasma concentrations may vary rapidly in response to several stimuli[9]. Moreover AVP in urine is more stable than in plasma[10] and there is a highly significant correlation between urinary AVP excretion rate, plasma AVP levels and urinary osmolality[9,10].

MATERIAL AND METHODS

63 metabolically stable nonazotemic type 2 diabetic patients of comparable urinary osmolality (Urine osmolality range 500 $\pm$ 200 mosmol/Kg H_2O) were studied. The subjects were matchable for sex, age and duration of diabetes. Diabetic patients free of nephropathy and with incipient nephropa-

thy were included. Patients with urinary albumin excretion rate (AER) above 200 μg/min. (urinary Albustix positive), with other diabetic complications, blood pressure higher than 160/90 mm Hg, manifesting disease of any kind or nicotine and alcohol abusers were excluded. All the subjects were admitted into hospital and gave their informed consent to the study. All the drugs were discontinued at least two weeks prior the study except for the antidiabetic therapy (diet and/or hypoglycemic drugs). The patients were subdivided into two groups according to level of albuminuria identified on the basis of albumin excretion in repeated 24-hrs urine collections performed during normal physical activity. The two groups were defined as follow:

Group 1. Forty type 2 patients (age 55 $\pm$ 15 yr; duration of diabetes 14 $\pm$ 6 yr) with normal AER ($<$ 15 μg/min.).

Group 2. Twenty-three type 2 patients (age 59 $\pm$ 14 yr; duration of diabetes 16 $\pm$ 4 yr) with elevated AER in the range of 15 to 200 μg /min., i.e. patients with persistent microalbuminuria (incipient diabetic nephropathy). The daily intake of sodium, potassium and protein was fixed at 150 mEq/die, 60 mEq/die and 1 g/Kg/body weight respectively, and kept constant over the study. The patients were studied after diabetic control was stabilized as assessed by a five or six sample 24-hrs blood glucose profile, by haemoglobin A_{1c} (HbA_{1c}) and glycosuria measurements. On the day of study blood pressure (BP) and heart rate (HR) were measured in the supine position after overnight rest. Blood samples were taken from an antecubital vein to determine glucose, sodium (P-Na), potassium (P-K), urea and creatinine plasma levels. HbA_{1c} and plasma osmolality (pOsm) were also determined. In the same day a 24-hr urine collection was performed to assess AVP and albumin excretion rate, sodium (U-Na), potassium (U-K), creatinine concentrations and urinary osmolality value (uOsm).

Urinary AVP (uAVP) was extracted from 1 ml aliquotes of acidified urine and estimated by employing a sensitive and highly specific radioimmunoassay[11]. This method has an estimated detection limit of $\simeq$ 0.8 pg of AVP/ml. The intra-assay and inter-assay coefficient of variation was 6.9% and 7.6% respectively.

Urinary albumin concentration was measured by a radioimmunoassay using a double antibody method (Sclavo); the inter-assay variation was 5.9%.

Haemoglobin A_{1c} was detected by a HPLC tecnique (the normal range was 4.3-6.1%).

Plasma and urinary sodium and potassium were determined by flame photometer, creatinine and urea by Greiner autoanalyzer and glucose by a glucoxidase method.

The osmolality of each plasma and urine sample was determined by freezing-point depression on a Fiske OS™ Osmometer.

Diabetes was classified by the criteria of the National Diabetes Data Group[12]. Blood pressure was measured by standard mercury manometer, cuff width 12 cm., after the patient had rested for at least 20 minutes in the supine position. Diastolic pressure was recorded as phase 5; mean blood pressure (mBP) was taken as diastolic + 1/3 (systolic - diastolic) blood pressure.

STATISTIC

Results are expressed as mean $\pm$ SD. Statistical evaluation was performed by Student's t-test and linear regression analysis.

RESULTS

The clinical characteristic and laboratory measurement of the subjects studied are reported in Table 1.

Table 1. Clinical charateristics and laboratory measurements of 63 Type 2 (non-insulin dependent) diabetic patients.

DIABETICS	GROUP 1 (n=40, AER < 15 μg/min.)	GROUP 2 (n=23, AER=15-200 μg/min)
Sex (m:f)	18 : 22	11 : 12
Age (years)	55 ± 15	59 ± 14
Duration of diabetes (years)	14 ± 6	16 ± 4
mBP (mm Hg)	90 ± 2	91 ± 1
Fasting plasma glucose(mg/dl)	155 ± 62	148 ± 57
HbA_{1c} (%)	7.4 ± 1.9	7.1 ± 1.1
Creatinine Cl. (ml/min.)	99 ± 15	102 ± 14
Plasma urea (mg/dl)	35.7 ± 5.7	38.7 ± 4.1
AER (μg/min.)	6.7 ± 4.3	48.3 ± 37

The two groups were comparable for sex, age and duration of diabetes. Height, wheight and surface area were matchable in the subjects studied (data not shown). Long term metabolic control (HbA_{1c}) was similar in group 1 and 2, as well as fasting plasma glucose on the day of study. No difference was found in mean blood pressure between diabetic patients free of nephropathy and with incipient nephropathy. Creatinine clearance and plasma urea resulted similar in the two groups. The urinary albumin excretion rate was 6.7 ± 4.3 and 48.3 ± 37 in normoalbuminuric and microalbuminuric patients respectively.
Daily urinary AVP excretion rate (pg/min.) resulted significantly higher in microalbuminuric diabetic patients as compared to normoalbuminurics ($p < 0.01$) even if within the same urinary osmolality range (Table 2) (Fig.1). Sodium excretion, plasma sodium and potassium were similar in the groups (Table 2).
The urinary AVP excretion rate was correlated to the urinary albumin excretion rate in normoalbuminuric diabetic patients (n= 40, r= 0.40, $p < 0.01$), but not in microalbuminurics (r= 0.09) (Fig. 2).
Mean blood pressure was not correlated to urinary AVP nor to albumin extretion rate whether including all diabetic patients or analysing them separately. No correlation was found between AVP excretion rate and creatinine clearance.

Table 2. Daily urinary AVP excretion rate, urinary and plasma electrolytes in 63 Type 2 (non-insulin dependent) diabetic patients.

DIABETCS	GROUP 1 (n=40, AER < 15 µg/min.)	GROUP 2 (n=23, AER=15-200 µg/min.)
uAVP (pg/min.)	46.9 ± 39.6	84.2 ± 35 *
pOsm (mOsm/Kg)	280 ± 71	278 ± 6
uOsm (mOsm/kg)	500 ± 238	533 ± 263
P-Na (mmol/l)	142 ± 6	139 ± 4.5
P-K (mmol/l)	4.3 ± 0.9	4.1 ± 1.0
U-Na (mEq/die)	152 ± 60	184 ± 77
U-K (mEq/die)	65 ± 24	73 ± 32
C_{water}	-0.64 ± 0.6	-0.95 ± 0.1

*$p < 0.01$

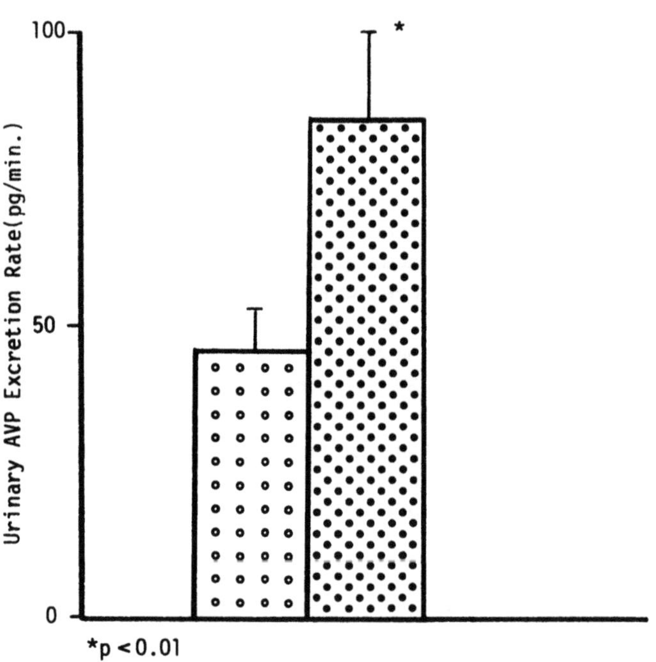

Fig. 1. AVP excretion rate in normoalbuminuric ⁘ and micro albuminuric ⁙ diabetic patients of comparable urinary osmolality (range: 500 ± 200 mOsm/Kg).

DISCUSSION

Our data indicate that, despite comparable urine osmolality value, the daily urinary AVP excretion rate is significantly higher in diabetic with microalbuminuria (i.e. incipient nephropathy) as compared to normoalbuminuric patients.

The cause of the increase in renal AVP excretion cannot be stated with certainty and some hypotheses can be considered.

Plasma osmolality, the predominant regulatory factor of vasopressin secretion in healthy adults[13], had not markedly increased in either group of diabetic patients. On the other hand the subjects under investigation had good metabolic control, no differences in urea values and above all, pla-

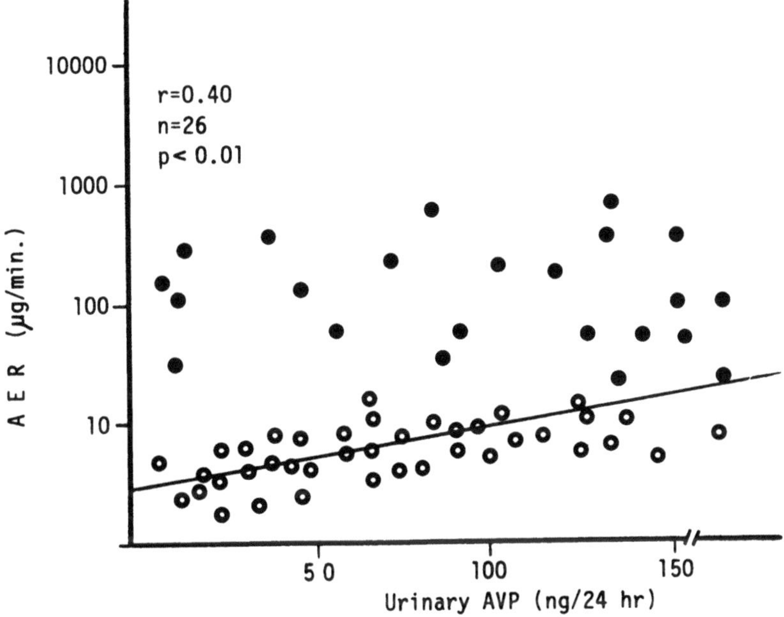

Fig. 2. Relationship between AVP excretion rate and AER in normoalbuminuric and microalbuminuric diabetic patients.

sma sodium, was comparable in diabetics with and without microalbuminuria.

Thus other possible causes must be considered. Hypotension can be excluded because blood pressure was normal both in group 1 and 2.

Hypovolemia would be expected to result from an intermittent solute diuresis, but microalbuminuric patients had long records of good metabolic control with persistently negative tests for glycosuria. In addition plasma urea and hematocrit were similar to those of normoalbuminuric diabetic patients.

The renin-angiotensin system itself could have provided a direct stimulus to vasopressin release[14]. The present studies do not permit any conclusion concerning the role of the renin-angiotensin system in the observed elevation in urinary AVP, but previous reports indicated that PRA is frequently low in diabetics and especially in patients with renal damage[15].

None of the patients experienced nausea or hypoglycemia at any time during these studies.

It is necessary to consider other factors that might elevate vasopressin in microalbuminuric diabetic patients.

Increased clearance of the hormone in our patients could conceivably result in increases in urinary vasopressin. This explanation seem unlikely, however, because clearance of the hormone in anephric patients is nearly normal[16].

Nonspecific stress must be considered, since it is a stimulus to hormone release[17]. Hence, it is highly questionable whether nonspecific stress contributed in any way to the increase observed in microalbuminuric diabetic patients.

The most likely explanation is that the early renal damage of diabetic kidney involves, other than the glomerular, also the tubule function. Changes in proximal tubule function is indeed well documented [18].
Our finding suggest that also change in distal tubule and/or collecting ducts consisting in vasopressin-resistant impairment of renal concentrating ability may exist in microalbuminuric diabetic patients. On the basis of this suggestions the increase in urine AVP output may be primarily interpreted as an effort (but relatively ineffective) to enhance the urinary concentration capacity of AVP hyporesponsive nephron.

The hypothesis of the reduced biological AVP activity is hardly tenable.

A correlation between AVP and albumin urinary excretion rate is apparent only in the normal range of urinary albumin concentration; this finding suggest that AVP can influence the permeselective characteristic of the glomerular basal membrane. The incipient diabetic nephropathy avoids or masks this relationship probably because other factors (hormonal, haemodynamic, biochemical abnormalities of basal membrane mesangial matrix), are involved and induce disregulation of the mechanism responsible for the relations observed above.

Whether the increase in AVP urinary output can be a mandatory factor or a consequence of microalbuminuria cannot be established, however a contributive role in the progression of incipient diabetic nephropathy may likely be postulated.

REFERENCES

1. SCHOR N., ICHIKAWA I. and BRENNER B. M.: Mechanisms of action of various hormones and vasoactive substances on glomerular ultrafiltration in the rat. Kidney Int., 20 , 442-451, 1981.

2. BOHRER M. P., DEEN W. M., ROBERTSON C. R., BRENNER B. M.: Mechanism of angiotensin II induced proteinuria in the rat. Am. J. Physiol., 233 , F 13 - F 19 , 1977.

3. ZERBE R. L., VINICOR F. and ROBERTSON G. L.: Regulation of plasma vasopressin in insulin-dependent diabetes mellitus. Am. J. Physiol., 249, E 317 - E 325 , 1985.

4. ZERBE R. L., VINICOR F. and ROBERTSON G. L. : Plasma vasopressin in uncontrolled diabetes mellitus. Diabetes 28 , 503-508 ,May 1979.

5. ICHIKAWA I. and BRENNER B. M.: Evidence for glomerular action of ADH and dibutyryl cyclic AMP in the rat. Am. J. Physiol., 233, 102-117, 1977.

6. MYERS B. D., WINETZ J. A., CHUI F. and MICHAELS A. S.: Mechanism of proteinuria in diabetic nephropathy : A study of glomerular barrier function. Kidney Int., 21 , 633-636 , 1982.

7. DE FRONZO R. A.: The effect of insulin on sodium metabolism. A review with clinical implications. Diabetologia 21 , 165-171 , 1981.

8. WEITZMAN R. E., FISHER D. A. , DI STEFANO J. J. , BENNET C.M.: Episodic secretion of arginine vasopressin. Am. J. Physiol., 233 , E 32 - E 39 , 1977 .

9. SCHRIER R. W. , BERL T. and ANDERSON R. S.: Osmotic and nonosmotic control of vasopressin release. Am. J. Physiol., 236 (4), F 321 - F 332 , 1979 .

10. KHOKHAR A. M., SLATER J. D. H. , FORSLING M. L. and RAMAGE C. M.: The physiological significance of urinary vasopressin and its relationship to plasma levels in man. Clin. Sci. Mol. Med., 49 , 14-15 , 1975 b.

11. TAUSCH A., STEGNER H., LEAKE R. D., ARTMAN H. G., and FISHER D. A. : Radioimmunoassay of arginin vasopressin in urine. Development and application . J. Clin. Endocrinol. Metab., 57 , 777-781 , 1983 .

12. National Diabetes Data Group. Classification and diagnosis of diabetes mellitus and other categories of glucose intolerance . Diabetes 28, 1039-1057 , 1979 .

13. ROBERTSON G. L. and ATHAR S. : The interaction of blood osmolality and blood volume in regulating plasma vasopressin in man. J. Clin. Endocrinol. Metab., 42 , 613-620 , 1976.

14. BONJOUR J. P. and MALVIN R. L. : Stimulation of ADH release by the renin-angiotensin system . Am. J. Phisiol. , 218 , 1555-1559 , 1970.

15. RASMUSSEN B. F. , MATHIESEN E. R. , DECKERT T., GIESE J. ,CHRISTENSEN N. S. , BENT-HANSEN L. and NIELSEN M. D.: Central role for sodium in the pathogenesis of blood pressure changes indipendent of angiotensin, aldosterone and catecholamines in type 1 (insulin-dependent) diabetes mellitus. Diabetologia ., 30 , 610-617 , 1987.

16. MAXWELL D. , Mc MURRAY S. , SZWED J., SHELTON R. and ROBERTSON G.: The effect of distribution and clearance on plasma of vasopressin in man. Clin. Res., 24 , 407 A , 1976.

17. WILLIAMS R. H.: Textbook of Endocrinology Philadelphia. W. B. SAUNDERS, 1974 , p. 84.

18. MOGENSEN C. E. : Maximum tubular reabsorption capacity for gluocose and renal haemodynamics during rapid hypertonic glucose in normal and diabetic subjects. Scan. J. Clin. Lab. Invest., 28 , 101-107 , 1971.

CAVH IN MYORENAL SYNDROME

Bernd Winterberg, Werner Tenschert,
Norbert Rolf, Katrin Ramme, Gisela Winterberg,
Michael Wendt, Konrad Teerling, Arno Lison, and
Heinz Zumkley[+]

Medizinische Poliklinik, Klinik für
Anästhesiologie und Operative Intensivmedizin
Medizinische Klinik und Poliklinik C
Universität Münster, F.R.G.

INTRODUCTION

Rhabdomyolysis describes the damage of striated muscle cell membranes which leads to fluid and electrolyte imbalances and to liberation of muscle components. The causes leading to rhabdomyolysis are numerous. The renal tubular overload with myoglobin can induce acute renal failure. The acute myoglobinuric renal failure in patients with crush-syndrome has been known since the first description by Bywaters and Beall (1941). This description gave rise to numerous reports on cases of acute renal insufficiency after traumatic or nontraumatic rhabdomyolysis. In about 8-20% of patients with rhabdomyolysis an acute myoglobinuric renal failure is observed. Myoglobinemia, toxic muscle cell membrane components, and alteration of renal perfusion lead to acute tubular necrosis. Circulatory collapse and shock represent additional factors in the pathogenesis of the acute renal failure (Bogaerts et al., 1982; Colombo et al., 1985; Grossmann et al., 1974; Hamilton et al, 1971; Hamilton et al., 1972; Kathrein et al., 1983; Koffler et al., 1976; Rowland and Penn, 1972; Sidorara et al., 1985). The usual therapy consists of adjustment of volume depletion and balancing of acid-base-electrolyte metabolism. If necessary, a renal replacement therapy is applied. Intermittent hemodialysis was shown to be an efficient therapeutic approach to uremia, but did not lead to elimination of myoglobin (molecular weight 17200 D) (Hart et al., 1982). In the study presented patients with myoglobinuric acute renal failure were treated with hemodialyisis and with continous arteriovenous hemofiltration (CAVH).

PATIENTS AND METHODS

Nine patients (mean age 40.7 years, range 6 to 72 years, female: n=5, male: n=4) with acute renal failure secondary to

rhabdomyolysis were accepted to the study (table 1). Diagnosis of rhabdomyolysis was based on the clinical characteristics of etiologically variable damage of striated muscle tissue, on extensive elevation of serum-CPK-activity and on the serum and urinary level of myoglobin. In one patient with a short course of the disease myoglobin derminations were not performed. In addition to the usual conservative therapy all patients were treated by intermittent hemodialysis for the acute oliguric renal failure. After the initial hemodialysis treatment because of hyperkalemia seven patients were submitted to CAVH. In one patient CAVH could first be installed in the later course of the disease due to a clotting-disorder.
For hemodialysis a parallel plate dialysator was used, (Gambro Lundia 5 N), CAVH was performed by the hemofilter PAN 250, Fa. Asahi and by the Ultraflux AV 600, Fa.Fresenius. Anticoagulation was achieved by 750-1000 I.E. heparin per hour. The laboratory, hematological, hemostaseological and hemodynamical parameters were determined by standard methods during the usual intensive care. The myoglobin levels in serum filtrate, dialysate and urine were determined by an immunological method (Rapitex-Myoglobin, Behringwerke).

RESULTS

All patients suffered from damage of striated muscles of the extremities and in some cases of the trunk with swelling and - in alert patients - pain. In one patient (pat.1) signs of a peripheral nerve lesion of the right leg secondary to muscular swelling were observed. However, a fasciotomy could be avoided since the swelling decreased rapidly. All patients were found to have a hyperkalemia of 5,5 to 9,0 mmol/l, a hyperphophatemia of 5,4 to 5,8 mg/dl and a hyperbilirubinemia of 1,4 to 12,4 mg/dl. The results of the other laboratory data are shown in table 1.
Patient 3 (malignant hyperthermia), patient 5 (staphylococcal sepsis) and patient 7 (shock) died shortly after onset of rhabdomyolysis.
Temporary arteficial renal substitution (hemodialysis, CAVH) led to complete recovery of renal function in the other patients. On dismission the altered laboratory parameters were almost normalized in all patients.
In patient 1 a significant decrease of serum creatinine and increase of urine output was observed 8 days after onset of CAVH. Thus, hemofiltrations could be discontinued after 10 days (Fig.1). In patient 2 hemodialysis could not be replaced by CAVH before normalization of a clotting disorder. After onset on CAVH serum creatinine decreased rapidly to normal values. Intermittent hemodialyisis was the only renal substitution therapy applied in patient 4. It took more than 60 days until recovery of renal function.
In order to assess the myoglobin clearance the myoglobin levels in serum, hemofiltrate and dialysate levels were determined under stable circulation. The hemofilter PAN 250 was found to have a myoglobin-clearance of about 32 ml/min, the hemofilter Ultraflux AV 600 had a myoglobin-clearance of ca. 42 ml/min. However, no myoglobin could be detected in the dialysate.

Table 1. Clinical manifestations in nine patients with myorenal syndrome

Pat.	Age	Sex	Diagnosis	max. CPK (U/l)	max. CPK-MB (U/l)	max. S.-Myo-globin (ug/dl)	K (mmol/l)	Ca (mmol/l)	max. S.-Creati-nine (mg/dl)	duration of renal insuff. (days)	
1	26	f	heroin	22400	544	>12800	6.2	2.2	4.4	20	
2	50	f	trauma	7100	380	>12800	5.9	2.2	6.0	46	
3	6	f	mal.hyper-thermia	8760	210	-	9,0	1.62	2.4	1	a
4	19	m	myolysis after march	65500	250	>12800	6.5	2.0	14.1	60	b
5	58	m	staphylo-coccal sepsis	15400	150	>12800	5.5	1.79	5.6	4	a
6	58	m	diphenhy-dramine	7938	72	>12800	5.7	2.22	6.4	3	
7	72	f	shock	3228	42	10000	6.0	1.8	7.2	2	a
8	27	f	Legion-naire's disease	1970	53	8000	5.9	1.9	7.0	14	
9	51	m	ethylene glycol	1462	41	4000	5.9	1.8	14.0	30	

a died, b hemodialysis only

Table 2. Etiology of acquired rhabdomyolysis (Glassock, modif.)

1. Increased energy consumption:
   Severe exercise
   Hypothermia
   Status epilepticus
   Heat stroke

2. Decreased energy production:
   Potassium depletion
   Ethanol
   Myxedema
   Phosphate depletion

3. Primary muscle injury:
   Polymyositis
   Trauma
   Severe burns

4. Decreased muscle blood flow:
   Compressive vascular occlusion
   Arterial thrombosis or embolism
   Shock
   Sickle cell trait

5. Infection:
   Viral influenza
   Legionnaire's dis.
   Infectious hepatitis

6. Miscell. toxins:
   Snake bite

   Diazepam
   Heroin
   Clofibrate
   Barbiturates
   Amphetamines
   Methadone
   Amphotericin B

   Ethylene glycol
   Haff disease

DISCUSSION

Acute myoglobinuric renal failure is most probably more frequent than often assumed. The combination of muscle swelling and pain with a dark coloured urine is suspicious for rhabdomyolysis. However, these symptoms are not obligatory

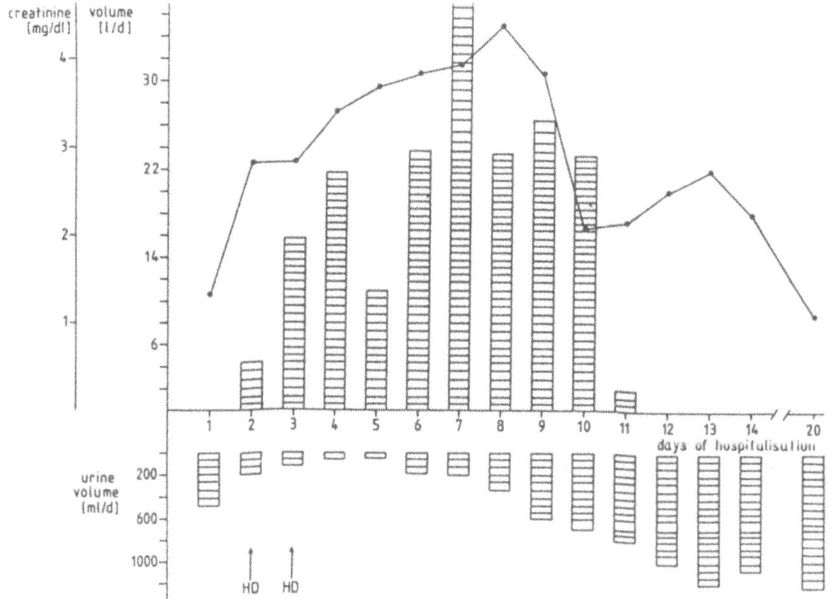

Fig. 1. Course of serum creatinine, urine output and hemofiltrate volume per day in a patient (no.1) with myoglobinuric renal failure (HD = hemodialysis).

and can therefore easily be overlocked in comatose patients. The urinary heme-pigment is detectable by means of a dip-stick-test, hematuria is ruled out by microscopy of the urinary sediment. Elevation of serum-CPK activity and serum and urinary myoglobin levels are evidential for a rhabdomyolysis. Simultaneous increase of the serum-activity of the muscular enzymes SGOT, SGPT, SLDH and aldolase and an elevation of myocardial enzymes such as CK-MB, a-HBDH are typical features (Glassock, 1983). The accelerated metabolism of heme lead to bilirubinemia (Rumpf et al., 1983).

The rise of serum creatinine in rhabdomyolysis induced renal failure is more rapid than in acute renal insufficiency of other origin. Thus, the ratio urea/creatinine usually is less than 60 (normal: 60 to 100). Rhabdomyolysis can be caused by various physical, chemical, immunological, infectious or ischemic etiologic factors (Glassock, 1983; Colombo et al., 1985) (Table 2).

It has been demonstrated in animal models (rat) that myoglobin does not have a direct toxic impact on renal function. In the animal model, dehydration represents a precondition for a myoglobin-induced impairment of renal function. Consequently, the decrease of the tubular urine flow and the lowering of urinary pH lead to formation of hematine and deteriorate the tubular transport mechanisms. This, together with obstruction by uric-acid cystals and pigmental cylinders gives rise to tubular necrosis. Reduction of cortical perfusion represents an additional pathogenetic factor in this process (Ayer et al, 1971; Oken et al., 1970; Richter et al., 1971). The release of intracellular potassium-, hydrogen- and phosphate ions after rhabdomyolysis leads to a marked metabolic acidosis and a hyperphosphatemic hypocalcemia. Soft-tissue calcifications, such as the calcifications of the myolytic muscle groups in patient 1, have been demonstrated in rhabdomyolysis (Akmal et al., 1978; Llach et al., 1981; Mc Carron et al., 1979).

Patients with wide-spread rhabdomyolysis often develop a hypercalcemia during the polyuric phase of acute renal failure which is most probably due to reabsorption of precipitated calcium ions (Koffler et al., 1976). In patient 1 the serum calcium increased up to 2,9 mmol/l. Alkalisation of the urine represents an effective measure to interrupt the pathogenetic process, since it inhibits the formation of hematine. If urine output can not be increased by conservative methods in the early phase of acute renal failure an arteficial renal replacement therapy (hemodialysis, CAVH) should be installed, let alone severe electrolyte imbalances such as hyperkalemia. After initial intermittent hemodialysis, renal substitution was continued by continuous arterio-venous hemofiltration, since the hemofilters were found to have a myoglobin clearance of 32 ml/min and 42 ml/min., whereas there was no myoglobin detectable in the dialysate (Hart et al., 1982). Thus, hemofiltration allows an additional elimination of myoglobin (Winterberg et al., 1987) exceeding that achievable by enzymatic metabolism (Massry, 1984). The excessively elevated serum myoglobin levels (>12800 ug/dl) in five patients were below 50 ug/dl (normal: < 10ug/dl) after two days of CAVH-treatment, whereas in patient 4 (hemodialysis only) myoglobin levels remained elevated for a longer time (4 days).

The results demonstrate that the duration of acute myoglobinuric renal failure can be distinctly reduced by early treatment with CAVH. Thus, CAVH represents an effective therapeutic approach to support recovery of renal function and to reduce the frequency of secondary complications in rhabdomyolysis induced acute renal failure.

LITERATURE

Akmal, M., Goldstein, D. A., Telker, N., Wilkinson, E., Masory, S.G., 1978, Resolution of Muscle Calcification in Rhabdomyolysis and Acute Renal Failure, Ann.intern.Med., 89:928

Ayer, G., Grandchamp, A., Wyler, T., Truniger, B., 1971, Intrarenal hemodynamics in glycerol-indurced myohemoglobinuric acute renal failure in the rat, Circulat. Res., 24:128

Bogaerts, Y., Lameire, N., Ringoir, S., 1982, The compartmental syndrome: a serious complication of acute rhabdomyolysis, Clin.Nephrol., 17:206

Bywaters, E. G., Beall, D., 1941, Crush injuries with impairment of renal function,, Brit.med.J., 1:427

Colombo, A., Briner, V., Truniger, B., 1985, Rhabdomyolyse, Dtsch. Med. Wschr., 110:1461

Glassock, R. J., 1983, Hematuria and Pigmenturia, in: Textbook of Nephrology, S. G. Massry, R. J. Glassock, ed., Williams and Wilkins, Baltimore/London

Grossmann, R. A., Hamilton, R. W., Morse, B. M., Penn, A. S., Goldberg, M., 1974, Nontraumatic rhabdomyolysis and acute renal failure, New Engl.J.Med., 291:807

Hamilton, L. L., Ramsey, W. H., 1971, Acute myoglobinuria associated with heroin addiction, J.Amer.med.Ass., 291:1172

Hamilton, R. W., Gardner, L. B., Penn, A. S., et al., 1972, Acute tubular necrosis caused by exercise-induced myoglobinuria, Ann.intern.Med., 77:72

Hart, P. M., Feinfeld, D. A., Briscoe, A. M., Nurese, H. M., Hotchkiss, J. L., Thomson, G. E., 1982, The effect of renal failure and hemodialysis on serum and urine myoglobin, Clin. Nephrol., 18:141

Kathrein, H., Kirchmair, W., König, P., v.Dittrich, P., 1983, Rhabdomyolyse mit akutem Nierenversagen nach Heroinintoxikation, Dtsch.Med.Wschr., 108:464

Koffler, A., Friedler, R. M., Massry, S. G., 1976, Acute renal failure due to non-traumatic rhabdomyolysis, Ann.intern.Med. 85:23

Llach, F. A., Felsenfeld, A. J., Haussler, M. R., 1981, The Pathophysiology of altered calcium metabolism in rhabdomyolysis-induced acute renal failure, New.Engl.J.Med., 305:117

Massry, S. G., 1984, Rhabdomyolysis: a clinical entity for the study of role of proteases, Adr.Exp.Med.Biol., 167:581

McCarron, D. A., Elliott, W. C., Rose, J. S., Bennett, W. M., 1979, Severe mixed metabolic acidosis secondary to rhabdomyolysis, Amer.J.Med., 67:905

Oken, D. E., DiBona, G. F., McDonald, F. D.,1970, Micropuncture studies of the recovery phase of myohemoglobinuric acute renal failure in the rat, J.clin.Invest., 49:730

Richter, R. W., Chellenor, Y. B., Pearson, J., Kagen, L. J., Hamilton, L. L., Ramsey, W. H., 1971, Acute myoglobinuria associated with heroin addiction, J.Amer.med.Ass., 17:1172

Rowland, L. P., Penn, A. S., Myoglobinuria., Med.clin.N. Amer., 56:1233

Rumpf, K. W., Kaiser, H., Leschke, M., Scheler, F., 1983, Diagnostik bei Myoglobinurie, Dtsch.med.Wschr., 108:266

Sidorara, L. D., Ierusalimskaia, L. A., Valentik, M. F, Razenko, T. N., Bedikhin, A. V., 1985, Porazhenie pochek pri alimentarno - toksicheskoi paroksizmal'noi mioglobinurii, (Iuksovsko-Sartlanskoi bolezni), Ter.Arkh., 57:120

Thomas, M. A. B., Ibels, L. S., 1984, Rhabdomyolysis acute renal failure (RMARF), Kidney Int., 26:241

Winterberg, B., Tenschert, W., Niederlein, G., Rolf. N., Ramme, K., Wendt, M., Lison, A. E., Zumkley, H.†, 1987, Akutes myoglobinurisches Nierenversagen, Fortschr.Med., 105:689

EFFECT OF IMIDAZOLE 2-HYDROXYBENZOATE ON ERYTHROCYTE CHARGE: A POSSIBLE EXPLANATION OF ITS HYPOALBUMINURIC ACTION

G.Gambaro, E.Cicerello, S.Mastrosimone, D.Del Prete, T.Lavagnini, G.Briani, and B.Baggio

Institute of Internal Medicine, Institute of Metabolic Diseases
University Hospital, University of Padova, Padova, Italy

INTRODUCTION

Recently in insulin-dependent diabetic (IDD) patients with incipient nephropathy we observed that a new non-steroidal anti-inflammatory drug (NSAID), imidazole 2-hydroxybenzoate (ITF-182), induced a reduction of the urinary albumin excretion rate (1). Since this drug did not determine any significant variation of blood pressure and of glomerular filtration rate, we suggested the hypothesis that this drug exerted its hypoalbuminuric effect modifying the glomerular charge permeaselectivity similarly to other NSAIDs (2), instead of acting on intrarenal hemodynamic.
This hypothetical effect could be due to a modification of structure and/or content of renal glycosaminoglycans (3), major determinants of anionic glomerular charges. This idea was in part suggested by the observation that the drug was also capable of lowering the urinary excretion rate of glycosaminoglycans (1).
Moreover in these patients we found a significant reduction of erythrocyte anionic sites (RBCCh)(4) which, from clinical and animal studies (5,6), could mirror the electrostatic charge of the glomerulus, a very important determinant of glomerular membrane selectivity for proteins. In these subjects, in fact, a negative relationship between RBCCh and albuminuria exists (4).

From this background, at the aim of testing if ITF-182 exerts its hypoalbuminuric action modifying the glomerular charge permeaselectivity, we evaluated the effect of this agent on RBCCh in a group of IDD patients

PATIENTS AND METHODS

The study was carried out in 16 IDD patients with albuminuria (RIA) lower than 300 mg/24hr randomly selected from a previously described group of diabetics (1)(6 females, 10 males; age 25-46 yrs; duration of the disease 5-20 yrs). The mean daily blood glucose level was 148.2±37.3 mg%, and glycosylated hemoglobin (HbA1c) was 7.3±3.1%.
The drug was administered for 30 days (750mg t.i.d.). At the beginning and at the end of the study period, we determined the erythrocyte anionic

charge using a cationic dye (Alcian Blue, AB) as previously described (4). Statistical analysis was carried out using the Student's "t" test for paired data.

RESULTS

During the trial, similarly to a previous study, ITF-182 did not induce any significant change in glucose blood level and HbA1c.
The drug produced a significant increase of RBCCh (85.80±5.23SD mgAB /10^6RBC vs 103.17±4.11SD ; t=8.32; p<0.001).

DISCUSSION

Our study shows that ITF-182 is capable of normalizing the RBCCh in diabetic patients. RBCCh is a mirror of the electrostatic charge of glomeruli, a finding supported by animal and clinical studies (5,6).
It has been shown to be reduced in proteinuric kidney diseases such as minimal change glomerulopathy and incipient diabetic nephropathy probably mirroring a similar derangement of glomerular charge (4,5). These observations obtained in diabetic patients (4) indirectly confirm the hypothesis that the onset of microalbuminuria, a marker of incipient diabetic nephropathy, is associated with loss of anionic glomerular charges (7).

Therefore, the effect of ITF-182 on RBCCh and possibly on the anionic glomerular charge, and consequently on charge selectivity of glomeruli, could justify its hypoalbuminuric action which could not be explained completely by its hemodynamic activity. This idea is in agreement with previous observations with other NSAIDs (2).

REFERENCES

1. B.Baggio, G.Briani, E.Cicerello et al Effects of imidazole 2-hydroxybenzoate on glycosaminoglycan and albumin urinary excretion in type 1 diabetic patients. Nephron (in press).
2. R.Vriesendorp, A.J.M.Donker, D.de Zeeuw et al Effects of non steroidal anti-inflammatory drugs on proteinuria. Am J Med 81 (s2B): 84 (1986).
3. R.Arumugham, S.M.Bose. Effect of indomethacin and naproxen on the metabolism of glycosaminoglycans. Scand J Rheumatol 11: 225 (1980).
4. G.Gambaro, B.Baggio, E.Cicerello et al Abnormal erythrocyte charge in diabetes mellitus. Link with microalbuminuria. Diabetes (in press).
5. M.Levin, C.Smith, M.D.S.Walters et al Steroid-responsive nephrotic syndrome: a generalized disorder of membrane negative charge. Lancet 2: 239 (1985).
6. J.M.Boulton-Jones, G.McWilliams, L.Chandrachud. Variation in charge on red cells of patients with different glomerulopathies. Lancet 2: 186 (1986).
7. T.Deckert, B.Feldt-Rasmussen, E.Mathiesen et al Pathogenesis of incipient nephropathy: a hypothesis. Diabetic Nephrop 2: 83 (1985).

INDEX

GPSR Compliance
The European Union's (EU) General Product Safety Regulation (GPSR) is a set of rules that requires consumer products to be safe and our obligations to ensure this.

If you have any concerns about our products, you can contact us on

ProductSafety@springernature.com

In case Publisher is established outside the EU, the EU authorized representative is:

Springer Nature Customer Service Center GmbH
Europaplatz 3
69115 Heidelberg, Germany

www.ingramcontent.com/pod-product-compliance
Ingram Content Group UK Ltd.
Pitfield, Milton Keynes, MK11 3LW, UK
UKHW051131260726
13967UKWH00010B/2975

* 9 7 8 1 4 6 8 4 8 9 5 4 5 *